Procreative Ethics
*Philosophical and Christian Approaches
to Questions at the Beginning of Life*

FRITZ OEHLSCHLAEGER

CASCADE Books • Eugene, Oregon

PROCREATIVE ETHICS
Philosophical and Christian Approaches to Questions at the Beginning of Life

Copyright © 2010 Fritz Oehlschlaeger. All rights reserved. Except for brief quotations in critical publications or reviews, no part of this book may be reproduced in any manner without prior written permission from the publisher. Write: Permissions, Wipf and Stock Publishers, 199 W. 8th Ave., Suite 3, Eugene, OR 97401.

Cascade Books
An Imprint of Wipf and Stock Publishers
199 W. 8th Ave., Suite 3
Eugene, OR 97401

www.wipfandstock.com

ISBN 13: 978-1-60608-230-0

Cataloging-in-Publication data:

Oehlschlaeger, Fritz.

    Procreative ethics : philosophical and Christian approaches to questions at the beginning of life / Fritz Oehlschlaeger.

    vi + 374 p. ; 23 cm. — Includes bibliographical references and index.

    ISBN 13: 978-1-60608-230-0

    1. Medical ethics—Religious aspects—Christianity. 2. Christian ethics. I. Title.

R725.56 .O38 2010

Manufactured in the U.S.A.

Procreative Ethics

Contents

Introduction / 1

1. Can the Use of Artificial Contraception within Marriage Be Consistent with the Natural Law? / 19
2. Abortion, the Sacred, and Sacrifice: Or, What's At Stake When Life Has Dominion / 47
3. In Defense of the "Conception Criterion" / 72
4. Abortion as Letting Die, Bad Samaritanism, or Just War: Why We Should Reject the Analogies / 104
5. Why David Boonin's Defense of Thomson Fails to Persuade the Abortion Critic / 145
6. The Ethics of Genetic Enhancement: A Test of Pragmatism as Democratic Tradition / 170
7. Why Designing the Subjects of Justice Is Likely to Be Unjust / 196
8. Giving Our Children Bread: Why the Harm Conundrum Is Not Such a Conundrum / 232
9. Why Genetic Therapy May Need Something "Very Much Like the Church" / 268
10. On Peter Singer's Silencing in Germany: Or, What's Wrong with Asking "What's Wrong with Killing?" / 299
11. Repugnance, *Frankenstein*, and Generational Injustice: A Consideration of Reproductive Cloning / 319

Bibliography / 349
Index / 365

Introduction

RECENTLY AN ENGLISH DEPARTMENT friend of mine whom I had not seen for a while asked me what I had been working on lately. When I responded that I was writing a book on bioethical issues at the beginning of life, he gently asked a question that I had myself been considering and avoiding: "What's your claim in that field?" Now there are conventional ways of my answering his question: I have been interested in ethics ever since I was an undergraduate at Michigan listening to William Frankena and admiring the clarity of his *Ethics*;[1] I have very largely foregrounded ethical matters in both my study and teaching of literature for the last thirty years; I have written on the relationships of theology, ethics, and literature and on the literature concerning one famous medical case and human sufferer, Joseph Carey Merrick, the "Elephant Man."[2] Since 1986, when I had the good fortune to participate in one of James Childress's NEH seminars on bio-medical ethics, I have given as much time as I could steal from other enterprises to reading in the field. This would be to give a professional answer to my friend's question, but it would leave many important things unsaid.

In *Playing God?: Human Genetic Engineering and the Rationalization of Public Bioethical Debate*, John Hyde Evans has charted the professionalization of bioethics over the past thirty years.[3] In the infancy

---

1. Frankena, *Ethics*.

2. See Graham and Oehlschlaeger, *Articulating the Elephant Man*, and Oehlschlaeger, *Love and Good Reasons*.

3. Evans's argument draws largely on the public debate over HGE, Human Germline Enginering, from the 1960s to the present. His claim is that bioethical debate has become increasingly "thinner" during that period, with a shift from a substantive conception of rationality to a formal conception in which discussion is largely limited to estimating the comparative effectiveness of means to already-accepted ends. Evans gives a central role in this process to government advisory commissions established to advise scientists on the "broader ethical implications of their work." The federal government

of biomedical ethics, contributions came from a wide variety of disciplines: theology, philosophy, literature, law, medicine itself. As the field has evolved, however, it has become increasingly, and now almost exclusively, dominated by professional bioethicists.[4] Partly this development seems inevitable. As the science has itself become ever more complex and specialized, so do those who reflect on the ethical issues it presents. Nevertheless it seems unhealthy to me for bioethics to become exclusively the province of ever-more-specialized practitioners. No field or practice, with the exception of theology, concerns us all in the way that medicine does. The revolution in genetics brings this emphatically to light. The routine question of genethics—"What kind of people should there be?"—is one calling for broad political reflection.[5] It's difficult to

---

tended, in turn, to accept the advice of these commissions in deciding the ethical status of experiments for funding. The commissions emerged as decision-makers, and the bioethics profession gained "jurisdiction" over the terms of debate, employing primarily the language of "Principlism" with its stress on autonomy, nonmaleficence, beneficence, and justice. See Evans, *Playing God?*, 36. "Principlism" has, of course, been associated with the middle-level principles articulated in the several editions of Beauchamp and Childress, *Principles of Biomedical Ethics*. Evans has recently addressed the way religious convictions do or should contribute to bioethics in "Who Legitimately Speaks for Religion in Public Bioethics?" in *Handbook of Bioethics and Religion*, 61–79. Part of the answer to his title's question depends upon "what we think public policy bioethics *is* or what we think it should be" (75). Evans develops several models of public bioethics and suggests how religion can or does contribute to each.

4. For three important responses to Evans's work, two by theologians with significant experience on government commissions, see Stout, "Comments of Jeffrey Stout," 187–91; Meilaender, "Comments of Gilbert Meilaender," 191–95; and Childress, "Comments of James F. Childress," 195–204. The most substantial of these is by Childress, who points out numerous problems in Evans's argument: the problematic quality of Evans's "implicit and explicit criteria for identifying bioethicists" (196); the oversimplifying of "principlism" and concomitant failure to consider alternative bioethical approaches of wide use in the public realm (particularly casuistry); and the underestimation of the continuing influence of theologians on government commissions, as illustrated by the 1997 NBAC report on cloning humans.

5. The relationship between bioethics and religion has been the subject of considerable scholarly activity in the last decade. The interest in this question no doubt derives from the growing academic consensus that there simply is no tradition-free account of reason in the Enlightenment sense. If all arguments always already depend upon particular convictions, warrants, class biases, unrecognized assumptions, etc., then it no longer seems legitimate to single out religious discourse for exclusion from the public square. In addition to the books cited in note 3, a partial list of studies devoted to religion and bioethics would include Verhey and Lammers, *Theological Voices in Medical Ethics*; Meilaender, *Body, Soul and Bioethics*; Meilaender, *Bioethics*; Chapman, *Unprecedented Choices*; Banner, *Christian Ethics and Contemporary Moral Problems*;

see how any degree of particular expertise could rightly answer such a question, and I hope there will be those who insist that it's a question—perhaps the question—we ought not to ask.

My first claim, then, is that it is healthy for bioethics to be in conversation with informed nonspecialists who will raise questions often lost in the detailed considerations of specialized bioethical issues.[6] My second claim is that this kind of interaction between nonspecialists and specialists will become even more imperative as the genetics revolution progresses—precisely because genethical questions are political. My third point is that the appropriate answer to my literary friend's initial question would have to allude to a variety of my roles, not simply my professional activities. I write as a child with allegiances to my parents, one now dead, the other aging; as a husband of thirty-seven years; as a father of two children and recently a grandfather; as a patient myself, sufferer of two major depressive episodes; as a long-time volunteer in service to persons disabled by serious mental illness; as a teacher of the humanities for more than thirty years in secular universities; as one who, for much of his life, was without formal religious affiliation but who now hopes he is a Christian; as one who shares the goals of feminism and has great respect for his secular feminist colleagues but who also thinks that we cannot accept many current arguments for abortion without profoundly distorting our politics and our souls. And finally I write as a citizen of the United States and patriot of sorts but also as one who believes that the boundaries of the community to which he most deeply belongs are those established by Jesus Christ—and that that name must never be appropriated by any nation for its own inevitably idolatrous purposes.

Rae and Cox, *Bioethics: A Christian Approach in a Pluralistic Age*; Pellegrino and Faden, *Jewish and Catholic Bioethics*; Davis and Zoloth, *Notes from a Narrow Ridge*; Deane-Drummond, *Genetics and Christian Ethics*; Cahill, *Theological Bioethics*; Gill, *Health Care and Christian Ethics*. In addition, the journal *Christian Bioethics*, edited by H. Tristram Engelhardt Jr., began publication in 1995.

6. For an excellent account of the way "standard bioethics" has managed to exclude voices, traditions, and accounts that challenge contemporary medicine's "Baconian project," see McKenny, *To Relieve the Human Condition*, 1–38. In an attempt to, among other things, enlarge the agenda of bioethics, McKenny considers the work of theorists who have been largely excluded from standard bioethical discussion, each of whom raises significant questions about the medical-technological project of eliminating suffering and overcoming death: Hans Jonas, James Gustafson, Leon Kass, Stanley Hauerwas, Drew Leder, Richard Zaner.

Medicine concerns us all because we all live under what Wendell Berry has called the "sign of mortality." In a story called "Are You All Right?," Berry's narrator, Andy Catlett, accompanies his middle-aged friend Elton Penn as they go to check on the safety of their common friends, Art and Mart Rowanberry, during flood time on the Kentucky River. As Andy and Elton reach the place where the Rowanberrys live, they realize they can come no closer than a quarter of a mile. Between them and their friends stands the shining and impassable backwater, to be crossed only by Elton's troubled cries. Finally the Rowanberrys do respond and Elton asks, "Are you all right?"—a question that brings an emphatic "Yeeeaaah!" Andy, narrating this retrospectively, adds what Elton did not know: "But now I know that it was neither of the Rowanberrys who was under the sign of mortality that night. It was Elton. Before another April came he would be in his grave on the hill at Port William. Old Art Rowanberry, who had held him on his lap, would survive him a dozen years." The title of Berry's story points to what I will call the general burden of risk-sharing. We ask each other that simple question, "Are you all right?," perhaps a dozen times each day, and the appropriate answer, unless the questioner is a very close friend, is "Yeeeaaah!"[7] That affirmation means nothing less than that one is confident that she can carry her share of the general human burden for that day and the foreseeable future, even though she "knows"—in the same theoretical way that we all do—that one day her ability to do so will end in death.

A good part of the modern medical and bioethical project seems devoted to a forgetting of the sign of mortality. In a response to Ronald Dworkin's book on abortion and euthanasia, *Life's Dominion*, Frances Kamm asks a startling question designed to challenge Dworkin's view of how works of art, or lives, become what he calls "sacred." Making her case that "many things (e.g., persons)" can have value "independently of their history," Kamm asks rhetorically, "If Rembrandt had created 'The Nightwatch' under coercion, would the painting have been any less valu-

---

7. Berry, "Are You All Right?," 198–200. In a recent novel, Berry's Hannah Coulter remarks that the "proper answer to 'How are you?' is 'Fine.'" This is true for her even, perhaps especially, when "the thing you have most dreaded has happened at last." The response indicates both an honest "unwillingness to act as if loss and grief and suffering are extraordinary" and "an honoring of the solitude in which the grief you have to bear will have to be borne." For Berry, these commonplace assurances reflect the "consent" we must give to time or to life in the mystery of time. See *Hannah Coulter*, 61–62, 148, 163.

able? I do not think so."⁸ What startles me here is Kamm's assumption that somehow "The Nightwatch" was not created under coercion. There are, after all, kinds of coercion other than having a gun to one's head. Rembrandt worked under the coercion of death, the curse of limited time. What we honor in his great painting is the wonderful thing he was able to create in the face of coercion. We can, of course, look at, analyze, and admire the painting as an art object, but its wonder for us, its ability to captivate, can never be fully separated from its history as the response of a unique human being to limits we all understand abstractly but experience passionally only as ourselves. "Nightwatch" speaks to us, somehow, from and as Rembrandt's freedom from coercion—freedom made meaningful precisely because it cannot banish the coercion that brings it into being. The painting gives us the sense—neither completely true nor completely illusory—that we, too, are free.

Kamm seems to have forgotten the coercion of time and mortality. Her well-known counterfactuals—in which "persons" seem capable of being produced by every conceivable process—suggest the degree to which bioethical reasoning seems sometimes to inhabit a world where neither medicine nor morality have much to do with the actual experience of embodied human beings.⁹ Much of the writing in bioethics, particularly genetics, testifies to what Gerald McKenny has called "the [contemporary biomedical] imperative . . . to eliminate suffering and to expand the realm of human choice—in short, to relieve the human condition of subjection to the whims of fortune and the bonds of necessity."¹⁰ McKenny insightfully argues, too, that the "moral commitments to expanding choice and eliminating suffering" depend on the formation of subjects—us—who monitor and exercise vigilant control over our bodies. Our moral identities, then, become abstracted from our bodies, which "in turn become (through technology, it is hoped) simply the object of one's choices and desires" (216). Modern medicine becomes

---

8. Kamm, "Ronald Dworkin's Views on Abortion and Assisted Suicide," 220. Kamm has written extensively on Dworkin and abortion in "Abortion and the Value of Life: A Discussion of *Life's Dominion*," 160–221.

9. Kamm, *Creation and Abortion*, 3–19. Kamm asserts her method is to "present hypothetical cases for consideration and seek judgments about what may and may not be done in them. The fact that these cases are hypothetical and often fantastic distinguishes this enterprise from straightforward applied ethics, in which the primary aim is to give definite answers to real-life dilemmas" (8).

10. McKenny, *To Relieve the Human Condition*, 2.

increasingly, in Stanley Hauerwas's words, "the Promethean project to get us out of life alive."[11]

I heartily endorse the first principle of Tristram Engelhardt's *Foundations of Bioethics*: "moral diversity is real."[12] In a modern liberal society, we each exist together with "moral friends," who share our comprehensive views of life, and "moral strangers," who do not. We must, at all times, seek peace between these groups, and for me, as for Engelhardt, this means we must be very reluctant to use the law in service of morality whenever there is substantial reason for some to consider the use coercive. Engelhardt's principle of permission must provide the very limited but still sufficient foundation for a secular bioethics, and Christians should welcome the freedom made possible by postmodernity—the freedom to make their convictions plain without reliance on the force that inevitably distorts them.[13] But there is great

---

11. Hauerwas, foreword to Shuman and Meador, *Heal Thyself*, xii.
12. Engelhardt, *Foundations of Bioethics*, 3.
13. As moral authority in a secular society "cannot be derived from rational argument or common belief," permission or consent must provide the authority to resolve moral disputes, and "respect of the right of participants to consent is the necessary condition for the possibility of a moral community." See *Foundations of Bioethics*, 123 and *passim*. Engelhardt makes a similar argument in *Bioethics and Secular Humanism*. There he provides a richly historical treatment of the various ways in which both the secular and humanism have been understood in the West. Ultimately the search for a universalistic secular humanism—the Enlightenment project—fails. Indeed "it would seem that secular humanism leads dialectically to its own self-destruction": the unsuccessful attempt to ground a common secular morality calls the whole "project of morality into question" (111). Still secular humanism provides a kind of default basis for morality since it leaves individuals free to "choose where there is no authority for others to intervene." The procedural morality of consent and permission that remains will be "secular" in that it shows no preference for any of the content-full moralities held by particular communities and "humanist" in that it will be "grounded in what we share as persons: the project of the peaceable resolution of moral disputes with moral strangers"(130). If there is a weakness here, it would seem to lie in Engelhardt's indebtedness to Kant, particularly if Kant is read as Engelhardt has more recently in "Public Discourse and Reasonable Pluralism," 169–94. If Kant's project is to reformulate Christian morality as the morality of reason itself, then Engelhardt's appeal to a Kantian "will to morality" (*Secular Humanism*, 122) is a second-hand appeal to the particularist, content-full morality of Christianity. To put the relevant question in lay terms: why should today or tomorrow's Nietzschean self-maximizer—armed perhaps with the technology of genetic enhancement—care about "peaceable resolution of disputes with moral strangers"? For more on this later essay of Engelhardt's, see note 19 below. For a critique of Engelhardt's work from a Christian perspective, see Gill, *Health Care and Christian Ethics*, 177–79, 205–9. Gill finds Engelhardt's analyses and language too

wisdom in Jeremiah's insistence that a profound obstacle to peace is to believe that there is peace "when there is no peace" (Jer 6:14). We will not approach any closer to peace by obscuring the distinctions between us and our moral strangers. Moral friends must seek to articulate both their moral positions and the reasons for holding them; they must listen carefully and respectfully to the arguments of their moral strangers; and they must look for every possible area of overlapping concern between members of various groups. This is why I listed earlier the various roles from which I approach questions of bioethics. Moreover, it seems to me that this is something all people concerned about such matters might usefully do: to think through the variety of positionings from which they regard moral questions in the search for overlap with others whom they might typically consider strangers. If a particular position I take as a Christian seems unreasonable to you, consider it as a position taken also by a parent. Perhaps we can meet from within that identity description and begin to talk fruitfully. Perhaps we can discover that we share at least what Kevin Wildes has called moral acquaintanceship.[14] This does not

---

divisive and polarizing, too likely to fuel the culture wars in ways neither necessary nor justified. He objects, for example, to Engelhardt's suggestion—made in a piece on the dechristianization of hospital chaplaincy—that a more faithfully Christian hospital chaplain might, among other things, encourage "health care professionals and health care institutions not to participate in interventions forbidden by traditional Christian norms (including refusing to refer to those who would provide such interventions)." Gill points out that doctors accepting these claims would be "unemployable in many clinical settings of both hospitals and general practice in the British National Health Service" (178). But that is precisely what Engelhardt believes ought to be the case and would be if the state acknowledged the limits of secular reason. For the quote from Engelhardt, see "Dechristianization of Christian Hospital Chaplaincy," 145–46.

14. Wildes argues that it is "too simple" to divide bioethics into two species: one of "different communities" based on substantive agreements and another a "minimalist, procedural bioethics for secular societies." He notes that "women and men, from different communities are able to reach agreements at different times. They can engage in discussion and give reasons to one another. Further, most men and women do not live in a single moral community but in many" (164). Wildes proposes the category of "moral acquaintances"—people who share some overlapping areas of agreement despite different community memberships—to supplement Engelhardt's "moral friends" and "moral strangers." For Wildes, even the most minimalist of procedural bioethics requires some degree of "acquaintanceship" among players. See *Moral Acquaintances*, 136–83. For an engaging appraisal of Wildes's work by one who is both a theologian and the pastor of a fourteen-member Wesleyan church in rural Kentucky, see Thobaden, "Pleased to Make your Acquaintance," 425–39. Particularly instructive are Thobaden's examples of how his parishioners manage the tensions of living both in and out of the world in accord with their Holiness tradition.

mean we will agree, but perhaps we can begin to see how and why we each take the positions we do from within the comprehensive views of life to which we are committed.[15]

The eleven chapters that follow this introduction are devoted to issues of biomedical ethics at the beginning of life. For the most part, their point-of-view is philosophical, but when it is important to articulate how one might see a particular matter Christianly, I have tried to do that. I hope the arguments here will be of interest to people from all traditions. Chapter 6 expresses my criticisms of the way pragmatism works in arguments for genetic enhancement of children, but I nevertheless hope to be considered one who takes seriously Jeffrey Stout's recommendation of pragmatism as the argumentative style most suitable to the tradition he calls democracy. Stout's model of ethical deliberation and political discussion involves the public exchange of intelligible reasons, a holding of one another accountable, and cooperation "in crafting political arrangements that promote justice and decency" in our relations with one another.[16] I have tried, in all of my arguments, to conform to the first two of these criteria and to indicate my willingness to abide by the third. When I have suggested the way Christian convictions would function in discourse about particular issues, my arguments are, in no way, prescriptive. I have no interest in coercion of any sorts. Like Thoreau, "I was not born to be forced."[17] But I do want to explicate the kinds of difference Christian convictions make. If I accept Engelhardt's description of a secular bioethics, on one hand, I also accept Hauerwas's description of the task of Christians as that of "be[ing] an alternative" to the world.[18]

---

15. The language here of "overlapping consensus" and "comprehensive views" obviously derives from Rawls, *Political Liberalism*, 133–72. For Engelhardt's argument that Rawls's formulations of consensus depend on a good bit of question-begging and silent exclusion of positions not deemed "reasonable" or "just," see "Foundations of Bioethics and Secular Humanism," 270.

16. Stout, *Democracy and Tradition*, 298.

17. "Civil Disobedience," 403. The passage continues: "I will breathe after my own fashion. Let us see who is the strongest. What force has a multitude? They only can force me who obey a higher law than I. They force me to become like themselves. I do not hear of *men* being *forced* to live this way or that by masses of men. What sort of life were that to live?"

18. Hauerwas, "Not All Peace Is Peace," 122. Hauerwas offers a sustained critique of the second edition of *The Foundations of Bioethics*. He argues that the privatization of particularistic convictions called for by Engelhardt cannot help but produce a "distortion" of Christian convictions, "for when Christians allow their faith to be privatized,

My obligations both as a Christian and as a participant in democratic

we soon discover that we can no longer maintain the disciplines necessary to sustain the church as a disciplined polity capable of calling into question 'the public'"(116). Being Christian "means that we must be embedded in practices so materially constitutive of our communities that we are not tempted to describe our lives in the language offered by the world, that is, the language of choice"(117). Hauerwas further suspects that Engelhardt conceives of "witness" as "what you need when your position cannot be rationally defended" rather than as "one of the most determinative forms of rationality" (117). He claims, too, that Engelhardt's vision is rather one of order than peace, and that that order is sustained by forms of violence that Engelhardt overlooks: that of the market and of the pervasive techniques of surveillance that Foucault has taught us to identify. Perhaps the heart of Hauerwas's critique lies in his sense that Engelhardt makes being a Christian too much a matter of "choice," whereas for Hauerwas it's more "like being Texan," an identity they share and one that comes first "as gift, not as choice" (114–15).

I would defend Engelhardt against this last claim by suggesting that Engelhardt has no more chosen to take the positions he does than Hauerwas has chosen to be Texan. Rusty Reno has said that Hauerwas's work "is overdetermined by a reaction against 'Americanism.'" (I'd challenge the "over," preferring simply to say that "Americanism" has had a very strong effect on it.) Engelhardt's work, on the other hand, reveals the determining influence of twentieth-century totalitarianisms. Writing about the drafting of *Foundations* and *Bioethics and Secular Humanism*, he has said: "The manuscripts took shape in a city destroyed through the evils of National Socialism. They took on their unity when Berlin was still divided by an international socialism which had in its own right killed tens of millions. Given the moral catastrophes of this century and the tens of millions slaughtered by both national and international socialism, it will not do simply to acquiesce in a contingency of sentiments with which we may agree, or in a *de facto* consensus that appears to be prevailing. No account of moral philosophy or bioethics can be complete without taking cognizance of the service philosophy provided for these tyrannies, or of the ways philosophy supported the proclamation of 'truths' that were empirically false about matters of global significance." The vocation of proclaiming liberty against state coercion backed by reason has chosen Engelhardt just as surely as Hauerwas has been chosen by the church's need to become visible after the long invisibility of Constantianism—caused, as he puts it, by the assumption "that God is governing the world through Constantine." As an American Christian born five years after the Second World War ended, and as a son and son-in-law of men who saw extensive service in the Pacific theater of that war, I cannot help but honor the positions taken by both Engelhardt and Hauerwas. We must proclaim liberty against state tyranny of all kinds, particularly that justified by appeals to reason insufficiently aware of its own contingency, and, as Christians, we must witness to an alternative way of being—one determined by faithfulness to God. Engelhardt's remarks are in "Foundations of Bioethics and Secular Humanism," 273. Reno's comment is from a letter quoted in Hauerwas, "Postscript," 236. Hauerwas on Constantine is from a comment of his on John Howard Yoder in "Explaining Christian Nonviolence," 173.

Engelhardt returns to these matters in "Public Discourse and Reasonable Pluralism,"169–94. Here he begins by asking whether it is "licit" for Christians to remain silent about "the truth of Christianity" and concludes that Christians "have no secular ground for hesitation when advancing their moral and religious views in the public forum" discourse involve engaging others in every way possible from the conviction that such engagement is itself part of practical peace-making. If the "public exchange of reasons" Stout calls for is ever to involve more than the barest cost-benefit calculations, it will require people of every standpoint to explain the way their public positions derive from their comprehensive views of life. Only by doing so can we begin to discern the places where some overlapping consensus might lie.[19]

---

(186). In telling the history, Engelhardt stresses the secular Enlightenment project of neutralizing "religious discourse" by "recasting its substance into moral commitments materially equivalent to those of secular morality so that it will no longer pose a sectarian threat to" universalist aspirations (175). The key figures in this process are Kant and one of his contemporary inheritors, John Rawls. Committed as ever to resisting totalitarianism, Engelhardt criticizes the "totalizing" claims of moral rationality in the later Rawls, where it "is hidden in a notion of the reasonable" that "thickly incorporates particular social democratic ideals." Rawlsian rationality thus requires the refashioning of all social structures "in the image and likeness" of justice as fairness (181). Over against this ideal of "totalizing social democracy" (179), Engelhardt continues to argue that the only legitimate source of secular moral authority is the permission of peaceable collaborators. He has also turned, in his writing for *Christian Bioethics*, to ever more sharply articulating Christian differences, insisting that Christianity implies a "moral epistemology"—nurtured by liturgy—that is quite different from secular understandings premised on giving an account of the good, the right, and the virtuous apart from the holy. A succinct way of putting this complex matter is to say that, created being will inevitably misunderstand and distort its circumstances when it tries to understand them "apart from Uncreated Being, Who can be experienced but not understood." See "What Is Christian about Christian Bioethics?," 241–53. Engelhardt's fullest statements on all these matters are in *Foundations of Christian Bioethics*. That volume would seem to answer Hauerwas's earlier criticisms, as it clearly articulates an alternative bioethics rooted in what Engelhardt likes to call "traditional Christianity," largely identifiable with the Orthodox tradition.

19. Cahill claims a vital role for theology in breaking out of what she sees as the stalemate of bioethical discussion in the public square as conceived by liberalism. For her, bioethics is primarily about practices, behaviors, institutions—national or international, just or unjust—and about how these might be transformed in accord with social justice. Theological language can play many roles in creating the kinds of consensus necessary for change. A "theological bioethics" should be "participatory" in the processes of change toward social justice. In her comments on Evans's *Playing God?*, what Cahill offers is not so much a criticism as an acknowledgement that Evans has rightly depicted the stalemate together with an argument that the real action for theological bioethics must be elsewhere. See *Theological Bioethics*, 1–69. Robert Song similarly argues for a rejection of the "contrast between thick, tradition-rich identities in private, and thin, tradition-free identities in public." I find both his and Cahill's approaches very appealing, although I also believe, with Engelhardt, that Christians must be aware and wary of the dangers of translating Christian language into even such admirable goals as "social justice." Song's Barthian insistence on the church's role in unmasking the idols of the secular would seem to provide protection against the loss of Christian difference.

The first chapter here attempts what seems semantically impossible, a natural law defense of artificial contraception within marriage. In its engagement with the Roman Catholic tradition, it may seem the most consistently "religious" chapter in the book, and I do write as a Protestant Christian specifically hoping to initiate conversation on this issue with Catholics. But the analysis of Martin Rhonheimer's understanding of natural law and its possible consequences for thinking about contraception is purely philosophical.[20] The second through fifth chapters consider the much-vexed matter of abortion. Their strategy is to maintain that we need not accept many of the seemingly most persuasive arguments for abortion. Chapter 2 takes up the call for "public argument" issued by Ronald Dworkin in *Life's Dominion*. Chapter 3 critically examines a series of prominent pro-abortion positions: one by Daniel Dombrowski and Robert Deltete whose central argument is that the Catholic tradition is more consistent with mediate than with immediate hominization; a second, by Peter Wenz, argues that the abortion choice should be understood as an exercise of the freedom of religion; and a third, by David Boonin, attempts a systematic refutation of the important anti-abortion argument by Donald Marquis that has come to be known as the "future like ours" position. Boonin claims to have refuted the critic of abortion on grounds the critic already accepts. I believe he does not accomplish that aim.[21]

Chapter 4 examines two prominent versions of the "bad Samaritan" defense of abortion: one perhaps the most famous of all articles on the subject, that by Judith Jarvis Thomson, about which I hope to have some new things to say; and a second by Donald Regan. These arguments freely grant the personhood of the fetus but claim that it can be killed anyway because to require a woman to carry to term is to ask a degree of good Samaritanism from her that we do not insist on elsewhere. Also considered in this chapter is Lloyd Steffen's attempt to articulate principles of "just abortion" based on just war theory. Steffen's position should also be considered an "abortion despite personhood" one, as the turn to just war thinking necessarily implies that the issue at hand is the killing

See "Christian Bioethics and the Church's Political Worship."

20. I draw particularly on Rhonheimer, *Natural Law and Practical Reason*.

21. Dombrowski and Deltete, *A Brief, Liberal, Catholic Defense of Abortion*; Wenz, *Abortion Rights as Religious Freedom*; Boonin, *A Defense of Abortion*; Marquis, "Why Abortion Is Immoral," 320–37.

of human beings.²² The fifth chapter again engages the work of David Boonin, in this case his defense of Thomson's famous violinist argument. My effort here, too, is to show that Boonin does not successfully answer the critic of abortion on grounds the critic already accepts.

I hope these chapters on abortion will not seem to my readers to be too much going over old ground. Although I do not insist on the point specifically, several of my later chapters will suggest my anecdotal conviction that abortion continues to be the issue that most poisons our political life. Abortion has the potential to divide as it does for the simple reason that hardly anything is more central to who we are than the way we understand the place of children in our lives—even when we decide not to have any. Decent political discussion—free of lies, subterfuge, and the carefully managed denial of reality—can hardly exist where some citizens regard others of their fellows to be murderers and those others regard their opponents to be, at best, misogynists bent on punishing women and, at worst, potential terrorists. I would describe myself as a critic of abortion, although for much of my life I was an uncritical supporter of the practice. Surely nothing has been so important to my own changed point of view than the rearing of my children, whom I have come to understand as gifts beyond any conceiving. What it means to be a "critic of abortion" is partly that I have seen no arguments for the practice that cannot be answered—as I hope to demonstrate here, at least for some of the best. Moreover, if it is primarily the uniqueness, the irreplaceability, of human beings that matters most to us, then conception seems, to me, to be the most reasonable place to think of a new and precious being beginning his or her life.

Nevertheless for many years my wife and I used an interuterine device for contraception. I consider that to have been an uninformed choice, and I wish that we had not done so. But I certainly do not consider the contraceptive effects of an IUD to be the equivalent of mass murder, and I think that references to abortion as murder lead not only to division but to serious confusion about the practice.²³ "Murder" is a description

22. Thomson, "Defense of Abortion," 131–45; Regan, "Rewriting *Roe v. Wade*," 1569–1646; Steffen, *Life/Choice*.

23. Analogies between the regime of abortion and the Holocaust are also both inaccurate and unhelpful, in my view. On the other hand, I do believe, with Dale Aukerman, that we must always be prepared to examine the possibility of the "dark continuity" between our own practices—and ourselves—and the worst of human evils. See *Darkening Valley*, 18–23. Understanding where our practices are mired in sin or given over to

that implies certain things about motive that are completely irrelevant to abortion. Those who use the term to describe the supporters of choice inadvertently make discussion of the matter nearly impossible. The description has the effect of pressing pro-choicers to cease attempting to discern "what is going on" in abortion and to begin justifying a practice about which they cannot really ask. Justification of abortion leads to its routinization, which, in turn, leads to ever easier, partly because more necessary, justification. Misdescription of abortion as murder promotes this seemingly unbreakable cycle.

I offer no ways to "break the abortion deadlock" here, as a number of books have sought to do. My purpose is the more modest one of showing how the critic of abortion can respond to major pro-abortion arguments. The most useful thing I can say toward promoting renewed conversation about abortion is that it can be helpful to think about pro-life language, particularly that about the status of conception, as meant to transform us toward a higher regard for the uniqueness of human life than is carried by our ordinary moral intuitions. Ronald Dworkin and a host of choice proponents rest part of their claim on what seems to me the indubitable fact that we commonly attribute increasing moral status to the fetus as it develops. We think of the fetus as acquiring more protection against being killed the more it comes to be "like us." This perfectly reasonable intuition is, in some ways, what the claim for protection from conception is meant to counter. That claim forces us to ponder both what is most distinctive about us and what is involved in killing another human being.

If we recognize that what is most distinctive about "us" is that "we" are unique, embodied beings, each of whom lives out an unrepeatable history experienced from a point-of-view never fully commensurate with that of others, we will conclude that conception is the most reasonable point to consider that history as beginning. Part of what is wrong with killing is that it deprives each of us of the ground of human dignity—i.e., that we each live out a unique story whose end, though the fate of all, is experienced by each of us in a way incommensurate with the way it is experienced by all others. We have a right to life because we cannot give it to ourselves, we cannot finally secure it, and we cannot be compensated for its loss. The meaning of our lives derives from the way we make

---

falsely created "necessities" is something Christian faith can enable, for it allows us to examine what we are doing from the confidence that we are already forgiven in Christ.

something of them despite the fact of their limitations. It is not our part to close definitively the possibility of meaning for another by depriving him or her of the horizon of understanding from which meaning is created. If we come to understand the process of meaning-making in this way, we will want to protect any being capable of it at every stage of its life. But it should also move us toward changing whatever unjustly limits all human beings from living out their stories. Thus it should make us particularly sensitive to the aspirations of women, which seem often dependent on the availability of abortion. Suggesting how to reconcile these claims is beyond my intention. What I do hope to have indicated is that desire to protect the fetus from conception can be consistent with support for the aspirations of women. Two things are certain. First, women's need for abortion is directly related to the systemic gender inequality that has marked, and continues to mark, this and nearly every other human society.[24] Second, meaningful change on the abortion question can be brought about—immediately and perhaps even most efficiently—by the transformation of men's attitudes toward children.

Chapters 6 through 11 of this volume concern issues occasioned by the current revolution in genetics. Chapter 6 addresses the matter of genetic enhancement of children, seeing in the question also a place to test the viability of pragmatism as a public philosophy. Chapter 7 challenges claims that justice may demand far reaching genetic interventions. I carefully engage the arguments of the authors of *From Chance to Choice*, questioning their attempted redemption of eugenics, their blurring of the distinction between therapy and enhancement, and their understanding of the model of justice implicit in their discussion.[25] Chapter 8 treats the problem sometimes called the "harm conundrum," which concerns how we are to understand "harm" to a child occasioned by parental action or neglect when that particular child had no way of being born free of the condition. The chapter examines attempts to understand this paradox by numerous writers—among them Peter Singer, Derek Parfit, and Jeff McMahan—and proposes a commonsense alternative rooted in justice understood as the fair sharing of risk.

---

24. For the argument that issues involving sexuality must always be considered within the context of systematic gender inequality, see MacKinnon, *Feminism Unmodified*, 85–102.

25. Buchanan et al., *From Chance to Choice*..

Chapter 9 addresses two related and very difficult matters regarding disability or differential ability. In his fine book, *The Future of the Disabled in Liberal Society*,[26] Hans Reinders considers the way disability and the disabled will be regarded in a society like ours as the revolution in genetics makes it increasingly possible to eliminate disabling conditions. One position he repudiates is the so-called Distinction Between Persons and Conditions argument, or DPC, which maintains that we treat conditions, not persons, and that therefore elimination of disabling conditions can be accomplished without implying a very negative judgment about the lives of those now suffering from the conditions in question. While I agree with most of Reinders's concerns and argument, I try to rescue a nuanced version of the DPC, and I argue—after the manner of Stanley Hauerwas's "Salvation and Health: Or Why Medicine Needs the Church"[27]—that something very like the church is needed to keep the distinction between person and condition clear and to enable us to fully honor the lives of those disabled by conditions that we simultaneously seek to eliminate. The second part of the chapter addresses the issue of designing for disability and Dena Davis's courageous—but, in my view, finally unsuccessful— attempt to come to terms with it by positing the child's "right to an open future."[28] Again I suggest that something like the church can provide a helpful context for the discussion of what seems irresolvable in the terms offered by liberal society. Issues concerning disability are also the focus of chapter 10, which focuses on the work of Peter Singer. Beginning with Singer's objections to being "silenced" in Germany for broaching the subject of euthanasia, I examine his claims that his ethical positions should be of no special concern from the disabled.[29] I disagree. Singer's silencing is certainly deplorable, but distress at his positions among the disabled seems at least partly justifiable. My last chapter turns to the matter of reproductive cloning, or SCNT. It begins by considering why we find cloning repugnant and then explores the relevance of Mary Shelley's *Frankenstein* specifically to issues raised by SCNT. The chapter concludes with a purely secular argument against widespread use of SCNT.

26. Reinders, *Future of the Disabled*.
27. Hauerwas, "Salvation and Health," 63–83.
28. Davis, *Genetic Dilemmas*.
29. Singer, "On Being Silenced in Germany," in *Practical Ethics*, 337–59.

Clearly there are other issues equally worthy of treatment: the ethics of embryo research and implantation, the claims of germ-line versus somatic gene therapies, the moral questions raised by therapeutic or research SCNT. All I can say is that any book represents only the tiniest part of what can be done. I hope readers will find what this book has done to be helpful in their thinking about the matters addressed. I want to close here with some brief stories that I introduce as evidence for why reflection on questions of medicine and ethics can never become simply or wholly a professional as opposed to a personal matter. Joel Shuman begins a book I very much admire, *The Body of Compassion*, with a story about his grandfather, a countryman from West Virginia who, after enjoying good health all of his life, was diagnosed with leukemia—on one of his very few journeys away from the home place. The doctors proposed an operation and he went to Charleston to have it, only to "die alone in a hospital hours from home, denied an active role in the last days of his life and his death by a world that was almost completely foreign to him."[30] Shuman tells the story as a way of introducing what he calls "the irony of modern medicine": that "at the very time medicine has become more successful than ever as an enemy of disease and prolonger of human life, it has become increasingly incapable of contributing meaningfully to our living and dying well."[31]

Shuman calls for a renewal of our sense—for him grounded powerfully in Christianity—that medicine must involve a recovery of the wisdom of the body, that we must relearn the truth that we are not simply Cartesian angels manipulating a machine by means of the pineal gland.[32] I agree with him fully, but I want to insist also that we not set this understanding of medicine over against a scientific one. We need for medicine to be both art and science. We need contexts in which we can accept our limitations, learn to live with and into the unavoidable varieties of suffering, and know that the great dignity of human beings derives

---

30. Shuman, *Body of Compassion*, 4.
31. Ibid., 6.
32. In discussing the hypertrophy of the intellect and will in Edgar Allan Poe, Allen Tate quotes Jacques Maritain on the effects of Cartesian dualism: it "breaks man up into two complete substances, joined to one another none knows how: on the one hand, the body which is only geometrical extension; on the other, the soul which is only thought—an angel inhabiting a machine and directing it by means of the pineal gland." See Tate, "Angelic Imagination," 411–12. The quotation is from Maritain, *Dream of Descartes*, 179–80.

from living under the sign of mortality. But we also need to remember the extraordinary achievements of medicine as science, achievements made possible, to some degree, by the ability to objectify the body for examination and research.

When I think of my grandparents, I remember how three of the six children in my grandmother's family died in adolescence of diphtheria, no more than a hundred years ago, or how my grandfather's mother died young in an insane asylum. I think of that same grandmother caring for many years for her own mother, so crippled by rheumatoid arthritis that she was unable finally to use any of her limbs. One of my father's best family stories concerned what my great grandfather did immediately after her death. He closed the door of their room and spent a few minutes alone with her. When he emerged, he said that he had done what he promised her he'd do: to straighten her body so that she might be straight, once at least. I remember, too, the children in iron lungs in my neighborhood in the 1950s and the way parents greeted the news of the Salk and Sabin vaccines almost as blessings from above. Finally, I remember most vividly of all my mother's telling me after school one day when I was eight that my nine-year-old first cousin had been taken to the hospital in the middle of the previous night and died of a rampant intestinal infection.

Many of the students I teach have very little memory of stories like these I have just recounted. That they do not is a tribute to the success of modern medicine. It also means that many of them have not had the need for a serious story about the place of suffering in human life.[33] Medicine has been so successful, so fast, in erasing cultural memories of the ills flesh is heir to that one prominent bioethicist now proposes

---

33. Robert Jenson's description of those living with the *fact* of postmodernism fits many of my students well: they are "folk who simply do not apprehend or inhabit a narratable world. Indeed, many do not know that anyone ever did. The reason so many now cannot 'find their place' is that they are unaware of the possibility of a kind of world or society that could have such things as places, though they may recite, as a sort of mantra, memorized phrases about 'getting my life together' and the like. There are now many who do not and cannot understand their lives as realistic narrative." Often their encounters with the medical system encourage their sense of the senselessness of things, for if there is one medical memory that many of them do share, it is of some elderly person, often a grandparent, whose life has been extended beyond the point where it could be said to possess any reasonable quality. I do not want to overgeneralize here, though, as some of my students have suffered, often very deeply, with family and friends going through major illness. See Jenson, "How the World Lost Its Story," 21.

that we think of medicine as just what we do in hospitals[34]—without reference to any norms about the cure of disease or bodily health. With so little appreciation for the therapeutic tasks of medicine, it is little wonder that the distinction between therapy and enhancement comes to seem tenuous. Now research into the human genome seems to promise unprecedented mastery over our limitations, at least for the affluent in the developed world. At the same time, health care in large parts of the developing world bears almost no resemblance to that taken for granted by the North Atlantic bourgeoisie, and the evils that afflict human beings have familiar faces: epidemics, poor sanitation and living conditions, childhood diseases, parasites, insect-borne fevers, and completely treatable yet ultimately lethal infections. Surely there will be an unending series of complex questions to be addressed by those engaged in bioethical reflection. These questions are far too important to be left only to a cadre of ethicists with very specialized expertise. We need reflection that combines solidarity with the body of compassion and a deep respect for the therapeutic purposes of medicine. To attempt to write from that combination has been my goal here.

---

34. McGee, *Perfect Baby*, 126.

1

Can the Use of Artificial Contraception within Marriage Be Consistent with the Natural Law?

THE PROHIBITION OF ARTIFICIAL contraception occupies a central place in Pope John Paul II's morality of the acting person and his critique of the contemporary "culture of death."[1] Discussing John Paul's anthropology and theology of marriage, William E. May, in fact, refers to artificial contraception as the "gateway" to the culture of death.[2] For John Paul, the development of a "contraceptive mentality" represents a grave symptom of a falsely dualistic understanding of the human being and a distorted emphasis on subjectivity alone as the defining mark of the person. The danger of artificial contraception lies in its breaking the unity of the person by instrumentalizing the body, which then becomes merely a subhuman means to goods assumed to be personal. What is compromised, perhaps even "annihilated" in the process, is man's "au-

---

1. On John Paul II's morality of the "acting person," I have found extremely helpful MacIntyre, "How Can We Learn What *Veritatis Splendor* Has to Teach?," 171–95, and Rhonheimer, "'Intrinsically Evil Acts' and the Moral Viewpoint," 1–39.

2. May, "Contraception, Gateway to the Culture of Death." In the interpretation favored by May, the connection between contraception and the culture of death lies in the development of a contraceptive or contralife will in those who use artificial contraception. On this view, the contraceptor first projects a child who might come to be as a result of intercourse and then rejects the child. On this point, see Grisez et al., "Every Marital Act," 40–47 et passim. For a thorough critique of their understanding of the wrong of contraception, see Smith, *Humanae Vitae*. Smith argues the evil of contraception lies not in its involving a contraceptive will but in the intrinsic quality of the act itself. For Grisez et al., contraception "presupposes and is closely related to sexual acts" (43). For Smith, this is not enough: contraception "is a perverse sexual act" (361). See also Grabowski, *Sex and Virtue*, especially chapter 6.

thentic personal dominion over himself."[3] Implicit in the contraceptive mentality is a falsely dualistic or mentalistic understanding of personhood. Personal autonomy becomes associated with emergence from all dependence; personal dignity is too narrowly associated with "*the capacity for verbal and explicit*, or at least, perceptible, *communication*"; and freedom loses its "*inherently relational dimension*," becoming instead "absolute in an individualistic way." "On the basis of these presuppositions," John Paul argues in *Evangelium Vitae*, "there is no place in the world for anyone who, like the unborn or the dying, is a weak element in the social structure, or for anyone who appears completely at the mercy of others and radically dependent on them, and can only communicate through the silent language of a profound sharing of affection."[4] John Paul's alternative to the false subjectivist and dualistic assumptions of modern notions of autonomy has been to insist on personhood's involving the embodied human being in its entirety. In regard to marriage, this has meant his development of a theology of "mutual donation," one that treats sexuality as the mutual bodily self-giving of persons-in-love.

Let me begin by saying how thoroughly I accept certain features of John Paul's description of the contemporary situation, even though I am going to offer a defense of artificial contraception within marriage as consistent with the natural law. The broadly Enlightenment conception of personhood as autonomous from all determining contexts does seem inherently threatening to those "radically dependent on others"; artificial contraception has seemingly given rise to a "contraceptive mentality," which too often sees children as burdens to be avoided; the aspiration to a comprehensive medical control over all natural processes does tend to devalue suffering and undermine human solidarity in suffering. Suffering becomes simply a problem to be solved, a scandal that ought not to exist, rather than a mystery that must be confronted and lived through in mutual dependence. Against this so-called "culture of death," recent Popes have sought to build a civilization of love, one of whose most basic affirmations insists that sexual acts must be "open," in all cases, to children. The fact that we even contemplate genetic engineering of children for enhancement suggests the degree to which children have become projects of their parents' wills, acceptable only on condition of

---

3. Wojtyla, "Anthropological Vision of *Humanae Vitae*," 19.

4. *Gospel of Life: Evangelium Vitae*, 36–37. Further references will be given in the text with the abbreviation EV.

their meeting certain standards of quality. This commodification of children lends weight to John Paul's contention that sexuality has become "depersonalized and exploited: from being the sign, place and language of love, that is, of the gift of self and acceptance of another, in all the other's richness as a person, it increasingly becomes the occasion and instrument for self-assertion and the selfish satisfaction of personal desires and instincts" (EV 43). It is of immeasurable importance for Christians to insist on parenthood as a matter of self-giving, of fundamental generosity. The child who understands herself as the free gift and outpouring of her parents' generosity is one who will be able to freely give herself in love. The free gift of self from parent to child will be, for many, the realest analogy of—and pointer to—God's free gift of himself in Christ.

Thus it is with the greatest respect that I hope to enter into dialogue with the Catholic tradition on the matter of artificial contraception. I do so as one who is not a Catholic but as a Protestant Christian who confesses faith in "one holy, catholic, and apostolic church" and also, I hope, as one of good will. I mention this last point because the encyclical *Humanae Vitae* addresses itself specifically to "all Men of goodwill," and discussion of that encyclical must, of course, be at the heart of any consideration of contraceptive matters.[5] The point I will attempt to make is that artificial contraception within marriage can be consistent with the natural law understood as *opus rationis*, a work or ordering of the practical reason. For this understanding of the natural law as articulated by Thomas Aquinas, I am indebted to Martin Rhonheimer's magisterial *Natural Law and Practical Reason*. Thus it is crucial here to explicate briefly Rhonheimer's understanding of natural law as practical reason. I should say, in advance, that Rhonheimer does not draw conclusions similar to mine from his understanding of natural law. Indeed he specifically examines the teaching of *Humanae Vitae* and Pope John Paul II and concurs fully with it. Nevertheless I believe his understanding of natural law does make dialogue possible with the tradition regarding artificial contraception, and this I will attempt to foster.

A critical point to understand is that the "natural law is not primarily and per se a collection of normative statements that the practical

---

5. References will be to the translation of *Humanae Vitae*, made from the Latin, in Smith, *Humanae Vitae*, 269–95. Further citations will be given parenthetically with the abbreviation HV.

reason simply finds 'already there' to 'follow.'"⁶ It is not simply a matter of our reading off laws that are somehow established in nature. Rather the natural law is constituted by acts of the practical reason as it pursues the good. The good is the "object of the practical reason," which "*constitutes* commands, norms, duties, and so on under the aspect of the good, that is, it forms statements in the form of 'ought' or 'should'" (59). The "application (*applicatio*) of this normative knowing to concrete behavior" involves acts of the conscience ("*con-scientia*, 'knowing-along-with'"). These acts of practical judgment and conscience take place on one level, one directly concerned with the carrying out of acts; the natural law is formulated at a second level of reflection upon the acts of the practical reason in pursuit of the particular goods within various "field[s] of action" (58). "The acts of the practical reason itself do *not* have the natural law for their object"; rather they provide the subject matter for reflection, thus "in fact *constitut[ing]* the natural law" (58). Perhaps it will help to clarify what this means by considering the status of statements like the "'good is to be done' (*bonus est faciendum*)" or "'evil is to be avoided' (*malum est vitandum*)" (59). These clearly are not statements "made by the practical reason at the level where it actually *makes*" precepts or commands; rather they are the fruits of "*reflection upon*" particular "preceptive act[s] of the practical reason" (59). Rhonheimer is very concerned to prevent a reading of Thomas that "establishes the 'autonomy' of the natural law in contradistinction to the so-called 'natural order'" (63). Thomas's *Lex naturalis est aliquid per rationem constitutum*—"the natural law is something constituted by the reason"—does not point to "a full metaphysical disjunction between nature and reason," as it might in a Kantian sense. Such a disjunction "has its ultimate origin in an attempt to *oppose* reason to a thoroughly naturalistic ("physicalistic") interpretation of the 'order of nature.'" "Such a reason would have the character of unlimited freedom vis a vis the natural" and would make impossible the establishment of natural law norms.⁷

Rhonheimer discusses the "model of married love" at length both in order to "illustrate the comprehensive personal structure of human

6. Rhonheimer, *Natural Law and Practical Reason*, 61. Further citations will be given parenthetically.

7. Ibid., 63–64: *Lex naturalis est aliquid per rationem constitutum; sicut etiam propositio est quoddam opus rationis* ("The natural law is something constituted by the reason, just as the *proposition* is a work of the reason"). See Thomas, *Summa Theologiae*, I-II, q. 94, a. 1.

willing or loving" and to defend the prohibition of artificial contraception affirmed by *Humanae Vitae* and John Paul II. He insists first that the "natural inclination toward the 'joining of male and female'" is not to be understood as "an 'incarnation' of human love": to do so is to suggest that human love is originally a spiritual phenomenon that only secondarily becomes bodily (96–97).[8] Neither is the "marital act" simply an "act of the power of procreation" or generation that can also serve "as an expression of love" (100). Married love unites "sensuality and spirituality" as the act of bodily entities "'ensouled' and endowed with reason, according to the classical and precise formulation: *animal rationale*" (97). The *inclinatio naturalis* lies at the basis of married love, but that love comes about only when this inclination is carried out in a specifically human manner, in accord with the natural law. To ask about the "object of the 'marital act,'" then, is to "inquire into the object or 'objective significance' of the love between husband and wife, and not into the 'natural end' (*finis naturalis*) of the procreative power" (100). Thomas presents a "personal and integral anthropology and ethics" that recognizes "bodiliness and sensation" to be the "*foundation* for all spiritual acts" (102) but which also sees these as ordered to fulfillment in distinctively personal acts and consistent, in the case of sexuality, with responsible parenthood and the dignity of the human person (personal "love between man and woman" being "the only form of the transmission of human life that is worthy of the human person" [101]). We must not understand the natural law to be simply the moralization of certain laws of nature in a biological or scientific sense. *Humanae Vitae* opposes artificial contraception not in order to maintain the "integrity of the 'natural order'" but rather to preserve "the integrity of human love, which is at once an *ordo rationis*, as well as an *ordo virtutis*" (114).

Rhonheimer points out the wrongheadedness of criticisms of the encyclical that claim its argument for the immorality of artificial contraception "rests upon preserving the biological integrity of the act, and upon the (likewise biological) laws of cyclical fertility" (113). He finds instead the central statement of *Humanae Vitae* to be the teaching on the "inseparable connection, willed by God and unable to be broken by man on his own initiative, between the two meanings of the conjugal

---

8. On this point, see also Grisez, "New Formulation," 343–61. For Grisez, a realistic Christian personalism depends absolutely on our recognizing that man is a rational animal, not an incarnate spirit.

act: the unitive meaning and the procreative meaning."[9] For him the "key to the argument" lies in the "concept of *responsible parenthood*" (114). The difference between natural and artificial birth control is not simply a difference in method. Responsible parenthood is present only where the limitation of the number of children has its "origin in an act of the virtue of chastity" (114). The *ordo virtutis* is closely connected to the *ordo rationis*, as noted above in Rhonheimer's language about preserving the integrity of human love. Developing the *habitus* to integrate action from moral precepts with reflection on the natural law involves also understanding the virtues involved in particular actions and arriving at a rational ordering of them. Marital chastity or continence is the virtue particularly suited to responsible parenthood, and to rely on artificial contraception is to destroy the very conditions within which this virtue can be developed. In *Familiaris Consortio*, John Paul draws a very strong distinction between periodic abstinence and artificial contraception, arguing that the difference "is much wider and deeper than is usually thought" and ultimately connected with "two irreconcilable concepts of the human person and of human sexuality."[10]

In her study of *Humanae Vitae: A Generation Later*, Janet E. Smith has drawn attention to the stress John Paul lays on the virtue of self-mastery in his interpretation of the encyclical. The narrow meaning of self-mastery pertains to chastity, but the broad designation points to that "mastery of any passion" that is essential to the development of the moral virtues and thus "to the perfecting of the human person." Chastity is "essential to the true expression of love" (and thus to justice as well), for "if one is driven by one's passions one will treat one's spouse as an object designed to satisfy those passions, not as a person deserving to be loved."[11] The practice of abstinence can be an enriching feature of the dialogue between married persons, "purifying it, deepening it, and at the same time simplifying it."[12] The crucial point is that the human being must "'have possession' of himself in order to express himself authenti-

---

9. *Humanae Vitae*, article 12, quoted here from Rhonheimer, *Natural Law and Practical Reason*, 113.

10. John Paul II, *Familiaris Consortio*, Article 32, p. 21.

11. Smith, *Humanae Vitae*, 235. Further citations will be given parenthetically. For a brief history of Catholic thinking about chastity and its place in the thought of John Paul II, see Grabowski, *Sex and Virtue*, ch. 4.

12. Pope John Paul II, *Reflections on Humanae Vitae*, 64.

cally and in accord with objective truth and to give of himself fully" (Smith, 237). Artificial contraception substitutes technological control for the right ordering of the passions in the self-mastery of continence. The specific immorality in artificial contraception, to cite Rhonheimer, lies not in its being an "improper means of exercising procreative responsibility, but rather in the willing refusal of procreative responsibility *as such*" (132). There can be no justification, according to Rhonheimer, "for exercising one's moral responsibility in a certain field of behavior by simply *removing* this field from the need to be governed" by will, reason, and virtue. To do so is to violate "human dignity, which consists in living *secundum rationem*" and to refuse "to be human, and this is so even if the exercise of human dignity requires sacrifice, discipline (*askesis*), and self-denial," which, in "true love," "are always a source of joy, fulfillment, and inner peace" (137–38).

To establish the background for my later argument, it will be helpful to stay with Rhonheimer's analysis a little longer, particularly on the correlation of marital chastity and procreative responsibility. In a piece on the "Philosophical Foundation of the Norm of 'Humanae Vitae,'" Rhonheimer reaffirms his argument that the perspective of the encyclical is "*not to defend the demand of respecting natural patterns inherent in the biological or physiological constitution of man and his generative acts, but to stress what has been called the 'intentionalness of the thing one is doing' by contracepting, an intentionalness which relates to the virtue of chastity and to its specific requirements within the context of procreative responsibility.*" This, Rhonheimer thinks, "is the key to a proper understanding of the encyclical" and "probably the only way of explaining why contraception violates natural law."[13] The "*very core*" of his argument lies in "the analysis of the difference between contraceptive intercourse and intercourse in the context of a practice of a periodic abstinence." These he deems "radically different forms of sexual behavior," the one informed by responsibility, the other, a forsaking of responsibility (12).

The couple practicing abstinence engage in "a real *conjugal* act"; they maintain the procreative meaning of their actions while bringing their behavior under intentional control, guided by the virtue of chastity. "Acts of procreatively responsible continence" possess a "proper *marital* and even *parental* meaning," as they are "acts of bodily constituted loving

---

13. Rhonheimer, "Contraception, Sexual Behavior, and Natural Law," 4. Further references will be included parenthetically. Emphasis in original unless otherwise noted.

persons engaged in responsibly arising to the exigencies of their marital and parental vocation" (24). The chastity they exercise belongs to the virtue of temperance, which "tempers" the "sensual appetites according to reason" so as to enable those "appetites *themselves* to pursue what is according to reason." Rhonheimer stresses the way the virtues never simply repel or suppress "sensual inclinations and their proper goods or goals." Rather they redirect or modify those inclinations in order to bring them into accord with the whole person's "striving" for the goods pursued by the will under the guidance of practical reason. Because procreative responsibility is to be understood as an exercise of virtue, marital love must remain open to procreation not only in its totality but at "*the level of single performances of sexual acts*" (22). This is because "single acts and their corresponding choices are morally specified by their intentional contents which spring from the virtues" to which they belong. Conjugal acts "belong to" chastity/temperance; choices made about them are to be considered and understood according to these virtues.

Artificial contraception, however, "signifies that to avoid conception sexual behavior need not be modified." Rhonheimer notes that "*something* in the behavior must be modified," but this he limits to one spouse's "taking the pill, say, according to medical prescriptions." But "sexuality, the sensual appetite or drive precisely, need not be modified." Contraception is "not problematic because of its 'un-natural' character" but rather because it "render[s] needless responsible modification of sexual behavior." Moreover, it "*involves a choice against virtuous self-control by continence*," leaving sexual behavior to become "a pure act of deliberate will which treats sexuality and the body as its *object* (equal to a diseased liver, heart or digestive apparatus)" (25). Thus contraception represents "a fundamental attack on both the integrity of the human-person as a body-spirit unity and on marital love which expresses this unity." Contraceptive intercourse "*is not* an expression of *marital* love. *In itself* (disregarding the marital context), its point in nothing differs from the point of any other form of sexual activity, as mutual masturbation or sodomy" (26). Whereas the practice of periodic continence involves "an act *common* to both spouses," who become united "in one flesh and live a common vocation," the "contracepting couple undermines" this kind of "communion." A "principle of disintegration" is set to work in married life. A condition of "sensual heteronomy" obtains, one in which sensual appetite becomes "directed only to actual satisfaction and self-gratification" rather than integration "into the 'logic of the spirit.'" Spouses may become only "object[s] of sexual desire" experienced as "worthless in the same measure as sexual desire is satisfied." The result is "isolation and loneliness" rather than "communion" as spouses are transformed "into *accomplices* of common masturbation" (29). A "problematic gap" opens between the spiritual and the sexual, precisely because "the link established by the procreative task" is no longer there (30).

In the face of these arguments, a natural law defense of contraception may seem next to impossible, but I think this need not be the case. It may also seem inherently contradictory to attempt a *natural* law defense of *artificial* contraception, but, as we can see from Rhonheimer's analysis, this is only an apparent, not a real, problem. For, as we have seen, the natural law does not simply moralize natural processes in the scientific or, more specifically, biological sense. In fact, a natural law defense of artificial contraception within marriage might begin with the observation that Rhonheimer still seems more committed to a kind of "biologism" than he claims. That biologism is evident in his assigning sexual behavior to the virtue of chastity alone. I should say, at the outset, that I find compelling both Rhonheimer's account of temperance and his analysis of the way periodic continence serves the mutual self-giving of married love—although I suspect he underestimates the degree to which continence sometimes promotes disharmony rather than loving communion. He seems concerned that "an already deeply implanted contraceptive mentality" will find periodic continence "unreasonable"—something I have no wish to do.[14] My point is rather that Rhonheimer's account unnecessarily restricts the virtues under which decisions about marital sexuality must be made. Here I follow a suggestion made by Stanley Hauerwas in response to a commentary of Rhonheimer's on *Veritatis Splendor*. If "one has to analyze intentional contents as belonging to the structure of the virtues," Hauerwas comments, "then one has to consider why certain descriptions are privileged."[15] Rhonheimer privileges chastity/temperance in relation to marital sexuality for obvious, largely biological reasons. This does not, however, close the possibility that a much thicker account of marriage—and particularly of parenthood—might cause us to situate the intentions involved in marital sexuality under other virtues. Decisions about sexuality and contraception might well be

14. Rhonheimer, "Contraception, Sexual Behavior, and Natural Law," 24.
15. Hauerwas, *Sanctify Them in the Truth*, 116.

formed as matters of justice, charity, and marital friendship. A decision for contraception might well derive from a very thoroughly and temperately achieved integration of spiritual and bodily love, both in the person and between spouses. This is perhaps particularly true *where there are already children*. In some ways, Rhonheimer's account underestimates the way marriage and child-rearing transform sexuality itself—its contexts, the relevant virtues, the intentions involved.

By way of thickening up this account, I ask a certain patience from the reader as I introduce some considerations from the world of historical demography that are relevant to the argument. These bear especially on the contexts in which married couples now make decisions about procreation and contraception. The key points are that these decisions are now made in the contexts of much longer life expectancies, much surer child survival, and greatly increased percentages of elderly in our populations. As Peter Laslett has maintained, the aging of societies over the past one hundred twenty years—since the so-called Demographic Transition—is so great that we can speak of these periods almost as two different worlds, as the Before and the After.[16] I hope the following reflection will contribute to what Laslett and others call "processional knowledge"—knowledge that takes into account how people think about practices in relation to reasonable expectations for those at their place in the procession.

Just how dire and different matters were in what we might call the Long Before is suggested by a passage cited by Peter Brown at the beginning of his study of "sexual renunciation in early Christianity." The passage is from a life of the virgin Saint Thecla written by a Christian priest from the southern coast of Turkey in the fifth century. In it Thamyris, rejected suitor of Thecla, arraigns St. Paul for his teaching on virginity and the abandonment of marriage:

> This man has introduced a new teaching, bizarre and disruptive of the human race. He denigrates marriage: yes, marriage, which you might say is the beginning, root and fountainhead of our nature. From it spring fathers, mothers, children, and families. Cities, villages and cultivation have appeared because of it. . . .

---

16. The terms "Before" and "After," Laslett explains, "were introduced in an attempt to distinguish aging from the other constituents of 'modernization' and the aging process from the demographic transition or transitions." They refer most specifically, then, to the enormous changes in phenomena related to aging rather than to the demographic transition from a pre-modern condition of high birth and death rates to a modern one of low birth and death rates. See "Necessary Knowledge," 68.

> What is more, from marriage come the temples and sanctuaries of our land, sacrifice, rituals, initiations, prayers and solemn days of intercession.

Brown uses the passage to stress the strangeness of Paul's teaching in a world "more helplessly exposed to death" than even the most "afflicted underdeveloped country in the modern world." The average life expectancy of citizens of the Roman Empire in the second century C.E. was "less than twenty-five years." According to Brown, "only four of every hundred men, and fewer women, lived beyond the age of fifty." The pressure to bear children in such a society was enormous; Brown concludes that maintaining even a stable population would have required each woman to produce "an average of five children."[17] The continuity and cohesion of society, indeed even its continued existence, depended on an extraordinary commitment of human energy to begetting and rearing children.

Laslett has argued that a knowledge of aging in the past is "necessary knowledge," a "body of information that all persons must have to understand themselves as they are today."[18] This is because the "populations of developed societies have grown old at an amazing pace." In the last one hundred years, and largely in the last fifty, the populations of "Europe, North America, Australasia, and Japan have become far and away the oldest human populations of which we have knowledge" (3). These populations are older, and continuing to get older, in two ways: "average individual lifetimes last for very much longer than they ever have before anywhere or at any time, and these populations have among them quite unprecedented numbers of elderly people." In Laslett's view, this situation is so "novel," the change so dramatic and rapid, that "there has not yet been time enough to take account of the transformation" (4). As a result, we are living in "a state of cultural lag," "continuing to make assumptions about age and aging that, though they had always been true before the present century, have incontinently disappeared" (4). What is more, this "demographic transition" that began in the developed world in the late-nineteenth century is now beginning to be evident in the de-

---

17. Brown, *Body and Society*, 5–6. Brown's citation derives from *Vita Theclae* 16 in Dagron, ed. *Vie et Miracles de Sainte Thecle*, 190–92.

18. Laslett, "Necessary Knowledge," 3. Further citations will be given parenthetically.

veloping world as well. What is occurring is truly a secular shift with which we must come to terms.

Understanding what is going on requires more than simply noting the greatly improved rates of infant mortality and much longer life expectancies. Obviously these circumstances have changed dramatically in our day, especially, of course, in the developed world. The life expectancy of American males and females is now seventy-five and eighty-one years, respectively, for those born in the year 2006.[19] This contrasts sharply with the figures for the 1880s: 42.5 years for U.S. males, 44.5 for females. Even in the 1920s, the expectancies were only 55 years for males and 57.1 for females. Expressed in terms of percentage, the rise in male life expectancy in the United States from the 1880s to the 1980s was 168%; for females, 173%. Percentage rises from some other countries are even more dramatic. Male life expectancy in Germany more than doubled from the 1880s to the 1980s, from 35.6 years to 71.8 years, or 202%. In Greece, Spain, and Italy both male and female life expectancy more than doubled during the period, the sharpest rise of all occurring among Italian women, who went from 33.9 years to 78.6, a jump of 232%.[20]

An accompanying change has occurred in the proportion of populations aged 60 or older. 5.4% of the U.S. population was over 60 in the 1880s, only 6.7% in the 1920s. The percentage in the 1980s–90s had risen to 15.9%, a percentage increase of 294% over the 1880 figures. Other countries with a greater than 200% rise include Canada, 5.4 in the 1880s, 11.3 in the 1980s–90s, or 209%; England and Wales, 7.4 and 17.0, 230%; Germany, 7.9 and 16.7, 211%; Greece, 4.6 and 15.2, 330%.[21] The curves for future projections continue the dramatic rise. The figures for England, for example, may rise from roughly 20% at present to somewhere between 30 and 40% by 2200.[22]

Clearly two strong trends with massive consequences have emerged during the last one hundred twenty years. People can reasonably and routinely expect to live much longer lives than in the past, and an ever-

---

19. These figures are from "The World Fact Book" at www.cia.gov/cia/publications/factbook/us.html.

20. For these statistics on changes in life expectancies by country, see Table 1.1 in Laslett, "Necessary Knowledge," 12.

21. For the percentages of persons aged 60 or older in various societies, see Table 1.2 in Laslett, "Necessary Knowledge," 13.

22. See Figure 1.1 in Laslett, "Necessary Knowledge," 15.

growing segment of the population will be over sixty years old. What exactly this latter phenomenon means is unclear, but surely it suggests that people's working lifetimes will be much longer and that ever greater numbers of people will become dependent and in need of care—from their children and a host of institutions—particularly as those already over sixty become those over eighty. In order to understand how such changes affect the kinds of decisions made over a life's course, however, it is necessary to consider some additional statistics. In the "high pressure" regime of the Roman Empire, only 37% of all infants born would live to twenty-five years of age, roughly only 26% to 40. Even if one lived to be fifteen, one had only a little more than a 50% chance to live to 45. If we assume relatively equal death rates for males and females over that stretch of the life's course, then the chance of a marriage surviving until both partners were 45 is only one in four. In fact, since each fifteen year old had only about a 70% chance to live to 35, it is likely that half of marriages were ended by the death of one or both spouses before age 35.[23]

Any couple engaged in child rearing would simultaneously face the grim facts of infant and childhood mortality. Nearly 36% of infants died before age 1, more than 50% of children, by age 5. Even if a child was among the 49% who reached age 5, parents still faced a one in nine chance it would not reach 15 and a one in six chance it would not make 20. Finally, as some 54% of children died before age 10, it seems very likely that many couples must have lost all or nearly all their children. Just as a matter of statistical average, they could expect to lose more than half. As a matter of horizon of expectations, however, surely many must have approached conception with the not wholly unreasonable apprehension that they might conceive five, six, or seven children and yet still be left alone if they had the "good fortune" to live to thirty themselves.[24]

Even as we bring the story up from the Roman period to times closer to our own, we must be struck by the extraordinary difference between the Before and After. Average expectation of life at age 15—an especially useful statistic for thinking processionally—remains around forty, or just above, in England from the middle of the sixteenth century

23. Figures on Rome are from Parkin, *Demography and Roman Society*, Appendix B, Table 6, 144. Parkin presents an adapted version of the data from Frier, "Roman Life Expectancy," 213–51.

24. The speculations are mine here; they are based on Parkin, *Demography and Roman Society*, 144.

until the middle of the nineteenth century. It must be remembered, too, that this does not mean that every fifteen year old could expect to live into the early forties. There have been very old people in every society, and the figures for their ages at death will, of course, press the life expectation figure upward. What is critical to note is that "very few could expect to live to the later decades on the lower plateau." Of the men who reached age 25, "something over a quarter" could "expect to live until age 70." That prospect today—that a man would survive from age 25 to age 70—is "over 80 percent."[25] As late as the 1930s, English working-class people saved very little for late life, "but they did save penny by penny for their funerals, which could of course come at any age for them as it could for all their predecessors." In doing so, they were "acting rationally," Laslett remarks, and "as if prompted by processional knowledge." They had little reason to prepare for an old age they did not expect to experience, particularly if there was "public money" available to support them on the odd chance they would need it (62).

It is impossible to sketch out all the changes brought by the transition to the After. Indeed, as we are in the midst of them, it is impossible even to understand them fully as yet. But several are noteworthy. First, "the immemorial association in family time between the exit of the parental generation and the beginnings of the independent family life of the child generation has gone forever." "Proliferation and prolongation" of the empty nest stage ensues, along with increased "elongation of vertical kin links"—links across generations. The latter results in changes "in flows of support between generations, particularly the appearance and spread of multiple dependency, in which a woman has at the same time to attend to the needs of her children or grandchildren and to those of her parents or even grandparents" (43–44). In addition, what has come to be known as the Third Age emerges, a development Laslett has called "the most important of the outcomes for the present and future of developed societies and the future of societies yet to develop" (42). This concept refers to a period of healthy, active life, "beginning for most people" at retirement and lasting until death or until the onset of the Fourth Age, marked by "final decrepitude and dependency." The possibility of Third Age living depends upon a variety of factors: adequacy of savings and social transfers, the wealth and development of a society, and the

---

25. Laslett, "Necessary Knowledge," 67.

availability and levels of education, including that "over the whole life course."[26]

The possibility for this Third Age of life did not exist—for any but the smallest numbers of people—until the middle of the twentieth century, when the necessary background conditions began to exist in Western Europe and "in countries with populations of European origins." Only at that time did survival rates meet the two criteria demographers use to identify the presence of the Third Age: half of a country's men must be able to expect to survive from 25 to 70 and at least a quarter of all adults—those over 25—must be 60 or older (51). The population of England met the first of these in 1951, the second, in 1961, and both numbers have continued to rise very significantly since those dates. Whereas 53.2% of twenty-five year old English men could expect, in 1951, to live to 70, that figure had risen to 69% by 1991 and is, as we have seen, as high as 80% today.[27] One final factor to take into account as we think processionally is the compression of morbidity: in short, that the secular shift in aging has brought a tendency for sickness to be concentrated in the later years rather than distributed over the (much shorter) life span. As people routinely look toward much longer life spans than in the past, they too can expect much longer periods of good health before final decline.

It is fascinating to speculate about how such facts have affected couples' lives and the understanding of sexuality. One thing to observe is how "heroic" it was for Roman couples to simply attempt to reproduce themselves, for there was surely a substantial and emotional disincentive to conception in the fact that one's child was more than likely to die. The inherent anxiety and distress occasioned by attempts to reproduce likely militated against intercourse's playing a significant part in the emotional bonding of the couple. This possibility should cause us to rethink the relationship between the two features of sexual experience emphasized in Catholic teaching: the procreative and the unitive. Surely the unitive potential of sexual experience is correlated to the probability that a child resulting from the union will survive and become not only a living exemplar of the couple's bond but a continuing responsibility for both parents. Apart from the reasonable expectation of reproductive success—not just conception but survival of children into adulthood—sexual experience, perhaps particularly for men, seems likely to be seen as a thing in itself,

---

26. Ibid., 50, 72.

27. For these figures, see ibid., 52, Table 1.4. For the 80% figure for today, see 67.

separable from enduring relationships with women. Once reproductive success becomes sufficiently certain, however, the procreative aspect of sexuality can begin to strengthen the unitive aspect—and the two can clearly work together. When children's survival and maturation become reasonably certain, parents and potential parents must come to think about sexuality in a different way. The joining of man and woman must now be thought within the context of prolonged commitment to nurturance and education of children—these being no less "natural" and embodied actions than the joining itself. Moreover, the unitive dimension of sexual experience receives a continuing source of strength from the very presence of children who embody and yet transcend the couple's own hopes, giving their unity a radically new basis and meaning.

One thing seems certain. As long as couples needed to produce more than five children simply to reproduce themselves and had simultaneously to reckon with the strong possibility that one or both of them would be dead by age 35, thinking about sexuality would, of necessity, be dominated by the overriding importance of procreation. It would seem utterly "natural" to think about sex only in its "natural" meaning. Refusals of that natural meaning could have profound social consequences. If enough young men followed the example of Onan—unwilling to do his levirate duty as brother-in-law to Tamar—societies would be unable to continue themselves (Gen 38:8–10). Or if enough young men became libertines on the order of the early Augustine, similar consequences might follow. Sexuality had to be disciplined toward its reproductive function, particularly because potential parents faced the demanding task of producing many children, in a short time, and with the near certain knowledge that they often would be giving birth to death. Spacing of children in the Before must typically have been dominated by life expectancy. When life expectancy at 15 was in the early 40s, a couple marrying at twenty had to conceive their children in a relatively short span of years if they were to have a reasonable chance to rear them to marrying age. A couple married, conceived children, reared them to the point where they could marry, and then departed. Such was that immemorial pattern of family time alluded to by Laslett.

A processionally-thinking hypothetical couple of the Before looked, then, with considerable uncertainty, on producing perhaps five children in the first ten years of marriage—that is, if they were to have any reasonable chance to see their youngest children to adolescence before their own deaths. During almost the whole of their marriage, perhaps twenty years, conception would be a possibility. Today, by contrast, a couple marrying in their mid twenties can look confidently toward the prospect of 50 to 60 years of marriage and nearly as long a period of sexual activity. Obviously judgments about the spacing of children become possible and necessary in ways they could not have been in the Before. Every decision to conceive becomes—necessarily and thankfully—a decision to rear the child to adulthood. Moreover, greatly extended life expectancy itself operates to loosen the "unitive and procreative" dimensions of sexuality—or to press these to take other, more complex forms. As much as twenty-five years of the sexual activity of our contemporary couple will not be open to conception simply because it will be post-menopausal (using fifty-one as an average age of menopause). Another ten years will be during a period of significantly reduced fertility. If we think of current life spans as somehow "natural," then it is difficult not to conclude that nature itself is loosening the strict bond between sexuality and procreation. This is not to deny, of course, that procreation is an important—even, the primary—natural end of the joining of man and woman. What I do want to stress, though, is that a couple confidently expecting fifty or sixty years of marriage will think about sexuality and child-bearing as aspects of a total relationship in a way that couples of the Before simply could not.

Rhonheimer has placed great emphasis on the way contraception "renders needless" the "responsible modification of sexual behavior."[28] But note that is precisely the effect of longer life spans and the extended period of sexual activity. Now presumably Rhonheimer would not want to say that the sexual activity of a post-menopausal couple loses its procreative meaning because it no longer needs to be governed by continence and chastity. It does seem to me he would have to account for why this is so. He would have to explain why we ought not to assume that a principle of disintegration is at work in this couple's marriage that will lead them to begin regarding one another as sexual objects rather than loving partners. Such an account would require a more developmental sense of the way chastity/temperance operates within marriage—not simply as restraint on sexual desire but as a virtue working together with justice, charity, and prudence within the context of ongoing and deepen-

---

28. Rhonheimer, "Contraception, Sexual Behavior, and Natural Law," 25.

ing marital friendship, the real guarantor that spouses will not objectify one another.

One of the first things that account might recognize is that artificial contraception and chastity/temperance are certainly not mutually exclusive. Contraception does not eliminate the need for responsible modification of sexual desire in marriage, and it certainly can be a matter of mutual discussion and responsibility. Much more important, however, is the consideration of how a couple's sexual behavior would retain its "procreative meaning" long after there is no possibility of their conceiving a child. Where there is a child or children, the answer to this question is, in my view, easy. What ensures the continued "procreative meaning" of sexual activity for the couple is the fact of the child as an embodiment of their love—along with their shared history of responsibility and care as parents. We might say that the procreative meaning of their sexuality has been established by God and in a way incapable of being broken by man—precisely by their having given birth to and reared children. This will be true both for practitioners of the periodic continence Rhonheimer endorses and for those who opt for artificial contraception. Those who use artificial contraception might be thought of as simply anticipating that time in life when they are no longer capable of conception. They begin even during the child-bearing years to integrate sexuality into loving marital friendship. This may involve a richer practice of prudence and temperance than that advocated by Rhonheimer, for whom temperance still seems primarily a matter of restraining bodily desire. Those practicing contraception will need the virtues of temperance and prudence as they go about seeing how to make sexual activity a part of their ongoing and deepening friendship. The popes and Rhonheimer seem to assume that only the openness of every sexual act to conception is capable of preventing the partners from objectifying one another. This underestimates the way marital love operates to restrain any objectifying tendencies on the part of the partners.

As we have seen, decisions about sexuality now take place, too, in societies that have become by far the oldest ever known. As societies attempt to care for greatly increasing populations of elderly, many more people will have to be engaged in either active provision of that care or in economic activity to produce the resources needed for appropriate social transfers. As this care and economic effort will largely have to come from people who are at some stage of their child-bearing and child-rearing years, decisions they make about procreation will often involve complex questions of justice—questions about the distribution of their energies in care and work. Today's processionally-thinking couple may be involved simultaneously in rearing and educating their own children, caring for elderly parents or kin, and educating themselves in order to be of significant service in the long period after their children have left the home. They will be doing these things while supporting the system of social transfers through work, saving and paying for their children's educations, and trying to save enough money themselves so as not to become inordinately dependent during their own Third Age. They may also be engaged in forms of continuing education of one kind or another: activity moved by the desire to "stay-in-touch" with one another after their children are grown. I mention this last point, in particular, because it bears on a way the couple nourish their friendship, itself the context of the continuing procreative meaning of their sexuality.

The natural law moralist may, at this point, contend that I am making a consequentialist rather than a natural law argument—that is, that I am suggesting couples may use artificial contraception to bring about a variety of good consequences, but I am doing so by dangerously separating what Elizabeth Anscombe has called the "intention *embodied in* an action" from the "further intentions *with* which the action is done." Whatever one's further intentions might be, the fact is that one has distorted the "intention embodied" in the particular kind of act that sexual intercourse is. Thus, to use Anscombe's language, "*considered as intentional actions*, artificially contraceptive acts of intercourse *are* intrinsically unapt for generation," and it is this intrinsic intention that must count for the moral evaluation of actions.[29] Anscombe makes a rich and important distinction, but there are at least four ways of responding to it. First, the lengthening of life spans is again relevant: the intention embodied in intercourse for those past child-bearing is not procreation. Our living longer makes those acts "intrinsically unapt for generation," and this is a natural-cultural fact that must be taken into account when we consider the intentions involved in sexuality. My second point, based partly but not exclusively on the first, concerns the contexts within which the intentions embodied in sexuality are to be evaluated. Sexual intercourse never takes place just in itself but rather within a context where the intentions of the participants are formed according to the virtues

---

29. Anscombe, "You Can have Sex without Children," 86.

guiding their understanding of the relationship. Third, the exercise of intention in sexual intercourse cannot be limited strictly to the "joining of man and woman" in itself. It may have been possible to do so in the Before when child survival was chancy, but it is no longer so. To engage in intercourse open to conception is necessarily to exercise the intention to rear a child to maturity. Fourth, to separate the intention embodied in intercourse from the intention to rear represents a particularly male way of thinking that fails to do justice to the woman's experience. When a woman engages in intercourse that leads to conception, she begins the process of rearing the child in her own body without the exercise of any further intention whatever.

Anscombe asserts that contraceptive intercourse "is not even a proper act of intercourse, and therefore is not a true marriage act." She judges it a "greater offence against chastity than is straightforward fornication or adultery," presumably because it undermines the seriousness of marital acts themselves. I heartily endorse two of the general points Anscombe wishes to uphold with this analysis. First, that "we don't invent marriage, as we may invent the terms of an association or club . . . [that] It is part of the creation of humanity and if we're lucky we find it available to us and can enter into it." Second, if marriage is to be at all meaningful, it has to be a "mutual commitment in which each side ceases to be autonomous, in various ways and also sexually."[30] But identifying contraceptive intercourse and adultery distorts contraception's place within many marriages, again perhaps most especially those of couples who do already have children, even several of them. Such people very likely know that marriage is not simply something whose terms can be invented and that it requires the sacrifice of autonomy. They have become "one flesh," quite literally, in their children. Their mutual commitment will have been ensured by the strongest possible bond—care and nurture of the child or children. The complete separation of procreative and unitive meanings of sexuality will never be possible for them, for intercourse will always be the act that has bound them most fully to one another. In fact, opponents of artificial contraception should consider the degree to which its use can actually strengthen the procreative intention in some marriages—as well as the commitment to care for children. The mutual acceptance and affirmation communicated by intercourse within marriage—freed from care about pregnancy *at this time*—can certainly

---

30. Anscombe, *Contraception and Chastity*, 21.

nourish love that later becomes procreative or is needed, at the moment itself, for the nurture of children. Again, we must remember to evaluate such acts within the very long period of family nurture made possible by today's improved early mortality and longer life spans—perhaps greater than thirty years of very direct child care to rear, say, four children. To describe the use of artificial contraception within such a relationship as a graver sin against marriage than "straightforward" adultery seems a serious misdescription.

Those of us who now conceive children, at least in the developed world, exercise an intention that will likely involve at least twenty years of concerted care and education and a much longer period of relationship and involvement beyond that. Thus the turn to the greater certainty of control over fertility offered by artificial contraception may not indicate the development of a widespread "contraceptive mentality" (though I think John Paul is right to point to this danger in the culture of extreme consumerism).[31] Couples may use artificial contraception simply because the whole range of intentions involved in rearing a child are too difficult, at a particular moment in the marriage, to envision. It must be said, too, that use of artificial contraception is not necessarily related to the broadly dualist splitting of body and soul that John Paul connects to modern Gnosticism and falsely mentalistic versions of autonomy (though again I think these real dangers of modern technological society). If we think about the decision to procreate together with the decision to rear, then we are once again back in the world of fully embodied realities. Rearing children involves very intense embodied activity, much of it directed to caring for bodies, and it involves the economic wage

---

31. Those who have had children but then use artificial contraception are also unlikely, I believe, to find anything like their own thought processes in the analysis of the "contraceptive will" advanced by Grisez et al. I share Smith's reservation about the way Grisez's analysis posits the contraceptor's projection of a possible child only to reject it. For her, "the most challenging counterexample to the position of Grisez" is "that of contraceptors who truly want another child and would welcome a child but who for some reason decide that it would not be good to have another child at a certain time." See *Humanae Vitae*, 363–64. Smith's characterization of what the contraceptors' decision means can be nuanced further. Couples using contraception—maybe especially those with children—might well think it good to have another child at any time but that it is also good, particularly at this time, to be certain there is enough attention and care for the children already born or to attend to all the other responsibilities one has taken on in justice and love. The analysis of Grisez et al. referred to here is that in "Every Marital Act Ought to be Open to New Life."

earner's distribution of the energies of his or her body over the long period of time in which children need financial support. The improved early mortality rates and extended life expectancies of the After make it possible for people to develop much more complex and disciplined forms of caring for one another. It becomes possible for people—in much larger numbers—to commit themselves reasonably to the kind of extended discipline involved in modern education.

Decisions about whether to have children, or how to space them, have now taken on complexities inconceivable in the Before. Consider, for example, a couple who would like to have four children and who are committed to seeing each of these children educated to the point of his or her maximum ability to make a contribution, in love, to the welfare of others (I do not mean to imply by this that others of less education are less able to contribute, in love, to others' welfare, broadly construed). Our couple could easily face supporting children through a total of seventy years of education, at least twenty of which might involve higher education. Clearly this couple is open to children, and yet it would seem eminently in accord with practical reason for them to choose the greater level of control offered by artificial contraception as they seek to space their children. The papal documents often stress the direct cooperation of parents with God in the "true practice of conjugal love"; thus Paul VI writes in *Gaudium et Spes*: "Parents should regard as their proper mission the task of transmitting human life and educating those to whom it has been transmitted. They should realize that they are thereby cooperators with the love of God the Creator, and are, so to speak, the interpreters of that love."[32] For the popes this cooperation has meant allowing God the possibility of bringing conception in every act of intercourse. Yet the couple of my example might well say that they, too, cooperate with God as they exercise practical reason and intelligence to rear and educate their children to contribute lovingly to the good of God's creatures. They do so as fully embodied beings prudently and justly distributing the energies of their bodies as they care for one another and for their children. They accomplish this care within the forms God has provided, marriage and family, in accord with the natural inclination of men and women toward one another and the extended period of dependency of children.

---

32. Paul VI, *Gaudium et Spes*, 28, section 50.

My contention is, then, that the choice of artificial contraception within marriage can represent an exercise of prudence in the service of love and marital friendship. If we understand chastity/temperance to involve the process of wisely learning to integrate sexuality within that friendship, then artificial contraception does not preclude chastity or temperance. Between the couple and in relation to their children, love and friendship are the primary virtues shaping the intentions behind the choice for contraception. As the couple make choices in relation to their broader obligations and commitments, justice is perhaps the primary virtue shaping their intentions.[33] What remains to be considered is the way the dynamism of marital love, and of child-rearing, can itself create the contexts in which artificial contraception becomes a wise and virtuous choice—in regard to spacing of children, provision of education, balancing of familial and extra-familial responsibilities. The popes have written movingly of this dynamism, particularly John Paul in *Familiaris Consortio*. What I would like to do with the remainder of this chapter, then, is to suggest a little of how it might work.

We might begin by reflecting imaginatively again on the Before and the After, particularly on the matter of parental vulnerability. Parents have always been vulnerable to the loss of their children; they have always been vulnerable in their children. Basic to parenting is the experience that one is now at least as endangered and vulnerable in the life of another as one is in one's own. Parents in the Before must surely have had to hedge against this vulnerability when child survival was so very unpredictable. As children's survival became much more likely, parents could afford to risk emotional exposure in the child to a greater degree. Yet this greater exposure also brings risk: of greater emotional loss if the child should die or even perhaps if the child turns away from the kinds of expectations parents have for him or her. These developments are taking place as modern life makes possible a vastly greater differentiation of roles and deepening individuation. One way parents can respond to this is by increasing control over their children's lives and identities. Thus they attempt to ensure a kind of return for the vulnerability they experience in the lives of their children. If they are to take such risks,

---

33. "Between friends there is no need for justice," Aristotle comments, and this would seem particularly true in marital friendship. Relationships between the married partners themselves and others outside the marriage would still be governed by justice. See *Nicomachean Ethics*, 259.

then at least their children should be representatives or images of them carried on into the future. It is easy to see how some developments in genetics—cloning or designing children—might spring from this parental desire for control induced by feared vulnerability (even if there is much less reason for this fear than in the past). Of course it is also easy to see how these developments—rooted in increased life expectancies and improved rates of child survival—may lead to vastly increased intergenerational tension.

But there is another possibility, and that is for the parent to give himself or herself to the vulnerability experienced in and through the child. The parent sees—in a continuing and ever deepening way—that it is good for the child to develop in his or her own right. Marriage is, of course, important to this process as well. In a loving marriage, one comes to see the rightness of becoming one flesh with his or her partner, of having one's center, so to speak, moved from within oneself to the bond with one's spouse. The poet, as Kierkegaard might put it, would here say that one comes to love one's spouse more than oneself; but Christian faith might simply say that one comes to love one's spouse as oneself—and as one does, one loves the spouse in the child as well, sensing also the spouse's vulnerability in the child.[34] The parents must learn to open themselves to increasing vulnerability in one another and their children without anxiously seeking to protect or shape their children's identities. They learn, in love, to let be. And there is no compensation for this, for they must learn that to ask or expect compensation from their children is inconsistent with love. In fact, if they truly love, they will desire only to love more. What they do learn cannot be reckoned as compensation, for it is beyond that: they learn to see the rightness of love as the form of that which enables them to rear their replacements with joy rather than resentment (though, on any honest accounting, there is much of this in the process). Even this formulation, however, needs to be modified, for it suggests that love is somehow there as the enabling force before

---

34. Kierkegaard, *Works of Love*, 35: "Should it not be possible to love a person *more than oneself*? Indeed, this sort of talk, born of poetic enthusiasm, is heard in the world. Could it then be true, perhaps, that Christianity is not capable of soaring so high, and therefore (presumably because it directs itself to simple, every-day men) it is left standing wretchedly with the demand to love one's neighbours *as oneself*, just as it sets the apparently very unpoetic *neighbour* as the object of love instead of a *lover, a friend*, the celebrated objects of lofty love (for certainly no poet has sung of love to one's neighbour any more than of loving *as oneself*)—could this perhaps be so?"

the process of rearing. What happens rather, it seems to me, is that love comes to be and is in the process of caring: one cares for the child simply because of its need and one receives a response without calculation. This is not to say that even loving parents and children are never manipulative: of course they are. But if they have come to inhabit the form of love, they will recognize their own acts of manipulation from a deep longing to return to love more simply experienced: as care given and returned from the recognition that it is good.

The movement of love I have described inevitably presses beyond the bounds of the family. Parents' sense of their own children's utter singularity can become a powerful source of compassion for others, shadowed always, as we are, by the possibility of losses for which there can be no compensation. The prolonged experience of vulnerability in the persons of others—their children—should tend to produce compassion as well. That kind of compassion can then become the motivating force for the acquisition—often through long years of discipline—of the knowledge and skills necessary for the service of others in modern societies. Part of my point here, then, is that the experiences of marital, parental, and familial love can themselves lead to the need to acquire complex skills and education for the loving service of others. Acquiring those skills within the context of a marriage is greatly facilitated by the increased control over spacing of children provided by artificial contraception.

To put a sharp personal focus on this point, I can say additionally that acquiring the skilled discipline that allows one to translate work into loving service can be a life-sustaining matter. "One is borne along only by one's responsibilities," Gabriel Seailles has said, and I would add to this only that one is borne along also by one's loves.[35] One is doubly privileged, as I have been, if one can blend one's responsibilities and one's loves. Being able to love others in work is—greatly but of course not exclusively—what bears me along from day to day. Let me put this point, too, in the context of greatly extended life expectancies. I took care of children for nearly thirty years, and now, though I may die this afternoon, my statistical life expectancy is another twenty years or so. My problem and task for the rest of life is to carry over into other contexts the love that I very largely learned through caring, with my wife, for our children. I do not wish to say that the ability to enact love in work is dependent on acquiring the discipline of one working in the symbol-making class of the information economy. I was privileged to grow up

---

35. Quoted in Marcel, "Mystery of the Family," 84.

in a working-class city and close enough to the immigrant experience to know many people who gave themselves, body and mind, to forty and even fifty years of work that they did with as much regard to love of the neighbor as conditions would allow. They were people who made the extraordinary seem ordinary. But for me, being able to love in my work as the singular person I am is bound up with the intellectual discipline I have acquired over a very long period of education. The same is true for my wife. Decisions we made about contraception and family size could best be described as judgments balancing and ordering a whole constellation of responsibilities rooted in love: to our children, to our parents and extended families, to our and our children's education, to my students and my wife's legal clients, to our friends, to neighbors, to volunteer organizations, to the local and also the broader church. (Needless to say, we often failed miserably in some or all categories.) My point is simply that in such a context, reliance on artificial contraception, with its greater control over the spacing of children, can represent an act of the practical reason in the right ordering of love. To say this is not, in my view, to encourage a dualism in which mind becomes excessively split off from the body it controls. All of the responsibilities enumerated above involve continual bodily activity. Judgments about the distribution of love are judgments about the distribution of bodily energy. They are grounded in our nature as embodied persons engaged with others in the world.

The analysis offered here seems consistent with many of the guiding principles of John Paul's analysis of sexuality and contraception. The analysis shares fully his insistence that "the personal order is the only proper plane for all debate on matters of sexual morality."[36] My intent has been to try to contribute to a reflection on what Paul VI calls "the full sense of mutual self-giving and human procreation in the context of true love."[37] I think there is some truth to Lisa Sowle Cahill's objection that sometimes John Paul's elaborate language of "self-gift" has the effect of "romanticiz[ing] sexual commitment."[38] Nevertheless what John Paul and Paul VI before him have said of the "fundamental and innate vocation" of love seems both enormously important and unimpeach-

---

36. Wojtyla, *Love and Responsibility*, 18. Further citations will be given parenthetically.

37. Paul VI, *Gaudium et Spes*, 29, section 51.

38. Cahill, "Catholic Sexual Ethics," 146.

ably grounded in scripture.[39] In *Gaudium et Spes*, Paul VI argues that man "cannot fully find himself except through a sincere gift of himself." His note to this observation links it to Luke 17:33: "Whoever tries to preserve his life will lose it; whoever loses it will keep it."[40] We discover life and our true selves in sincere giving of ourselves. In commenting on Yahweh's creation of Eve, John Paul has stressed the way man cannot realize his essence "alone" and without a "helper": "He realizes it only by existing *'with someone'*—and even more deeply and completely: by existing *'for someone.'*"[41] Smith has helpfully glossed John Paul's analysis here by saying that "the communion of persons means existing in a mutual 'for,' in a relationship of mutual gift"[42] (253).

Where I would want to engage the tradition is on the scope of this existence "for" the other. Surely marriage at its best becomes precisely what John Paul depicts it as: a communion of persons realizing ever more deeply their vocations to love as they give themselves in love to one another. But too much, in my view, of the papal teaching on contraception identifies sexuality and procreation—apart from child rearing—as the central defining acts of marriage. Certainly one discovers the way he or she exists "for someone" in the marital bond, but the phrase also points to what one learns in caring for children. Children are at the heart of our coming to understand ourselves as mutual gifts to one another. We give the gift of life to children and then realize that they become gifts to us in ways we could never even have imagined. In the process we come to understand that we could only give life as a gift because it is not our possession to give but rather the gift of God (if it were ours to possess, we could never give it freely enough). And we understand the rightness of receiving children as gifts from God, for that gives them the distance from us that allows us to relate to them in love and not possession. But, as I have argued earlier, it is the very leading beyond oneself of love that leads to the practical rationality of artificial contraception within marriage. The analysis offered here concurs fully with the language in

---

39. Grabowski notes "there is widespread agreement among both moral theologians and biblical scholars that a more thorough integration of biblical teaching is essential for the renewal of moral theology" (24–25). He contributes significantly to that needed integration in chapters 2, 3, and 5 of *Sex and Virtue*.

40. Paul VI, *Gaudium et Spes*, 13, section 24. The note is on 57.

41. *Original Unity of Man and Woman*, 107.

42. Smith, *Humanae Vitae: A Generation Later*, 253.

Familiaris Consortio that suggests the way "fruitful married love" leads to a "manifold service to life." There John Paul speaks of the way "every act of true love towards a human being bears witness to and perfects the spiritual fecundity of the family, since it is an act of obedience to the deep inner dynamism of love as self-giving to others." This "fecundity" must "have an unceasing 'creativity,' a marvelous fruit of the Spirit of God, who opens the eyes of the heart to discover the new needs and sufferings of our society and gives courage for accepting them and responding to them."[43] As I hope to have argued persuasively, perhaps nothing "opens the eyes of the heart" more effectively than recognizing the vulnerability of one's children and one's own vulnerability in them. The motivation to serve others, also so vulnerable, can lead the practical reason to decide for artificial contraception within marriage as a way to enable the acquisition of complex disciplines through which to love the neighbor in the contemporary world. Much improved rates of childhood survival and life expectancies make the acquisition of such disciplines possible for large numbers of people, at least in the developed world. If it is a matter of both reason and virtue that we be led beyond ourselves in the service of love, then it seems artificial contraception can be understood as a reasonable and virtuous choice in accord with the natural law.

---

43. John Paul II, *Familiaris Consortio*, 28, section 41.

2

Abortion, the Sacred, and Sacrifice
Or, What's At Stake When Life Has Dominion

ONE HESITATES EVEN TO address the subject of abortion and yet it seems that a bioethical treatment of matters at the beginning of life can hardly ignore the practice altogether. It is difficult to imagine that any subject has been so exhaustively written about to so little effect, if we judge effect by the numbers of people who have been moved to modify their points of view by one argument or another. In fact, there is now a sub-genre of works devoted specifically to breaking the abortion deadlock, to pressing the debate beyond the polarized positions of pro-choice and pro-life, or to reconstructing abortion as a more positive experience for women than it has often been thought to be by advocates on both sides of the issue.[1] Thus I approach and offer the next four chapters with a certain fear and trembling. I do not propose to break the abortion deadlock. Nearly all the attempts to do that have been written from the pro-abortion or, at least, pro-choice position. I write as a critic of abortion, though not as one who would advocate making abortion illegal. One thing I hope to do is to show why many of the best attempts to break the deadlock fail to understand the positions of the critic of abortion. Perhaps this can be a first modest step toward mutual understanding by people on both sides. Surely there can be no real reconciliation on this or any other matter without a full and respectful attempt to

---

1. A partial list would include Tribe, *Abortion: The Clash of Absolutes*; Lunnenborg, *Abortion: A Positive Decision*; Dworkin, *Life's Dominion*; Steffen, *Life/Choice*; McDonagh, *Breaking the Abortion Deadlock*; Boyle, *Re-thinking Abortion*; Sanger, *Beyond Choice*.

understand the way the matter appears to those whose convictions differ from one's own.

A second purpose of mine is to show why some of the best pro-abortion arguments fail. I do not know how to make a new, clear, and compelling argument that would cause people to become pro-life, or even critics of abortion. It seems to me that one cannot be moved by argument alone to relinquish a pro-abortion or pro-choice position in favor of one more nearly "pro-life." Pro-life convictions are part of a whole way in which one understands one's vocation as a parent, the role of children in our lives, and, for the Christian, God's sovereignty over life. What I can do, though, is to show how the best pro-abortion arguments can be challenged successfully. Sometimes this will involve challenging their logic directly; at other times, it depends upon bringing out the way pro-abortion arguments depend on background assumptions that it is not incumbent on us all to accept. My purpose here is to keep the issue open: to resist the conclusion that it has been settled definitively in favor of the justifiability of abortion on demand. Where it is possible, I try to engage the pro-choice or pro-abortion advocates in such a way as to open the possibility of our reasoning together more fully: by asking, for example, whether they want to endorse all of the consequences that may follow—at least as I see those—from their arguments and assumptions.

Something I have said just above requires fuller explication. Discussing why a question like when life begins may never really be settleable, John Noonan has remarked, "It depends on assumptions and judgments about what human beings are and about what human beings should do for one another. These convictions and conclusions are not easily reached by argument. They rest on particular perspectives that are bound to the whole personality and can only shift with a reorientation of the person."[2] I write as one who has undergone such a reorientation. At one time in my life, I would certainly have described myself as being strongly "pro-choice." The overriding considerations were, for me, the autonomy of the woman in determining the disposition of her own body and the sense that equality of the sexes was really not a possibility as long as women bore the consequences of unwanted pregnancy alone. I still believe these things. Women should be able, insofar as is humanly or technologically possible, to exercise bodily autonomy, but this consideration should not outweigh the claim of unique irreplaceable hu-

2. Noonan, *Private Choice*, 2–3.

man beings to be born once they are conceived. Nor should women bear the consequences of pregnancy alone: indeed this is a powerful reason to attempt to impress upon men the uniqueness and irreplaceability of the children whom they participate in conceiving. I suppose if I had to characterize my change of emphasis in thinking about the issue, I would say that I began to put the rights questions second and to think first, as Stanley Hauerwas puts it, about "what kind of attitude" we should "have toward the having of children and what kind of sexual behavior is most appropriate to that attitude."[3]

Clearly the most important influence on my reorientation was the rearing of my own children. Caring for children over an extended period of time, perhaps especially for a succession of children within a family, involves participating in and observing the development of unique, irreplaceable human beings, each with a history of his or her own. As children rear one in turn; pose problems, fears, and possibilities one never imagined; and carry one continually beyond oneself, one comes to understand what it means to speak of children as gifts. As I developed in chapter 1, part of this gift comes paradoxically in the form of a greater vulnerability for parents in the lives of their children than they ever could previously have predicted. That vulnerability is a gift because it can be an opening to a larger compassion and love—a care, for instance, for an ever-widening circle of children. In the process of caring for children, one comes also to understand the gift-language of Christianity as protection for children against parental will. One comes to see the rightness—for oneself and for one's children—of children coming to one as

---

3. *Community of Character*, 207. Guido Calabresi has characterized the abortion difference as one between "values and beliefs which would give primacy to equality (among men and women as to participation in sex) even occasionally at the cost of life-values, and values and beliefs which would give primacy to life-preservation (even of not fully developed life) over equality." See *Ideals, Beliefs, Attitudes, and the Law*, 99. The liberal side of me is sympathetic to this description; the parental, realist, Christian side is skeptical of the rhetoric here of "values" and "beliefs," with their strongly social-constructionist emphasis. Of course much, perhaps nearly everything, about the experience of sex, gender, reproduction, pregnancy, etc. is socially constructed and thus alterable. But one thing is not alterable: that everyone reading this was once utterly dependent on others for the preservation of his or her life. Young children *must* be cared for by somebody; in that sense, "life-preservation" must always have a certain kind of "primacy" over equality. Perhaps the fact we all share dependence as children provides a possible, and, to my mind, healthy corrective to the illusion that all values are "socially constructed," at least when that phrase is used rhetorically as a way of suggesting that every social arrangement is fully capable of de-struction and reconstruction.

gifts. To the degree, then, that one comes to understand a crucial part of one's vocation to be the welcoming and care of children, one will tend to resituate the question of abortion: away from one involving primarily a conflict of rights, and toward one involving primarily the kinds of sexual practices we should encourage if we are to cherish and rear children as the unique and irreplaceable beings parents come to know them to be. Women's bodily autonomy and equality with men do not cease to be important goals; it simply becomes unthinkable that abortion could be the means to assure these. We must think otherwise.

Another factor in my change on abortion has been wide reading in the sometimes extraordinarily alien world of bioethics. The sheer number of abortions since *Roe v. Wade* is sometimes cited as evidence by pro-life people that the decision for abortion is no longer the painful, reluctant one liberals once assured us it always was for women.[4] I reject this pro-life claim and continue to believe that the decision for abortion is almost never taken lightly. But the examples devised by philosophers to illuminate the abortion decision often seem calculated to routinize it. As I cite some of these examples at later points in the book, I will not develop the point here except to give an instance from Peter Singer's work. Singer defends his argument for children's "replaceability" by asking where the wrong lies if a woman who is two months pregnant decides to terminate her pregnancy in order to avoid rescheduling a mountain climbing excursion. As the woman is committed to having children and will later have one—one she would not have if she has the one she is carrying—Singer concludes there is nothing to object to in the pregnancy's termination.[5] The real import of Singer's example seems, to me, in the narrative itself, with its way of situating the abortion choice among other consumer choices. What will seem most alien in Singer's narrative to the critic of abortion is precisely what he finds mitigating of potential criticism: that the woman is open to children and will have a replacement.

The critic will wonder what such openness means if it does not entail postponing the mountain climbing trip in order to bear the child who is instead aborted. It seems frankly inconceivable that one who

---

4. One estimate puts this number as high as 36 to 53 million abortions worldwide each year. See Ewart and Winikoff, "Toward Safe and Effective Medical Abortion," 520–21.

5. Singer, *Practical Ethics*, 154.

could so light-mindedly weigh the fetus's value against a pleasure trip could ever manage the discipline, work, constancy, and sometimes suffering required to rear a child. The world in which fetuses are killed for the sake of mountain climbing cannot help but seem somewhat unreal to those for whom parenthood is a central vocation.

Singer's strategy is to entirely separate questions of sexual morality from other ethical matters, as he announces in chapter one of *Practical Ethics*:

> Even in the era of AIDS, sex raises no unique moral issues at all. Decisions about sex may involve considerations of honesty, concern for others, prudence, and so on, but there is nothing special about sex in this respect, for the same could be said of decisions about driving a car. In fact, the moral issues raised by driving a car, both from an environmental and from a safety point of view, are much more serious than those raised by sex. Accordingly, this book contains no discussion of sexual morality.[6]

One might think that sex raises some unique concerns precisely because it sometimes issues in children. Or that sexual fidelity between spouses is at least as important as driving a fuel-efficient car because it promotes the family stability and trust needed by children and nourishes the emotional depth and support needed by the parents themselves in order to sustain lasting commitments to their children. One might even question Singer's separation of sexual morality from environmental issues. The primary reason I drive a fuel-efficient car is that I want to contribute to the development of sustainable environmental practices for the sake of my children and those other children whom I have come to care for primarily through learning what it means to care for my own. I would like further for my children to be able to be friends with the children of other countries—Venezuela, for instance—and I recognize this can only happen if the United States curbs an appetite for cheap energy that increasingly drives it toward a policy of perpetual war required to control the flow of natural resources.

To return to my own "reorientation" on abortion, I would say that bioethical attempts like Singer's to separate sexual morality from the constellation of questions involved in parenthood simply came to seem untenable to me. If we are to rear children to become happy, secure, loving, and empathetic human beings, then we must order our lives in ways

6. Ibid., 2.

requisite to their care. This seems to me to require, at the very least, a strong presumption for life that is significantly at odds with much of the tone and many of the assumptions of the pro-abortion literature.

Developments in genetic technology and the accompanying bioethical reflection have also served to re-frame the abortion issue. No longer is abortion simply a requirement for women's exercise of bodily autonomy and equality with men. Rather abortion is one of a series of technologies—the crudest, if you will—whose goal is becoming increasingly transparent: the comprehensive shaping, control, and selection of the kinds of human life we will allow to be. One who recognizes this development is Mary Boyle, whose socially constructionist pro-abortion treatment seeks to reconstruct abortion as a positive experience for women. Boyle follows Foucault's analysis of the changing concept of power in the nineteenth and twentieth centuries. During this period, power ceases to be simply a matter of "deduction, the power to take away, to impose injury or death" and rather becomes part of a comprehensive machinery for life-enhancement. This new "bio-power," concerned "with the regulation of birth, health, welfare, and well-being" becomes, as Foucault argues, integrated into life itself.[7] Wars are thus no longer waged simply to defend a sovereign; rather

> they are waged on behalf of the existence of everyone; entire populations are mobilized for the purpose of wholesale slaughter in the name of life necessity: massacres have become vital. It is as managers of life and survival, of bodies and the race, that so many regimes have been able to wage so many wars, causing so many men to be killed . . . The principle underlying the tactics of battle—that one has to be capable of killing in order to go on living—has become the principle that defines the strategy of states.[8]

Boyle claims Foucault inadequately understood the gendered nature of the discourse of war, which itself has functioned to reinforce patriarchal hierarchies and to separate men and women physically and psychologically. Abortion on demand threatens this separation, as it means men cease being the only "socially sanctioned killers." As Boyle puts it, "If women, too, become killers on a large scale—even if only of 'potential life'—then the separation of male and female becomes more

---

7. Boyle, *Re-Thinking Abortion*, 54.
8. Foucault, *History of Sexuality*, 1:137.

difficult to sustain" (58). Since Boyle opposes the patriarchal "separation of male and female" and endorses abortion on demand, the conclusion suggested by the above seems obvious: integration of abortion discourse, along the lines of that about war, within the Foucauldian understanding of bio-power as that which enhances life. Abortion, like war, would be understood as advancing, enhancing, and improving life. Women would gain equal status with men by being allotted the power to kill for the health of the state.

Sensing the direction of her argument, Boyle maintains that her point is not to distinguish morally among the various kinds of "socially-sanctioned killing" or to offer a moral case for the justification of abortion. But the latter seems implicit in her argument. As long as the life of states depends upon war—upon the illusion of bringing enhanced life out of death—and unless women are admitted fully to power over life, then men will control the public life of nations. Even if one thinks Boyle's analysis overstated, she poses serious questions for those who consider themselves pro-life.

Pro-life people should take two criticisms of Boyle's with utmost seriousness. One is her claim that the support of many pro-lifers for capital punishment belies their opposition to abortion. Such critics of abortion should ask themselves whether their sometime support of capital punishment unwittingly assists the state in its drive to become ultimate arbiter over life. They should ask further whether support of capital punishment derives from real concern for justice in the most extreme crimes or from an unwillingness to relinquish the illusion of power over death. By converting death into a power used for good we mask the fact that death has power to deprive us of all. Such, at least, is the assumption of Foucault's analysis of a shift in the concept of power from that of detraction to that of enhancement. Pro-lifers should also ask themselves whether their opposition to abortion reflects assumptions about the strong separation of gender roles whose ultimate ground is the conviction that war is necessary, inevitable, and thus constantly to be anticipated. In a division of labor at least as old as Troy, women must bear and nurture within the city while men like Hector defend the walls. Critics of abortion should recognize that women's claim of abortion rights properly challenges this rigid division of roles. Our response should be to recognize the inherent injustice of separate-but-equal gender divisions and to grant the rightness of such analyses of sexuality and power as those of Catherine MacKinnon, who contends that these must be understood together in a society of systematic gender inequality. I agree with MacKinnon's claim that abortion would be seen very differently if there were greater equality between men and women in society.[9] But it's important to add that it would be seen differently primarily by those who are now pro-choice and who put the equality question before the life question. Those of us who are critics of abortion simply will not do this: the commitment to life must precede the commitment to equality, even as important as the latter is. But if we are truly committed to equality, we must question and transform the structures that undergird gender separation and inequality. If the Foucault-Boyle analysis is correct, this means questioning the assumption that war is necessary and integral to the life of states as the provider of a collective experience of life-enhancement that allows us to deny death's personal sting. For those of us who are Christians, this questioning is mandatory, for we are not permitted to assume that war is simply necessary or that life can only be sustained by our constant readiness to kill.

In the remainder of this chapter, I want to engage one of the most thorough and influential of the attempts to break the deadlock over abortion, Ronald Dworkin's *Life's Dominion*. My purposes are to show how several of Dworkin's key arguments are unsuccessful and how he sometimes frames the convictions of abortion critics in ways they would not endorse. When it is possible to engage in fruitful dialogue with Dworkin's views, I have tried to do so. This is not a simple matter of discovering "common ground." Rather it is a matter of reinterpreting Dworkin's arguments, bringing out assumptions on which they depend but which are invisible to him, and then showing how and why the abortion critic will draw different conclusions from those assumptions. This strategy will be particularly evident in the analysis of Dworkin's concept of the sacred and his discussion of the ways in which we respond differently to the deaths of others according to their ages. Finally, I suggest why abortion is as critical a political matter as it is by showing how

---

9. MacKinnon, *Feminism Unmodified*. See particularly "Sex and Violence," 85–92; and "Privacy v. Equality," 93–102. I would subscribe completely to Lisa Sowle Cahill's assessment: "Much needed, in my view, is an ethical discourse that examines in a more thoughtful and consensus-building way the status of the fetus, the practical demands of enacting real equality for women, and the function of law and social policy in enabling creative solutions to unplanned pregnancy or to pregnancies in which the child to be born is threatened with serious illness" (175–76). See *Theological Bioethics*, 169–93.

it undermines the concept of the "public," the very concept on which Dworkin's work depends.

Dworkin calls his book a "public argument," a representative of a genre he believes has unfortunately gone out of favor in America. Distressed by conflict over abortion, which he frequently likens to "war," Dworkin seeks "a responsible legal settlement of the controversy, one that will not insult or demean any group, one that everyone can accept with full self-respect."[10] Dworkin believes such a settlement is "indeed available" and can be reached by the identification and dispelling of "a widespread intellectual confusion" involving the nature of opposition to abortion. The unrecognized but "crucial distinction" in the abortion debate lies between what Dworkin calls the "derivative" and the "detached" grounds for protecting human life (10–11). The "derivative" objection claims "that fetuses are creatures with interests of their own right from the start." Thus "abortion is wrong in principle . . . because [it] violates someone's right not to be killed, just as killing an adult is normally wrong because it violates the adult's right not to be killed." Dworkin labels this the "*derivative* objection to abortion because it presupposes and is derived from rights and interests that it assumes all human beings, including fetuses, have." A second "very different" way in which to understand the familiar rhetoric opposing abortion is "that human life has an intrinsic, innate value; that human life is sacred just in itself; and that the sacred nature of a human life begins when its biological life begins, even before the creature whose life it is has movement or sensation or interests or rights of its own." On this view, abortion is "wrong in principle because it disregards and insults the intrinsic value, the sacred character, of any stage or form of human life." This "detached" objection "does not depend on or presuppose any particular rights or interests." Government has a "detached responsibility" for "protecting the intrinsic value of life," but it has no "derivative responsibility" to prohibit abortion—a responsibility that would derive from the assumption that fetuses possess the same rights and interests as other human beings (11).

Dworkin believes that nearly all who oppose abortion hold the detached rather than the derivative, objection, irrespective of what they think they believe. One of the maddening qualities of his argument is his penchant for dismissing the convictions of opponents by asserting that they do not know what they "actually" or "really" believe. Dworkin,

10. *Life's Dominion*, 10–11. Further citations will be given parenthetically.

of course, does not consider himself to be dismissive of those who hold pro-life positions. Rather he simply thinks that the "derivative" position is inconsistent with various other convictions of even the most ardent pro-lifers, and he also fears that holders of the "derivative" objection cannot be integrated into the state. In offering his own insight into the "intellectual confusion" surrounding this issue, he believes himself to be vindicating pro-lifers against the more extreme charges of their opponents—suggesting, for instance, that they need not necessarily be seen as "either acting in deep error or [as] sadistic, puritanical bigots, eager not to save lives but to punish women for what they regard as sexual sin" (10). If people of pro-life persuasion can be shown to hold the "detached objection"—just as pro-choice people putatively do—then a ground can be established for "reasoning together."

Dworkin exhibits intense concern about the threat to social unity posed by differing views on the morality of abortion. He argues, for example, that "self-respecting people who give opposite answers to the question of whether a fetus is a person can no more compromise, or agree to live together allowing others to make their own decisions, than people can compromise about slavery or apartheid or rape" (10). In developing this point, however, Dworkin seems to suggest that the threat really comes only from one side, pro-life: "For someone who believes that abortion violates a person's most basic interests and most precious rights, a call for tolerance or compromise is like a call for people to make up their own minds about rape, or like a plea for second-class citizenship, rather than either full slavery or full equality, as a fair compromise of the racial issue" (10). The "great tradition of freedom of conscience in modern pluralistic democracies" can be reconciled with a particular combination of views: "a profound conviction that it is intrinsically wrong deliberately to end a human life" together with the belief "that a decision to end human life in early pregnancy must nevertheless be left to the pregnant woman" (14–15). He does not ask whether that "great tradition" is consistent with allowing individuals to deliberately do what is "intrinsically wrong" in regard to the most sacred of matters.

Part of the reason Dworkin thinks the "derivative" objection to abortion untenable—and not really held by many people—is that he cannot reconcile it with tolerance. Those who oppose abortion in principle but believe that it should remain legal can do so, according to Dworkin, either from a respect for separation of church and state or from the conviction that "government should not dictate to individuals on any matter of personal morality." On the other hand, tolerance is not a possibility for those "who really consider a fetus a person with a right to live." Such people would have to endorse government prohibition of abortion, for "protecting people from murderous assault—particularly people too weak to protect themselves—is one of government's most central and inescapable duties" (31). Elsewhere Dworkin claims that "no one can consistently hold that a fetus has a right not to be killed and at the same time hold it wrong for the government to protect that right by the criminal law. The most basic responsibility of government, after all, is to protect the interests of everyone in the community, particularly the interests of those who cannot protect themselves" (14). But the Christian can certainly claim the following: that a fetus ought not to be killed because it is a person, one who will develop into a being who understands itself as living a continuous unique history ending only with its own unique death; that many people, perhaps the great majority, do not yet understand human life in this way, and thus ought not to be categorically forbidden abortion by the law; that respect for others with whom we live means allowing even such deplorable practices as abortion when there is no legitimate consensus about outlawing them; that the same respect also means that we must be allowed to witness to the truth as we see it—and that involves insisting 1) that God is sovereign over life, 2) that he has himself come to us in the shape of a specific human being whose history is recorded from conception to solitary death, 3) that he so mingles love and knowledge as to be able to number the hairs on the head of the child, and 4) that he invites and disciplines each of us to love all other children with that same intensity of regard for their specificity.[11]

Dworkin also believes opponents of abortion cannot really hold the "derivative" objection because they are generally unwilling to deny abortion in all circumstances: danger to the life of the mother, rape, and incest. "It is a very common view," he asserts, "that abortion should be

---

11. Frances M. Kamm suggests that Dworkin unfairly discounts what she calls a "Tolerance View." "Why," she asks, "is it not possible for someone to believe that the fetus is a person, on grounds that he thinks are reasonable but *that he recognizes may not convince every rational person*? Then, without abandoning his belief in fetal personhood, this person might hold that the state should not enforce his view because it is not based on reasons that demand universal assent and because enforcing it would greatly burden others." See Kamm's extensive analysis of Dworkin's book, "Abortion and the Value of Life," 168–69. Kamm also examines *Life's Dominion* in "Ronald Dworkin's Views on Abortion and Assisted Suicide," 218–40.

permitted when necessary to save the mother's life. Yet this exception is also inconsistent with any belief that a fetus is a person with a right to live." Dworkin acknowledges that in such a case self-defense can be offered as a reasonable defense of the woman's right to abort, but he argues further that "any safe abortion is carried out by someone else—a doctor—and very few people believe that it is morally justifiable for a third party, even a doctor, to kill one innocent person to save another" (32). Dworkin here obfuscates the issue through his use of "innocent." Of course the fetus is innocent of any intention to commit mayhem against its mother, but in those few cases where it poses a threat to its mother's biological life it might more appropriately be compared to a human but unintentional threatener. Let's suppose one is a sharpshooter employed by the government to guard a particular stretch of highway. From one's perch one sees a truck careening out of control, its exhausted driver asleep, about to cross the centerline and collide head on with a small car coming the other direction. The driver of the car, a solitary woman, has no chance to avoid the crash, which will surely result in her death. Would most people (since they are the source of Dworkin's standards) not be willing to approve the sharpshooter's shooting the sleeping truck driver on even the chance that the accident might be averted? If it were averted, would most people not hail the sharpshooter as one who took a courageous but necessary decision? Dworkin may be right that only a few people believe it justifiable to kill one innocent person to save another (actually it would seem easy to prove otherwise: we might simply poll Americans on their approval/disapproval of the bombings of Hiroshima, Nagasaki, and Dresden). But, in any case, his use of the word "innocent" distorts the situation in which the fetus poses a threat to its mother's biological life. The fetus is "innocent" of any wrongdoing but it still poses a mortal threat. To make a choice for the life of the mother is to acknowledge tragedy in the classical manner: that there are some situations in which the pattern of events forces us to choose and yet no choice is clearly desirable or even justifiable.

That "abortion conservatives" often will allow the rape or incest exceptions also means, to Dworkin, that they cannot seriously hold the "derivative" objection. What Dworkin fails to understand is that one can seriously hold a position and yet not desire or insist that it be written into law. Believing only in "law's empire"—to cite the title of one of his other books—Dworkin assumes that to hold a belief is to work for its institution as law and thereby to force it on others. He seems incapable of imagining a position I will call that of Christian liberty. This position would hold 1) that abortion in the case of rape or incest is a grave wrong; 2) that it is a grave wrong because God commands us not to kill and also to break cycles of violence by returning good for evil; 3) that Christian regard for the freedom of others insists on a renunciation of undue force in law-making; and 4) abortion should be legal in cases of rape or incest because carrying the children to term in these cases can only be designated supererogatory. We ought not to insist on supererogation, but that does not mean that Christian communities should avoid appealing to victims of rape or incest on the grounds of the Gospel. Women victimized by rape or incest can choose to return good for evil. Christian communities should do everything they can to make this choice possible for women. This means providing support during the period of pregnancy and a variety of options for the child's rearing, including adoption and orphanage care.

Several points regarding rape and incest need to be made here. First, to say that the woman victimized returns good for evil by carrying the child does not mean that the woman who chooses to abort returns evil for evil. Rather she defends herself against the evil perpetrated against her. Second, appealing to her according to the Gospel must not become a way to blame her, to judge her guilty if she chooses to abort. Indeed the Gospel makes possible an appeal to her freedom precisely by precluding any possibility of judgment by others. As we have all sinned and fallen short of the mark, none of us is in any position to respond to the victim who chooses to abort with anything except compassionate sorrowing. Nevertheless faithfulness to the Gospel requires our saying to the victim that her future can always be different from what the world will tell her it must be. The possibility of this difference can only be apprehended in faith, and Christians ought to recognize extraordinary witness to the Gospel in the victim of rape or incest who chooses to carry her child to term. This is quite true without regard to her status as a professing Christian. Third, at present one would have to say that the Christian church fails miserably to support women victimized by rape or incest. That we do so fail is a sure sign that we do not believe the Gospel, that we do not really believe good can come from evil or that the future is open or that there is any wisdom on such matters other than the world's. Remaining in such unbelief is comfortable, and we must be careful that our motivation for endorsing the rape/incest exception is not simply the wish to avoid confronting the whole ugly matter. After all, the exception allows the tidy, private resolution of such matters. It enables us to avoid confronting rape and incest as issues of violence, power, and sexuality.

Believing he has successfully discounted the "derivative objection," Dworkin develops what he terms the "fundamental unity of humane conviction" (71) underlying the divisions on the abortion issue. This conviction stresses the "intrinsic value" of human life, its sacredness—by which Dworkin means "it is *intrinsically* regrettable when human life, once begun, ends prematurely" (68-69). Part of what makes this premature ending regrettable is that it means the waste of creative "investment," natural and human. "Abortion," Dworkin argues, "wastes the intrinsic value—the sanctity, the inviolability—of a human life and is therefore a grave moral wrong unless the intrinsic value of other human lives would be wasted in a decision *against* abortion" (60). One curious feature of Dworkin's position is that he, a liberal, adopts a rhetoric usually associated with conservatives on this issue: the rhetoric of sacredness, or sanctity, of life. He grounds the liberal position in a quasi-religious regard for life's "sacredness," devoting an extensive chapter to defining the idea of the "sacred." This intuition of the "sacred" does not depend on any specific religious or theological convictions, but it does reflect the value we assign to "the complex creative investment" of evolution, history, culture, and language that each human being represents.

One confusing feature of Dworkin's case for life's sacredness is his tendency to make "intrinsic value" depend on something else—e.g., our investment in it. Discussing MacKinnon's argument that "if women were truly equal with men . . . then the political status of a fetus would be different from what it is now," Dworkin claims that this point becomes "powerful if we take her to be discussing a fetus's status in the detached sense I have distinguished. Then the crucial question is whether and when abortion is an unjustifiable waste of something of intrinsic importance, and MacKinnon's point is the arresting one that the intrinsic importance of a new human life may well depend on the meaning and freedom of the act that created it" (55-56). As I indicated earlier, I am sympathetic to MacKinnon's analysis of the connectedness of sexuality and power in a society marked by systematic gender inequality. The position I'm developing shares Dworkin's and MacKinnon's sense that it is desirable for each "new human life" to result from free, uncoerced, meaning-endowing sexuality between equals. Nevertheless the value of the human life being created cannot be made to depend upon the equality of those engaged in making it, as MacKinnon and Dworkin suggest. To do so is to deny life's "intrinsic" value, for it is to make it dependent on something else. To assert the new human life's intrinsic value is simply to assert that its importance does not depend on anything else. The fetus's intrinsic value depends rather on its form, if you will, as a unique, irreplaceable human life whose uniqueness begins at conception and arrives at a definitive shape (at least for our eyes) only in death. That supreme meaningfulness of what we are creating ought to cause us to order our sexual relations in such a way as to be certain that we will never destroy incipient human life.

If we understand "intrinsic" to mean of worth in itself, then Dworkin does not believe fetal life to be of intrinsic value. He reveals a fondness throughout for the locution "life in earnest," which signifies his Franklinesque sense that life is a very serious matter because it is an opportunity for work. Work is the way by which one "redeems" life, for Dworkin, but life that is in need of one's own redemption is not of intrinsic value: it is of value insofar as one makes something of it to repay the investment of others in it. Advocating a gospel of work, Dworkin argues "that we are ethically responsible for making something worthwhile of our lives, and that this responsibility stems from the same, even more fundamental idea that I argued is at the root of the abortion controversy as well, the idea that each separate human life has an intrinsic, inviolable value" (27).[12] Similarly, he repeatedly speaks of the need to "redeem" one's life, as in the following comment about the effect a child may have on its mother's life: "A child whose birth frustrates the chances of its mother to redeem her own life or jeopardizes her ability to care for the rest of her family is likely, just for that reason, to have a more frustrating life itself" (99–100). If the child's life is of intrinsic value, as Dworkin would have us believe, then how can it frustrate its mother's life or its own? Obviously the child is not of intrinsic value for Dworkin, but rather of instrumental value, as is also the mother, whose life must somehow be redeemed.

---

12. Against Dworkin's Franklinesque sense that life must be redeemed through work, we might set Thoreau's comment from "Civil Disobedience," one more indicative, I believe, of a sense of life's intrinsic value: "I came into this world, not chiefly to make this a good place to live in, but to live in it, be it good or bad" (396).

Dworkin's assertion of the inviolability of life seems undermined, too, by some of his examples of legitimate abortion. He cites approvingly a number of quotations by adolescent women contemplating abortion who were interviewed by Carol Gilligan:

> They sometimes talked of responsibility to the child, but they meant the future hypothetical child, not the existing embryo—they meant that it would be wrong to have a child one could not care for properly. They also worried about other people who would be affected by their decision. One, in her late twenties, said that a right decision depends on awareness of "what it will do to your relationship with the father or how it will affect him emotionally." They talked of responsibility to themselves, but they had in mind not their pleasure, or doing what they wanted now, but their responsibilities to make something of their own lives. One adolescent said, "Abortion, if you do it for the right reasons, is helping you to start over and do different things." A musician in her late twenties said that her choice for abortion was selfish because it was for her "survival," but she meant surviving in her work, which, she said, was "where I derive the meaning of what I am." (59)[13]

It seems they talked of everything except the inviolability of a life other than their own that was, nevertheless, entirely dependent upon them at this stage in its existence. It seems difficult to take seriously Dworkin's commitment to the sacred, inviolable, or intrinsic value of life when it can be set aside to prevent emotional turmoil for the father or to make something of one's life or to get on with one's music. I do not mean to make light of these considerations or aspirations, but if life is truly "inviolable," to kill it for the kinds of reasons given above seems scandalous.

We should ask, then, just how the idea of the "sacred" functions for Dworkin. I think it is clear his arguments do not support the "intrinsic" value of fetal life. He conceives of value in instrumental fashion throughout, as is indicated particularly by the pervasive language of investment. People make investments in order to realize on them, to see them increase in value. A basic rule of investing is to avoid throwing good money after bad. Human beings conceived as the products of investments will be forced to prove themselves worthy of the time and energy (money) expended on them. They will need to vindicate, through

---

13. For Gilligan's analysis of the abortion interviews, see *In a Different Voice*, 72–105. Dworkin's quotes are from pages 78 and 89.

their lives in earnest, the "earnest" (money) expended on them in advance. Investment provides a concept by which Dworkin can weigh the value of fetal life against that of the lives of others affected when a decision against abortion is made. If the calculus points to a greater "waste of intrinsic value" by a child's being brought to term—perhaps because its mother's chance to redeem her life through work is blocked—then abortion is justified.[14] Dworkin does not confront the more fundamental question of how intrinsic value can be wasted. Value can, of course, fail to realize itself, but then it is no longer intrinsic but instrumental.

Three points need to be made about Dworkin's analysis of the sacred and his metaphor of investment. First, the metaphor itself represents a kind of abstract generalizing that is likely to seem quite alien to the critic of abortion—and against which the critic's position is a kind of protest. Critics of abortion recognize that each human life is, of course, indebted to the efforts and contributions of others. But the critic is much more likely to see these in specific or particularistic ways—that is, that the life of each unique human being derives from the specific history of other unique unsubstitutable persons, whose contributions cannot be simply subsumed under the category of "investment." "Investment" is itself a category already in service of what Wendell Berry calls the industrial mind, one so thoroughly abstracted from all particularity as to be able to think of everything in terms of something else. In short, "investment" seems very like the kind of concept required by some central distribution agency, the state, charged with apportioning resources and rewards.[15]

My second point, then, concerns the way Dworkin's concept of sacred investment funds a very compelling sacrificial system in which abortion functions to sacralize the natural and social investment, the

---

14. A further difficulty in what she calls Dworkin's IWT (Investment Waste Thesis) is pointed out by Frances Kamm. Suppose two young women, both pregnant and wanting abortions; the first is poor, the second "a well-cared-for, highly educated young woman who wants an abortion because pregnancy would interfere with her life plans." The IWT seems to suggest it is worse if the second young woman does not abort, as more has been invested in her, "but the reverse assessment is also possible: since the first woman has had so much less invested in her up to now, it is more important that she have a better future. What people have had out of life as well as what has been invested in them are important" (Kamm, "Abortion and the Value of Life," 181–82).

15. For representative arguments by Berry on the way industrial habits of mind have squeezed out nearly every other kind of thinking in our condition of "total economy," see "Economy and Pleasure," "Two Economies," and "The Whole Horse," in *Art of the Commonplace*, 207–48.

"earnest" expended on each of us in advance. I do not believe Dworkin either intends or understands what he is doing in this way. But the killing of fetal life works, in his system, to impart value to other kinds of choices: getting on with one's life, one's music—and, above all, redeeming one's existence. These are now elevated to the condition of sacred responsibilities by the fact that abortion has made them possible. The idea that we are responsible for redeeming the earnest expended on us is extraordinarily compelling. Each of us is the recipient of an enormous natural and social investment from the past, particularly in the kind of comprehensive welfare states favored by egalitarians like Dworkin. Surely this must involve some kind of return on our part, but just as surely, it is critical to limit the nature of this return in order to have the space for our own lives and to insure that the return we make is strictly our own—not taken forcibly from others, as in abortion, where we purchase *our* redemption by *their* sacrifice.

One should note the terrible way in which the sacrifice of fetal life both heightens the need for women to redeem their lives and renders this increasingly impossible. Abortion adds immeasurably to the earnest expended on women and thus to their need and burden of redemption. If we are looking for an analogy to understand how this process works, we might turn to war, recalling how often we hear the argument that we must fight—that blood must be shed—because of the sacrifices made by those who have gone before us. Lives must be expended because lives have previously been expended by our predecessors.[16] Contra Foucault, perhaps wars of a sort are still waged for a "Sovereign." Dworkin has referred to equality as "Sovereign Virtue," and perhaps we should under-

---

16. On this point, I have been greatly influenced by the work of Stanley Hauerwas, particularly the piece, "Sacrificing the Sacrifices of War." The painful question I want us to ask here is whether abortion should be understood as analogous to war in being a sacrificial system: that is, as Hauerwas puts it, one in which "future generations feel the need to sacrifice their young to show they are worthy to represent those that sacrificed their youth to give the present life. It does not matter what the past war was about or what the present war concerns. What is important is the sacrifice be repeated to show we are the rightful heirs of the sacrifices that we believe have been made on our behalf." Does the destruction of fetal life give "sacredness" to the social investment that young women then feel they must somehow "redeem"? Or, to put this another way, are we prevented from asking about the justifiability of abortion precisely because there have already been so many? If abortion is producing the sacred that asks to be endlessly reproduced, how can we break from it? How can we escape the no doubt compelling logic of Dworkin—in our condition of near total economy—that each owes to all the productive use of past investment?

stand abortion as a kind of war waged for sovereign equality. Resource egalitarianism depends on enormous social investment and thus on extraordinary acts of redemption to bring about ideal conditions: the roughly equal distribution of resources, with universal satisfaction and thus elimination of envy. Unwanted children are obviously obstacles to these acts of redemption and equalization: Dworkin unhesitatingly speaks of women's lives being "wrecked" and "wasted" by child-bearing and rearing. Moreover, the goal of equalizing resources requires some measure or currency by which everything can be valued in order to be comparatively assessed. An extraordinarily abstract concept like investment, then, serves sovereign equality by being able to absorb and represent all particularities. To abort is to kill, reluctantly, for the sovereign, to exercise responsibility earnestly in the pursuit, and the currency, of equality.

My third point regarding Dworkin's analysis of the sacred opens the possibility of pushing his intuitions in a direction more critical of abortion. When Dworkin asks "What is Sacred?," he addresses such examples as works of art, human cultures, and animal species. The thought of a self-portrait by Rembrandt being destroyed "horrifies us," for example, even if there is very little chance we will ever see the painting. Similarly, "we think it a shame when any distinctive form of human culture, especially a complex and interesting one, dies or languishes" (72). We create museums to "protect and sustain interest in some form of primitive art . . . not just because or if we think its objects splendid or beautiful, but because we think it a terrible waste if any artistic form that human beings have developed should perish as if it had never existed" (72). The disappearance of traditional crafts troubles us "because it seems a great waste that an entire form of craft imagination should disappear" (72). We take a "parallel attitude" toward "distinct animal species," believing it would be "terrible," for example, "if the rhinoceros ceased to exist" (75). "Causing a species to disappear, wholly to be lost," (76) is what distresses us so greatly.

Dworkin's language suggests, in each case, that what really accounts for our sense of the sacred is the irreplaceability of what is lost. He attempts to account for the sacredness of works of art by arguing we admire them "because they embody processes of human creation we consider important and admirable" (75). But our especial horror at the destruction of a Rembrandt or Michelangelo surely involves the knowledge that the work represents the unique, unrepeatable creation of a particular moment in the artist's history. It cannot be again. The same is true of a lost culture or craft form, and, at the current stage of our thinking, of an animal species. When we think about irreplaceability in regard to non-human animals, we tend to consider it in relation to the species, assuming members to be somewhat interchangeable. My point is not to argue that this is the proper way to regard the non-human animals. Indeed, I think we must be willing to consider whether members of various non-human animal species should more properly be regarded as irreplaceable individuals. If there is evidence that members of a species regard one another as irreplaceable, then, I, for one, am perfectly willing to extend the designation "person" to these animals. It seems to me that grieving or mourning behavior would be a place to begin such an assessment. The more immediate point here, however, is that Dworkin's examples and language show something more specific than his analysis: that the defining mark of the kinds of things he calls sacred is their irreplaceability. In non-human animals, we think of irreplaceability in relation to species; for human beings, in relation to individuals. What is sacred about the human being is his or her representing an unrepeatable, irreplaceable history. As this is the history of an embodied being of specific genetic identity—an identity important to, though not determinative of, the history—it makes sense to locate the beginning of this being's sacredness at the point where it begins as a continuously developing organism: conception.[17]

At this point, I believe it is possible to suggest a beginning place for constructive discussion with Dworkin, but before suggesting what that might entail, I want to engage another intriguing aspect of his argument in order to suggest what I believe to be a more adequate account of evidence he cites. Crucial to Dworkin's argument, as we have seen, is the concept of investment, for it allows him to correlate losses to the fetus and to the mother through abortion—while still maintaining that we take fetal value seriously. What he needs, of course, is a way to claim there is an amount of wasted investment in the woman that overrides

---

17. Jeff McMahan has offered a thorough account of problems in Dworkin's view of the sanctity of life in *Ethics of Killing*, 329–38. Probably McMahan's most important criticism is that "it seems impossible" to "identify any intrinsic properties that could constitute a plausible basis for the sanctity of life that are possessed equally by all human beings, including fetuses, but are not possessed by any animals" (338).

any investment in the fetus. To bolster his argument regarding these possibly varying degrees of wasted investment, he gives an account of the different intensities of grief we feel when life is lost at different ages:

> It is terrible when an infant dies but worse, most people think, when a three-year-old child dies and worse still when an adolescent does. Almost no one thinks that the tragedy of premature death decreases in a linear way as age increases. Most people's sense of that tragedy, if it were rendered as a graph relating the degree of tragedy to the age at which death occurs, would slope upward from birth to some point in late childhood or early adolescence, then follow a flat line until at least very early middle age, and then slope down again toward extreme old age. Richard's murder of the princes in the Tower could have no parallel, for horror, in any act of infanticide. (87)

Dworkin offers this argument as evidence that our sense of degree regarding the waste of life involves the amount of investment already made in it and a judgment about that investment's realization or frustration. We have the greatest sense of loss where there's been a relatively high degree of investment with little realization—adolescence to early middle age (roughly). Frustration is less, on the other hand, either where investment has been thus far limited—young child—or largely brought to fruition—elderly person.

There are several serious problems with Dworkin's argument, but I think he is largely right in his characterization of people's reactions to the deaths of others—though I will try to account for these otherwise. First, the problems. One is his unrelentingly Gradgrindian insistence that life is a matter of achievement and accomplishment: for him the death of the adolescent is more tragic than that of the three year old because we've invested more and thus can expect more in return. Second, his graph fails to take into account *any matters of relationship*. Are we to assume that the death of a three year old is, to her parents, a matter of less grief than that of a twelve year old to those who know him only casually or read about the death in the newspaper? Similarly, do parents feel less grief when they lose a three year old than when they lose a twelve year old? If they lose twelve-year-old fraternal twins of widely varying ability (and thus potential to realize on investment), do they feel vastly more grief for the brilliant one than they do for her brother? It seems much more likely to me that parents will reject all of these comparative judgments, saying simply that the loss of any child is the worst thing that can happen to one. Third, it again seems extraordinarily dangerous to me for Dworkin to connect our sense of tragedy to realization on investment—which inherently varies according to people's abilities.

Age is not the only variable related to one's ability to make use of investment. Does Dworkin's schema imply that we should grieve less the death of the thirty-five-year-old retail clerk than the death of the thirty-five year old surgeon? I suspect most people do think there is a greater "waste of life" in the surgeon's death than in the clerk's. But fortunately, at least until recently, most people (I think) have understood that they must correct this judgment about waste of life—thus recognizing that the clerk's death is, for her, just as great a tragedy as the surgeon's is for him. Thus they have affirmed the ground of true equality: the recognition that each person's relationship to his or her own life is an absolute one. The three year old's life is as valuable to the three year old as the twelve year old's is to the twelve year old—and the eighty year old's is no less valuable to her. In each case, this is true irrespective of investment made in them or their accomplishments. No one needs to redeem her life—for others—because it is good enough in itself. It is because life is an absolute value for the one living it that we pursue the murderer of the eighty year old just as seriously as the killer of the adolescent.

Still, there does seem some intuitive rightness about Dworkin's description of the way we experience grief at the deaths of people of different ages—assuming we are considering our generalized sense of loss when people die whom we only remotely know and not those whom we know, or are related to, intimately. Our first reaction probably is to be more distressed at the death of the adolescent than at that of the three year old and more at the loss of the forty-five year old than the eighty year old. But I would account for these reactions quite differently than Dworkin and without reference to the notion of life as primarily achievement. If we grieve more for the twelve year old than the three year old, it is because we sense that the adolescent has had longer, on the one hand, to become individuated and, on the other, to become related to the various communities in which we live our lives. Because of his or her individuation, we have a sharper sense of the unique possibility that has been lost and we suspect that his or her fuller relatedness will also cause greater suffering than is the case with the three year old—precisely because those to whom the adolescent is related will have become more aware of his/her uniqueness as this person and not some other. Secondary reflection, however, will lead us to see that all of these factors are irrelevant to the ones who have died and that the three year old's loss is every bit as much to be grieved as the adolescent's. This will be especially true of those who, as parents, will have come to know their children, through love, to be absolutely unique and irreplaceable.

Now one might object that we know the eighty year old more fully than the forty-five year old and thus my logic should lead to our experiencing a greater sense of loss when we lose the eighty year old than the middle-aged person. But individuation really does not continue indefinitely throughout life as this argument implies: by mid-life most people have become the specific, identifiable, and irreplaceable human beings they are going to be. This is not to say that people do not continue to change and grow even till death. We all know older people who become more delightfully individual right up to their last days. But our feeling of loss when the very old die is tempered by our sense of the natural shape of a life and our sense of justice. As Christians we believe life is an extraordinary gift and opportunity for service and love. The eighty year old has had a fair shot at experiencing that gift and opportunity. The forty-five year old simply has not had the same kind of chance. The death of the old brings grief, but it can also bring a somber sense of completeness that is lacking when even the middle-aged die.

Dworkin says late-term abortion is worse than early-term abortion because we have already made greater investment. I'd argue our sense that late-term abortion is worse than early-term abortion (and infanticide very much worse than all abortion) derives from our being able to more fully imagine the later fetus (or infant) as both an identifiable individual and one more fully related to others. The older the fetus becomes, the more we understand it as one already received into the community—a matter that becomes one of plain fact at its birth. These perceptions need to be supplemented by secondary reflection of the kind we earlier entered into regarding the loss of the three year old and the adolescent. On reflection, those of us who have come to know children as unique individuals are less likely to see relevant difference between the early conceptus and the late term fetus: in each there is a unique and irreplaceable identity. What we need is to enlarge our imaginations in such a way as to know the number of hairs on the head of the conceptus. Secondary reflection will remind us that the life of the conceptus is *the condition on which all else depends* for him or her just as it is for the late term fetus, the three year old, the adolescent, and each of us.

Dworkin's "detached objection" to abortion includes the conviction that "human life is sacred just in itself." That innocent-looking statement is what the Christian critic of abortion can almost but not quite accept. If we believe human life is sacred independent of its relationship to God, we may be all too tempted to participate in sacrificial enterprises designed to demonstrate our worthiness of the sacrifice that has made us possible. Besides, for the Christian critic of abortion—as well as for many others—there just is no human life "in itself." Particularity or singularity is an in-principled feature of human beings. The Christian might say we encounter others christologically—that is, as always already related to the God whose love for each of us is inviolable. It is from that love that we *derive* our inviolability. Here we have a glimpse of that love that opens the way for us, and we extend to one another some measure of inviolability—dependent really on how much we recognize something like ourselves in those to whom we're extending protection and care. The more the fetus comes to resemble us, the more likely we are to consider it worthy of protection. Training in Christianity seeks to supplement and correct this seemingly natural way of valuing by teaching us to see others as simultaneously like us and uniquely particular in their own right. We are in training to see analogically. As we see the unique particularity of Christ's life, death, and resurrection, we are to see the particularity of each woman or man before us and the sacred in their sheer givenness as *this* woman or *this* man.

As we come increasingly to see ourselves and others as uniquely particular, we will come to be increasingly critical of abortion. For we will recognize that what we share, most importantly, with all others is not the general physical shape of *Homo sapiens* but the destiny of being on the road between an unchosen conception and an ineluctable death as the uniquely historical beings we are, here once for all only. If we come to accept ourselves as beings of this kind—no easy task—we will tend to place the beginning of human life at conception as the moment most easily identified as the beginning of a uniquely new being. For this Christian critic of abortion, our sacredness is something both derived and undetachable, but not from the human capital that has been invested in us, great as that has been. The sacredness of each and every human being—as the particular he or she is—derives from a relationship with God that cannot be detached precisely because it is initiated and established, once for all, by God. That He goes ahead of us on the road—feeding each of our individual bodies with the whole of His life in every host—enables us to understand and bear the singularity that leads to our recognizing the singularity of even the earliest conceptus. To acknowledge that singularity not only with our minds but in all of our practices would be to become fully pro-life. Opposition to abortion on these grounds is a difficult task, for they lead us to see how consonant that opposition is with resistance to all the kinds of violence on which we have come routinely to depend.

3

In Defense of the "Conception Criterion"

I BEGIN THIS CHAPTER with what I believe to be a pair of commonsense arguments for conception as the point at which fetuses become worthy of consideration. To begin, we should note how often arguments about fetal protection/abortion depend on judgments or claims about how the fetus is "like us." One prominent defense of a fetus's right to life from conception—treated at length later in this chapter—has been called the "Future like Ours" argument.[1] In short, the fetus possesses the right to life from conception because it will have a future like that of the rest of us, including experiences it will come to value. Often, of course, the comparison of the fetus to the rest of us is used to buttress a pro-choice rather than pro-life position. *Roe v. Wade* famously distinguished three phases of fetal development, assigning different degrees of protection to the fetus at each stage of its development into a being just like us. Comparative accounts of personhood routinely attempt to mark off some point in the fetus's development—based on sentience or potential—when it passes over a line from being the kind of being that can be destroyed to one who wants to believe, at least, that it ought not to be killed—one "just like us."

The curious thing, of course, is that none of us has ever been more like anyone else than we are like the fetus who has become us. Yet, on a pro-choice view, we could kill that fetus who has become us on the ground that, at some point in its development, it was not like us. Why this does not do more to give us pause puzzles me. It seems to me an

---

1. Marquis, "Why Abortion is Immoral," 320–37; and Marquis, "Future Like Ours," 354–69.

important, largely concealed fact of political life under pro-choice—that is, that I have not been welcomed into the polity as the being I am most uniquely, for my genetic inheritance partly constitutes that, and it was not enough to give me a claim against being killed (this is not, in any way, to engage in "genetic determinism"). I have entered into a kind of conspiracy with others who allowed a being like me to live not because I am the person I am but because I was judged to be like them (and, for the indirect utilitarians, because my being killed would have made them afraid they'd be killed). If we wanted to ensure that every person in the polity felt entirely secure in his or her own person—and thus maximally free to develop in his or her own unique way—it seems to me we would be not only opposed to abortion but committed to being "pro-life"—that is, to affirming freedom for all of us from the question itself of who shall be killed.

A second commonsense argument for fetal protection from conception begins with asking what it means to say the fetus is "like us." What does it mean to say that I am like others? I am like others in being alive, desiring life to continue, looking forward to a future, valuing experiences. Like all others, I will die. Yet I experience all of the above as the unique, historical, embodied being I am. I will die my own death, and that death will bring to an end a personal reality that is irreplaceable, unrepeatable, and incommensurate with any other reality. Surely what makes it wrong to kill me is not simply that it would frustrate my desires but rather that no other has the right to bring to an end the reality that is so uniquely my own.

Now curiously I share the condition of uniqueness with all others. We all live as uniquely embodied beings for whom death will bring to an end a personal reality utterly our own. We are together in being apart, to paraphrase Robert Frost's "A Tuft of Flowers."[2] If this uniqueness as embodied historical being is what is supremely valuable about us, then it makes sense to ask at what point in our development we begin to exist as this kind of being. The most reasonable answer to that question seems, to me, to be conception, for it marks the point at which, for nearly all of us, a continuously developing new being came into existence. It marks the point at which we become a genetic identity, which, though it does not determine us, does surely contribute to our particularity. We live and die as personal embodied realities. Our bodies differentiate us, limit us,

2. See "Tuft of Flowers," in *Poetry of Robert Frost*, 22–23.

identify us. If we work backward to the point at which that particular embodiment began—the one whose death will be my death—we again arrive at conception. This, then, seems to me the commonsense point at which to say that uniquely personal beings worthy of consideration begin to exist.

Despite its commonsense appeal, the "conception criterion" has, of course, come under attack from a variety of standpoints. In the remainder of this chapter, I explore three attempts to discredit the criterion, showing in each case how the argument fails. All three of the works are informed by fairly explicit political purposes. Daniel A. Dombrowski and Robert Deltete's *A Brief, Liberal, Catholic Defense of Abortion* seeks to give Catholics grounds for justifying a more liberal position on abortion than that of the Vatican. Peter S. Wenz's *Abortion Rights as Religious Freedom* argues that the personhood of young fetuses is not a "matter of ordinary secular fact" but rather a matter of "religious belief." Freedom from religious establishment, in Wenz's view, requires allowing for abortion of fetuses before they become sufficiently like us that their personhood "becomes secular" and thus worthy of protection (somewhere between twenty and twenty-eight weeks). Perhaps somewhat less political is David Boonin's recent philosophical work, *A Defense of Abortion*, but it, too, seeks to create consensus around the moral permissibility of abortion. Boonin repeatedly and strenuously emphasizes that his aim is to show the moral permissibility of abortion on grounds that the critic of abortion already accepts. I will show here, and in chapter 5 of this book, that he does not successfully answer the critic of abortion on the critic's own grounds.

༺༻

A Brief, Liberal Catholic Defense of Abortion contends that a "Catholic 'pro-choice' stance is at least as compatible with Catholic tradition as the anti-abortion stance" now advocated by Rome.[3] To make this case, Dombrowski and Deltete defend a version of delayed hominization that they identify with Augustine and Aquinas. The traditional Catholic view is

---

3. Dombrowski and Deltete, *Brief, Liberal, Catholic Defense of Abortion*, 1. Further references will be given parenthetically. The authors contend that pro-choice "may even be more compatible with Catholic tradition than the *current* anti-abortion stance defended by many Catholics and most Catholic leaders" (1).

> that what makes an organism a human person is a rational or spiritual soul that is "infused" into the body by God. If this occurs at the moment of conception, the theory of *immediate hominization* is correct; but if a human soul is infused into the body only at a later stage, for example, when the latter begins to show a human shape or outline and possesses the basic organs (especially a central nervous system), then the theory of *mediate or delayed hominization* is correct. Before hominization the embryo is alive, but only in the way in which a plant or, at best, an animal is alive. (26–27)

For the authors, the fetus becomes "morally considerable" some time between "twenty-four and thirty-two weeks when sentiency, and then the cerebral cortex, starts to function" (56). The "burst of synapse formation toward the end of the second trimester" (57) marks the critical point at which the cerebral cortex is formed and the fetus can become a moral patient, capable of feeling pain. With the beginning of sentience, ensoulment can occur and personhood status begins. "To put the matter in Augustinian or Thomistic terms," the fetus develops "from a vegetative state to a sentient one, *after which* (!) it is possible for human ensoulment (or personhood) to occur" (16).

Dombrowski and Deltete's argument consists essentially of four parts: 1) an analysis of the facts of fetal development that shows it to be inconsistent with immediate hominization; 2) a review of Augustine and Aquinas on abortion that reads their views as consistent with delayed hominization; 3) a brief argument that now-discredited seventeenth-century ideas of the homunculus and preformationism are responsible for the church's commitment to immediate hominization; and 4) an argument for an asymmetrical "non-strict" identity view of the self that is alleged to be more consistent with abortion than symmetrical views of identity. For the sake of clarity, I will address these arguments one at a time. Because there is considerable overlap between the arguments of Dombrowski and Deltete and those of Peter Wenz in *Abortion Rights as Religious Freedom*, I will examine Wenz's arguments here as well.

The uncertainty of embryonic and fetal development points, for Dombrowski and Deltete, to the unreasonableness of placing personhood at conception. They make the point that the zygote may split within several days to produce monozygotic twins or triplets. Implicit in their treatment are questions asked also by Wenz in his study of abortion rights as religious freedom. As Wenz puts the questions:

> Which of these is the "person" who came into existence at fertilization? Who are the others? Do they, too, have full human rights? If so, does their personhood come into existence not at fertilization (when there was only one) but at some time (possibly days) later when the zygote splits? How do we know which one became a person at fertilization and which one(s) attained personhood later? These are all ridiculous questions.[4]

I agree with Wenz that these questions are absurd, but I do not draw the same conclusions from this fact that he does. The absurdity of the questions lies in the way personhood has come to serve, as Stanley Hauerwas has put it, as a "regulative notion"[5] completely divorced from any of the practices that give it meaning. In the normal course of things, fetal division has occurred well before pregnancy is discovered: thus any question of abortion is about whether to terminate already established genetic identities. Moreover, it is important to assess Wenz's questions as part of his rhetorical strategy, which is to limit protection of fetuses. Does it make sense to deny protection to the embryo because it may become two or three identifiable fetuses rather than only one?

Wenz's argument, and similar ones by Dombrowski and Deltete, show only the vulnerability of the pure personhood abstraction to pro-abortion arguments. The rhetorical strategy is simple: to divorce personhood entirely from its rhetorical function as a means to defend developing fetal life and then show how this leads to an absurdity. Dombrowski and Deltete, for example, argue that if possession of human genetic material constitutes personhood, then a heart extracted for transplant or even a cancerous tumor ought to be afforded protection. To cite one of their more extreme formulations: "If some unique genetic information is a sufficient condition for deserving moral respect as a human person, then large amounts of tissue excised in operating rooms, which is normally seen as medical waste, is anything but this" (56). Such an argument points only to the absurdity and vulnerability of the personhood abstraction when completely divorced from its rhetorical context as a means to de-

---

4. Wenz, *Abortion Rights as Religious Freedom*, 61. Further references will be given parenthetically.

5. "Must a Patient Be a Person to Be a Patient?," 128. Elsewhere Hauerwas acknowledges the difficulty of doing without the concept of personhood "in a society such as ours," for the "idea of 'person' embodies our attempt to recognize that everyone has a moral status prior to any role they might assume. It therefore represents the profound egalitarian commitment of our culture" (*Community of Character*, 288 n. 3).

fend life. It sheds no light whatever on the question of abortion, which is not about what to do with human genetic material that has no chance of developing into a unique identifiable human individual.[6]

The developmental fact that seems most important both to Wenz and to Dombrowski and Deltete, however, is that only approximately "one third of all conceptions lead to a fetus that has a chance of developing until birth *quite apart from* human intervention" (D and D, 11). To say that Wenz, Dombrowski, and Deltete are obsessed with this fact is not an overstatement, for they return to it again and again. What it means for them is that regarding fetuses as persons from conception would require an enormous, all-out effort of medical intervention to guarantee as many successful fetal implantations as possible: If "moral patiency, much less personhood, were attributed to zygotes, then this failure [to implant on the uterine wall] would constitute the gravest moral problem facing humanity, and unprecedented expenditures of resources on medical research would be justified even if the most favorable result—saving the lives of these 'persons'—would increase by 800 percent or more the number of infants born with severe genetic defects" (D and D, 78). Surely it must seem suspect that our inability to do this practically becomes a reason to deny protection against killing to the fetus who successfully implants and is perfectly viable. Furthermore we are told that protecting fetuses as persons from conception would lead logically to our mourning "particularly heavy menstrual flow" (Wenz, 61). Complicating that mourning would be the horrendous fact that "over two-thirds of the human persons who have ever lived have never gotten beyond the first stage of human 'personhood'"; to accept this would mean "the already remarkable extent of human tragedy, quite apart from the issue of abortion, is far worse than even the greatest pessimist could have imagined" (D and D, 52). As we cannot accept this tragedy, we must reject the idea that conception marks the beginning of personhood. Why it would be

---

6. Cf. Allen Verhey's remarks on the use of "person" in bioethics: "A discerning judgment concerning who counts as a person will be suspicious not only of reductionistic accounts of 'person' but also of the question itself when it is used to discount the responsibility to care. In the beginnings of bioethics the notion of 'person' was invoked to protect the powerless and to protest against injustices done to them. Now it is more frequently invoked as a 'permissive notion,' permitting doctors and researchers and the rest of us to do as we wish with those members of the human community whom we judge not to count as persons." See *Reading the Bible in the Strange World of Medicine*, 96.

more difficult to accept this "tragedy" than the one we already accept—that one hundred percent of conceptions end ultimately in death—we are not told.[7]

I hope it's clear I am not trying to defend the personhood abstraction. Rather my contention is that the personhood abstraction lends itself to the kind of *reductio ad absurdum* cited above. As a Christian, I am more than willing to allow God to dispose of zygotes that fail to implant in whatever way He sees fit. The question of abortion concerns whether destruction of fetuses that do successfully implant can be justified. When people use the language of personhood to defend fetuses, they do so to insist that something unique and irreplaceable is lost when an implanted fetus is destroyed. Indeed we should reject, on rhetorical grounds, the designation of failures to implant as nature's "abortions." My primary point is that facts about non-implantation tell us nothing about the morality of destroying what does implant. Having said that, I wish to add that certain features even of the reductions of Wenz, Dombrowski, and Deltete need to be challenged.

First, we need to know what percentage of the failed implantations are caused by people's repeated attempts to have a child: medical care aimed to increase the success rate of attachment might drop that number of failures considerably. Second, we need to know how much failure to implant is related to the condition of women's health and how much that, in turn, is related to availability of health care, age, poverty, and other factors. If poverty and poor health care negatively impact the rate of implantation, then Wenz, Dombrowski, and Deltete seem unwittingly to be using women's current poor health care to undermine the status of fetuses. Raising women's general health might raise rates of implantation, which, in turn, would make the successfully attaching fetus seem less anomalous, more normal. Third, if raising the status of fetuses leads to more and better prenatal care for women, then that seems to me a good rather than a fearful thing—though I might share Wenz and Dombrowski-Deltete's fears if I thought "personhood" were really going to function in the context-free absolutist way they hypothesize. Fourth,

---

7. One further, and I suspect wholly unintended consequence, seems implicit, too, in these arguments of Dombrowski-Deltete and Wenz. If attributing personhood status to very early fetuses would mean our commitment of enormous medical resources to assisting their development, does pushing back the age of personhood to 24 to 32 weeks operate as justification for provision of often inadequate pre-natal care, particularly for the poorest people?

Wenz, Dombrowski, and Deltete's concern about greatly raised numbers of defective newborns can only seem problematic to non-normally abled people. Moreover, one might argue that greater numbers of differently abled people might well have a salutary effect on the rest of us. Regular encounters with, and care of, non-normally abled people might well lead to a reduction in the compulsive drivenness of normals. This is, of course, a speculative matter, but it does seem important to challenge the assumption that the potential increase in the number of disabled people means we cannot grant fetuses a status causing us to care for more of them.

Dombrowski and Deltete's identifying Augustine and Aquinas with delayed hominization involves a prior characterization of historic Catholic opposition to abortion as depending on two grounds: one, the ontological position—based on the "ontological status of the fetus as a human person"—and two, the perversity position, based on "the view that abortion is a perversion of the true function of sex regardless of the ontological status of the fetus" (2). The authors argue that Augustine distinguished clearly between unformed and formed fetuses, refused to consider abortion of unformed fetuses murder, and thought primarily of fetuses "in the early stages of pregnancy in vegetative terms" (25). His opposition to abortion in the early stages, then, is "based on the perversity view, not the ontological one" (24)—that is, abortion distorts the true purpose of sex, which is the creation of children, and leaves sex merely the operation of *libido crudelis*, cruel lust. Now that "very few contemporary Catholics" (2) hold the perversity view, Augustine's objections to abortion can be overlooked and his assessment of the unformed fetus as vegetative made the basis for a contemporary Catholic pro-choice stance.[8]

---

8. Without, in any way, wanting to link her directly to Augustine, one might say that Catherine MacKinnon's insight into the inseparability of sex and power shares something of Augustine's sense that sex apart from procreation can be simply the operation of *libido crudelis*. As long as there is systematic gender inequality, there is very little, if any, truly consensual sex, according to MacKinnon, which means most sex could be construed as men's use of women for gratification, cruel lust. Perhaps Augustine's willingness to expose his own motives to the light of that God who was closer to him than he was to himself led him to conclude that often what drove his own sexual experience was a concern for his own satisfaction quite apart from the consequences for his partner. See MacKinnon, "Sex and Violence," 85–92. In fact, it seems to me there is still considerable descriptive accuracy in the phrase *libido crudelis* applied to contemporary sexual traffic. If a man forces a woman to have an abortion about which she is

It seems dubious, however, that the unformed-formed distinction of Augustine can be made consistent with modern genetic knowledge. The authors repeatedly stress the developmental aspects of embryology and fetology yet never adequately recognize that what is developing from the time of fertilization is a *particular* embryo or fetus. The development of the fetus is *in-formed* by a specific genetic code from the beginning. A favorite metaphor of the authors compares fetal development to the assembly of a computer: "A pile of wires and switches is not an electrical circuit, and a collection of nerve cells is not a functioning brain. . . . In effect, before synapses are sufficiently formed the brain does not function because it is just a collection of nerve (and other) cells" (13). The metaphor seriously distorts the process of fetal development, for the fetal brain is already informed by genetic coding in a way that the computer parts simply are not. An extraordinarily masculinist view of creation is also evident in the metaphor: the fetus does not grow on its own but must rather be put together by some figure distanced and apart from it. As things put together in this fashion are assembled according to some idea already given, the metaphor carries with it strong suggestions of replicablility and conformity to type. Mary Shelley explored this masculine idea of "creation" nearly two hundred years ago when Dr. Frankenstein assembled his creature from a collection of parts, only to produce a "monster" forever unable to fit his creator's idea of him.

The authors' vegetative metaphors also seem problematic. Pointing out that "vegetation has no *moral* status in the Catholic tradition," they compare the fetus before the third trimester to a "rose bush," which is "neither a moral agent (since it lacks rationality) nor a moral patient (since it lacks sentiency per se)" (25). But surely there is something odd about comparing the rose bush—which represents the adult form of its species—to the fetus, whose development has just begun. The strangeness of this comparison should point to the fact that fetus and rose bush are surely more different than similar. Even in the authors' view, the fetus will develop into a being whose intentional killing we regard the most serious of crimes. Yet we assign no guilt to anyone who kills a rose bush at any stage of its development, seed or cutting to adult. Surely this difference is rooted partly in the fact that human beings suffer in a way that roses do not, but it also reflects our sense that human beings are

---

ambivalent—either by directly threatening her or withdrawing psychologically—can we think of a better retrospective designation of his sexual behavior than "cruel lust"?

unique in a way roses are not (a fact that itself makes our suffering more intense than that of any other species).⁹ And part of the condition for the uniqueness we value is already present in the earliest-stage fetus.

Given its obvious inadequacies, why do the authors adopt the vegetative metaphor they find in Augustine? I suggest the answer lies in the sharp difference they draw between activity and moral patiency, subject and object. Despite their depiction of the dynamism of fetal growth—evident in the "burst" of synapse formation, a metaphor strikingly at odds with masculinist computer construction—the authors remain committed to the view that fetuses are formless matter waiting to have form impressed on them from outside. We may here be able to identify a crucial imaginative difference between the authors and those who are pro-life, particularly those who have reared children. Pro-lifers may simply consider the fetus active from its earliest moments in a way the authors do not—for, in their receptivity to life, they have already included the fetus as an active participant in the moral community. After all, even long before birth, the fetus begins to affect the lives of those waiting to receive it. It is not simply matter waiting to be impressed with a form but rather a new beginning of the world, one that may change everything.¹⁰

Perhaps this is the place to bring out what I see as a critical difference between a pro-life position and that of Peter Wenz regarding the crucial concept of potential and its relation to the way one understands or imagines social differentiation. To put the matter simply, Wenz's Aristotelian

---

9. Perhaps we do feel some sense of guilt when we fail a plant like a rose bush, which might mean that it carries some kind of "moral status." I have felt something very like guilt when I have had to dig up established rose bushes, particularly when I have had to do so because they have been weakened by diseases such as blackspot that I have been too busy to adequately control. Moreover, the more I have come to live with a certain rose, the worse I feel about losing it, precisely because it has emerged from some background concept like "the vegetation" and become a particular bush with a history and identity of its own—and particular claims on me.

10. Cf. the last phrases of Hannah Arendt's *Totalitarianism*, 176–77: "But there remains also the truth that every end in history necessarily contains a new beginning; this beginning is the promise, the only 'message' which the end can ever produce. Beginning, before it becomes a historical event, is the supreme capacity of man; politically, it is identical with man's freedom. *Initium ut esset homo creatus est*—'that a beginning be made man was created' said Augustine. This beginning is guaranteed by each new birth; it is indeed every man." Arendt's quotation from Augustine seems to be from the end of Book XII, Chapter 21: "Hoc ergo ut esset, creatus est homo, ante quem nullus fuit." "In order that there might be this beginning, therefore, a man was created before whom no man existed." See Augustine *City of God* XII.21 (Dyson, 532).

account of potential does not do justice to the degree of human differentiation in modern societies. He does not, on a pro-life view, value the fetus sufficiently because his understanding of what fetuses become is very limited, partly by his Aristotelian approach. Consider, for example, the limited degree of social differentiation implicit in Wenz's argument that late-stage fetuses and infants must be considered to have actualized potential in a way that is untrue of early-stage fetuses (and thus are worthy of protection not merited by the younger fetus). Following Aristotle, Wenz distinguishes first from second potential: "A person who is not currently trained to build houses is potentially a builder in the first of Aristotle's two senses of potentiality. In order to build a house she would have to learn the trade and then employ her newly acquired skills. A person who is not currently building a house, but who currently has all the requisite skills, is potentially a builder in the second of Aristotle's two senses" (55).

Wenz uses this distinction to insist that Judge Blackmun was thinking of potentiality in the second sense when, in *Roe v. Wade*, he defined the viable fetus as one "potentially able to live outside the mother's womb, albeit with artificial aid" (55).[11] Wenz adds "this point requires emphasis" because "some current Supreme Court justices reject the viability criterion as a result of failure to appreciate the distinction between first and second potentiality" (56). He heavily criticizes Justice O'Connor for a dissent in *Akron v. Akron Center for Reproductive Health*, in which she wrote that "*potential* life is no less potential in the first weeks of pregnancy than it is at viability or afterward. At any stage in pregnancy, there is *potential* for human life."[12] Later Wenz uses the first potentiality-second

---

11. *Roe v. Wade* in *Abortion Decisions of the United States Supreme Court: The 1970's*, 29.

12. For the Court's opinion in *Akron v. Akron Center for Reproductive Health*, see *Abortion Decisions of the United States Supreme Court: The 1980's*, 71–104. Wenz's criticism of O'Connor seems misplaced, mostly because he insufficiently attends to the whole context of her argument. The overall emphasis of her dissent is that the majority opinion of the Court shows the unworkability of the trimester scheme of *Roe*. In *Akron*, the majority struck down a provision of an Akron ordinance that required all abortions after the first trimester to be performed in hospitals. Part of their reasoning stressed the fact that dilation and evacuation procedures (D and E) had now become very dependably successful for abortions of 12 to 16 week fetuses. Thus procedures in this period—during the second trimester—no longer required performance in hospitals. O'Connor's claim is that these kinds of medical assessment are both inappropriate and impossible for courts to make adequately, particularly as they must take into account continually

potentiality categories to distinguish young fetuses from "normal, but unconscious, children and adults." Young fetuses have only first potential, and no moral status; unconscious adults "have already developed and displayed their abilities, but happen not to be displaying them at the moment" (173). They have second potentiality.

One might object that becoming an infant (and thus worthy of protection) is utterly unlike becoming a carpenter or mechanic. It requires no training in a practice or authoritative guidance by a master craftsman. Absent human interference or natural destruction, every early fetus will become an infant whereas not everyone has or will become a craftsman. The particular, actualized skill of the craftsman sets him apart from others like him in all other relevant ways; what distinguishes fetuses and fetuses from infants is simply stage of development and genetic identity. Wenz acknowledges the objections of "advocates for the young fetus" who "point out that newborns are no more able than are young fetuses to engage in distinctively human pursuits"—and who hold, therefore, that aborting young fetuses should imply the legitimacy of infanticide. His "reply" to this position is "that newborns are significantly closer than are young fetuses to being able to engage in distinctively human pursuits" (174). But this is true only if one thinks of "distinctively human pursuits" as Wenz apparently does—as the performance of skilled roles like carpentry or auto mechanics relatively open to everybody. If one considers a much more widely differentiated society—one unimagined, of course,

---

improving technologies. Thus she sees the trimester scheme as on a "collision course with itself": technological improvements, on the one hand, will continue to make abortion procedures safer later in pregnancies while also pushing the point of fetal viability earlier (95). Thus, for her, the trimester scheme "cannot be supported as a legitimate or useful framework for accommodating the woman's right and the State's interests" (92). She sees the woman's right to an abortion and the "state interest in potential human life" as existing "throughout pregnancy" (97). In evaluating particular legislative restrictions on abortion, the Court should attempt to determine, in O'Connor's view, whether these are "unduly burdensome" (98) to the woman seeking abortion services. Thus it's difficult to see how her point bears in any fashion on Wenz's first potentiality-second potentiality distinction. If the State claims to have an interest in potential human life, O'Connor argues, then that interest must be there from the beginning, through all stages of fetal life. One might think of her line of reasoning as curiously similar to that of Catherine MacKinnon in that O'Connor asserts that the matter of pregnancy is a public one throughout its course and that the question of abortion cannot be solved by partitioning off some phase of pregnancy delimitable as "private" and then a later phase that is public. For MacKinnon on *Roe*, see "Privacy v. Equality," 93–102.

by Aristotle—then it no longer makes sense to say that fetuses are not as close to "distinctively human pursuits" as infants.

Infants may be marginally closer to "some distinctively human pursuits," but young fetuses are equidistant from, or even much closer to, other of those pursuits than infants—particularly where there is an important genetic contribution required for the pursuit. Given the extraordinary combination of eyesight, hand-eye coordination, strength, and explosive speed required to be a major league shortstop, for instance, it makes little sense to say that a particular infant is "closer" to that pursuit than an early fetus. This point about relative distances from fetus or infant to particular human pursuits holds for thousands of differentiable human abilities: solving advanced differential equations, doing microsurgery, playing in the NBA, being a female Supreme Court Justice (which is perhaps why Justice O'Connor saw little difference between early and late fetal viability).

Wenz claims ultimately that the debate about the personhood of young fetuses is "inconclusive because every argument on one side can be countered with an effective argument on the other" (175). Thus personhood of young fetuses is not a "matter of ordinary secular fact" but rather a "religious belief." But I believe the analysis offered here proves otherwise. His distinction between infants and young fetuses depends upon an outmoded paradigm of potentiality and actuality, one that cannot account for the rich differentiation of human pursuits in modern societies or the genetic differentiation among fetuses. This is not a matter of religious belief but one of secular fact. Instead of depending on Aristotelian paradigms drawn from societies where most of the people from particular classes were assigned roles and virtues all could be expected to master, and where women and slaves did much of the work that was too basic to yield meritocratic distinctions, we should recognize that modern societies attempt to harmonize the efforts of individuals widely differentiated in ability and function. Where there is such variety of distinctively human pursuits, it becomes impossible to say categorically that infants are closer to these pursuits than fetuses. The most we can say is that some infants are closer than fetuses to some pursuits whereas some fetuses are closer than infants to others.

Whether Aquinas should be read to support delayed hominization in the light of contemporary biology is also a matter of contention. Joseph Donceel, SJ, claims that he should be, arguing that Thomas's position contains "a mixture of erroneous biological information and sound philosophy." The sound philosophy lies in Thomas's "hylomorphic conception of man," which Donceel believes to be an important protection against the ever-present "danger of slipping into some kind of Platonic or Cartesian dualism"—dualism that he associates with theories of immediate animation or hominization and considers to be contrary "to the main trends of contemporary philosophy."[13] Thomas distinguishes three stages in the organism's animation: first, the vegetative; next, the sensitive or animal; and finally, the rational or human. This final human soul is infused from without by God, but only at the point at which the body has developed sufficiently to be "disposed to receive a human form."[14] The soul must be understood "as the substantial form of man," and as such, it "can exist only in matter capable of receiving it." In man's case, this means it can "exist only in a highly organized body."[15] Aquinas says, for instance, in the *Summa Contra Gentiles*: "Since the intellective soul is the most perfect of souls and its power the highest, its proper perfectible subject is a body having many different organs through which its multifarious operations can be carried out."[16] Immediate hominization—claiming that "the spiritual soul is virtually present in the fertilized ovum, or that this ovum is virtually a human body"—conceives of the "soul as an efficient cause" capable of producing the body or developing into the body by "an immanent activity" that is irreconcilable with Thomas's notion of formal cause as "itself the terminus of production" and not that which produces anything.[17]

A contrary reading of Thomas is offered by Stephen J. Heaney. The heart of his claim is that Aquinas's "acceptance of Aristotle's theory of a succession of souls is, in fact, totally dependent on his acceptance of the corresponding theory of generation," which insists that the semen provides the "active power" working on "the passive matter, organizing the body *throughout* the succession of souls. Without this organizing power,

---

13. Donceel, "Immediate Animation and Delayed Hominization," 79.
14. Dombrowski and Deltete, *Brief, Liberal, Catholic Defense of Abortion*, 28.
15. Donceel, "Immediate Animation and Delayed Hominization," 79.
16. Aquinas, *On the Truth of the Catholic Faith: Book Two*, 291.
17. Donceel, "Immediate Animation and Delayed Hominization," 83–84. The final three phrases are quoted from Henri de Dorlodot, "A Vindication of the Mediate Animation Theory," 282.

there is no way to explain the formation of the body." [18] For Heaney, "the power of the parents in the formation of the zygote and embryo" is "necessary to *any* theory of mediate animation under Thomistic metaphysical principles" (47–48). But this power simply is not present, and we might be fair to Aquinas to say that he came "to the conclusions he did, because he was never faced with the possibility that generation might take place in a way he had never even considered" (31). Heaney goes further, however, than simply saying that Aquinas should be excused for not knowing contemporary biology. Now we know "that the development of the organs is an activity *internal* to the embryo, not one being performed by an extrinsic power" (30). Thus the forming of the "organs necessary for the operations of the soul" seems most clearly attributable to power in the "embryo's own soul." The soul, then, must "be a human intellectual soul" from the very beginning; the "conceptus is matter properly disposed to be the subject of such a form as the rational soul"; and "infusion of this soul by God takes place at conception" (37). Readers who associate Thomas with delayed hominization miss the mark by suggesting "that we must *have* a human ontological individual before the soul comes," when, in fact, it is "the soul which *makes* this matter to be a human ontological individual" (48). Thus, in the light of contemporary knowledge, Heaney aligns Thomas with immediate hominization.

Dombrowski and Deltete's explanation for the Church's turn to immediate hominization emphasizes the seventeenth-century's fascination with the homunculus, a tiny fully formed little person that was thought to be present from the very beginning and needed only to grow larger. The associated scientific theory was "preformationism, a theory which asserted that each organism starts off with all its parts already formed" (37). The weakness of the authors' argument, in this section, involves not the discrediting of preformationism but rather their implication that association with the homunculus discredits immediate hominization. It

18. Heaney, "Aquinas and the Presence of the Human Rational Soul in the Early Embryo," 29–30. Further citations will be given parenthetically. For Thomas's remark on the way the semen contains "the formative power" based on "the vital spirit" that it "contains as a kind of froth," see *On the Truth of the Catholic Faith: Book Two*, 302. For more on the matter of hominization, see Donceel, "Abortion: Mediate v. Immediate Animation"; Diamond, "Abortion, Animation, and Biological Hominization"; Bedate and Cefalo, "The Zygote"; Suarez, "Hydatidiform Moles and Teratomas Confirm the Human Identity of the Preimplantation Embryo"; Bole, "Zygotes, Souls, Substances, and Persons"; Johnson, "Delayed Hominization"; Porter, "Individuality, Personal Identity, and the Moral Status of the Preembryo."

does not, for it is perfectly possible for immediate hominization to be credible even if some of the theory first giving it rise is now unacceptable. The authors also seem unaware of the implications of important features of their argument: thus they say that "what finally killed preformationist belief in a homunculus was the realization that organisms inherit characteristics from both parents" (38). In other words, what killed preformationism was the recognition that the fetus was a new creation, a new identity. If it is the genetic contribution of both parents that counts in creating this new being—as the authors recognize—then surely that new creation should be regarded to exist *from conception* and not from the burst of synapse formation at the end of the second trimester. One should note, too, how valorizing conception as the moment at which a new being exists has the effect of *equalizing* the contribution and status of both parents.[19]

Dombrowski and Deltete also offer a theory of personal continuity that they believe points to the superiority of delayed over immediate hominization. Their asymmetrical view of non-strict identity is presented as an alternative to two unacceptable alternatives, each symmetrical in its own right. The first of these is a Leibnizian view "that all events in a person's life are *internally* related to all the others, such that implicit in a fetus are all the experiences of the adult, and this is due to God's eternal 'foreknowledge' of everything that is to happen" (60). "An equally disastrous view," although it would permit abortion, is a view that denies

---

19. Here greater biological understanding enables us to hear something in Genesis 1 that we might not have heard otherwise and that perhaps represents an outworking of the text itself in biological knowledge: "So God created humankind in his image, in the image of God he created them; male and female he created them." (1:27) Here the balance of the lines suggests the perfect equality of men and women understood as, and deriving from, their being God's representatives. Both sexes stand in equal relation to God; the male is not, as in Aristotle, the norm of the human and the woman "misbegotten." If we see the form of the creation here—male and female as equal and new beings because they are equally from God—and apply it analogically to human procreation, we may be inclined to ask the critical question thusly: "At what point does a new being exist, equal to each of his or her parents, themselves the equals of one another and all others, including the child, by virtue of the one relationship that establishes the equality of all, their being from God?" Seeing procreation in this way will lead to our looking for that moment when male and female contribute equally—with the same beautiful balance that we hear in the line from Genesis—to the creation of a new equal, guaranteed that status not by gender or any other earthly attribute but by the qualitatively different relationship, shared by all, of being from God. Given current knowledge of genetics, it seems most reasonable to locate that moment at conception.

personal identity, claiming that events in a person's life are "*externally* related to the others," both past and future. On this view, also symmetrical, there is "strictly speaking ... no personal identity" (60).

The authors reject the symmetrical external view because it tends to undermine respect even for adult persons and the sense of moral responsibility—since it would allow, as in their example, a murderer to look "back on the killing he did and declar[e] that it was a different person who committed the crime" (66). The internal symmetrical view, on the other hand, denies "that with each change in life we have a partly new concrete reality." It would suggest that young persons must "identify themselves with the elderly persons they *may* eventually become" in a way that is untrue to experience (61). The authors' preferred view argues for an asymmetrical relationship between past and future: "a human person in the present is internally related to her past phases, but is only externally related to her future phases, if such there be" (60). It "makes sense to claim that a person in a later state includes that person in an earlier state, *but not vice versa*" (61). On this view, then, "Mary on Friday and Mary on Monday are somewhat different realities, both quantitatively (one is older than the other) and qualitatively (Mary on Monday has actually had experiences over the weekend that Mary on Friday could only imagine). The 'identity' between the two Marys is real, but it is an abstract reality rather than any concretely lived experience" (61).

The authors' primary purpose is to diminish the anti-abortion position by associating it with Leibnizian strict identity. The connection to pro-abortion of their own view is somewhat murky, but it would seem to lie in the assumption that the fetus-to-be-aborted has only an external relationship to the person it would otherwise become. The fetus has no claim, in a way, to a future not yet experienced and "indefinite."

The authors' position captures our commonsense view that we are differently related to past and future, but there are numerous problems with it as well, especially when used to justify abortion. First, it fails to consider the degree to which my future is dependent on my interpretation of it: I will understand my future experience, however different from my past, from within the categories, stories, beliefs, and history that I have lived to this point. It is, in short, not possible for the future to be as radically separated from the past, for me, as the authors wish to contend. I also carry into the future certain virtues, habits, settled dispositions, loyalties, and beliefs that ensure I will act in some ways and not in others—though surely these can be tested in extreme circumstances. Degrees of continuity in identity would also seem to be influenced by cultural factors: young people in very traditional cultures might well be able already to project what they will look like as elders. The authors' sense that young people cannot now do this may suggest less about the abstract theory of personal identity than it does about the fragmentation of contemporary life where everything comes to seem just one damn thing after another.

Moreover, the authors' theory may not allow for ascription of responsibility any better than the symmetrical external view they criticize. To use their example of Mary, cited above, let's suppose Mary commits murder on the Thursday before she has her life-changing weekend. What prevents her from claiming on Monday that it was not she who committed the murder? The authors will respond that, in doing so, she would be denying continuity with the past in a way inconsistent with their position. But she could say, in her defense, that the authors inadequately account for the way the future becomes the past. If the future is as discontinuous with the present as they suggest, surely there must be some degree of future discontinuity so great as to change the self sufficiently to make its past seem no longer its own. Of course we would commonly hold Mary accountable, but this is precisely because we do assume a greater continuity of past and present than the authors: we know that whatever Mary experiences over the weekend, she will do so as the particular being she is. The future does not simply "happen" to her: she experiences it as the being she is, and this limits its ability to render her other than she is. One of the factors that ensures this continuity is, of course, her body and genetic inheritance. Whatever I experience in future, I will experience it as the embodied being of particular genetic inheritance I am. The authors' position, in short, underestimates the importance of genetic inheritance (among other things) in ensuring personal continuity between present and future. Of importance to the Christian, too, is the claim that experience has already been storied by scripture. The very language we have for interpreting the future is not our own but Scripture: thus the continuity of self into the future depends not on us but on the God who sustains the world. God's future has come forward in Christ and thus, at baptism, the Christian begins to live proleptically in a future that is at least partially known through Jesus's cross and resurrection. Cross and resurrection provide the future's continuity with the present, for whatever happens in the future does so in the light of those realities.

If, then, there is greater continuity between I-present and I-future than the authors allow, their use of personal discontinuity to justify abortion seems weakened. Their own relatively strong view of continuity between I-past and I-present, however, also works against abortion in ways they do not develop. At some point in late-second to early-third trimester, the fetus gains, on the authors' view, moral status. When it does so, however, its present is, also on their view, strongly linked to its past. It seems counterintuitive, though, to say that a twenty-seven week old fetus cannot be killed, but that it could have been justifiably killed one day earlier—despite the fact that F27w and F27w-1d are continuous. The authors' way of obscuring this problem is by keeping the timing of sentience vague. We are told, for example, that "the fetus becomes morally considerable between twenty-four and thirty-two weeks when sentiency, and then the cerebral cortex, starts to function" (56). This may be good biology, but it also has the advantage of directing attention away from the difficulty of regarding the fetus as killable at one moment and protected at the next.

Peter Wenz employs a similar strategy in his defense of abortion rights as religious freedom. Wenz would protect the twenty-eight week old fetus, as differing from the newborn "primarily in their location, size, strength, and temporary need for support external to themselves" (178)—factors that do not affect the right to life of adults. Fetuses younger than twenty weeks deserve no legal protection, in his view, because the case for their personhood is inherently religious and thus irrelevant to secular law. But he keeps the status of the twenty- to twenty-eight-week-old fetus quite vague, saying even that he "cannot say exactly where between twenty and twenty-eight weeks the matter of fetal personhood becomes secular.... Even experts may not be able to agree on a particular week when the fetus differs from healthy newborns in no more than these four ways [location, temporary dependency, size and strength]" (180–81). This may again simply reflect an attempt to be biologically scrupulous, but its rhetorical effect should not be overlooked: it deflects the need to be precise about the time at which the fetus acquires legal status. Wenz adopts this strategy despite, or perhaps because of, his recognition elsewhere that the law must divide questions cleanly in order to allow people to use it as a guide. But if Wenz were to argue for a clean division in some particular week between twenty and twenty-eight, he would then have to confront the commonsense objection that the fetus he deems protectable is the same being he deemed killable one week earlier.[20] This is true both if we look backward from twenty-five weeks to twenty-four or forward from twenty-four to twenty-five, at least if embodiment and possession of a distinctive genetic identity are considered features of the continuity of a particular human being.

Reframing Peter Wenz's argument—and, to some extent, Dombrowski and Deltete's—we might, in the first and second persons, raise some challenging questions. Considering yourself as the particular embodied person you are—continuous with your past even on the asymmetrical view of identity—then to whom do you owe your protection during the first twenty-five weeks of your fetal existence (surely part of *your* past)? Of course the primary answer is to your mother, and perhaps also your father. But you do not owe it to the state. In fact, according to Wenz, you owe it primarily to the influence of religious beliefs in your society, for your status as a being worthy of protection was not a secular matter but rather one of religious conviction. You might ask further, then, what kind of thing this state is that did not consider you worthy of protection when you were most vulnerable. Or, what did you do, or must you do, to count in this state? Since what distinguished you in your pre-secular condition from you in your secular existence was that in the former you could be killed at will while in the latter you could not, then it seems possible that what the secular state is primarily about—regarding you and me—is distinguishing between who can be killed and who cannot (or when you or I can be killed legally). What you and I seem to have been allowed into is a kind of reciprocal pact based on our perceived mutual agreement on who can be killed and when. To be a critic of abortion, then, might be simply to insist that I want to be received into society just as I am and that I cannot be just as I am so long as the state accords me protected status only insofar as I assent to its definitions of who can be killed and when.

One of the most thorough rejections of the "conception criterion" in recent years is offered by David Boonin in *A Defense of Abortion*. Presenting a full response to Boonin is well beyond the scope of this chapter. Doing so adequately would require a book at least as long and

---

20. The inability to draw suitably "bright lines" about fetal viability and about the risks of abortion at various stages of pregnancy is pointed out strongly by Justice O'Connor in her minority opinion for *Akron v. Akron Center for Reproductive Health*. See *Abortion Decisions of the United States Supreme Court: The 1980's*, 93–95.

detailed as his. What I will do is to examine one of his most important refutations aimed at arguments attempting to defend the claim "that the human fetus acquires the right to life at the moment of its conception."[21] The argument in question, "The Future Like Ours" argument, has been put forth prominently by Don Marquis and discussed by several other writers.[22] My point will be that Boonin does not show the "Future Like Ours" argument against abortion to be invalid on terms that the abortion critic accepts. If this can be successfully demonstrated, it undermines the larger claim of his book. In the fifth chapter of this book, I will try to show also why some of Boonin's defenses of the Good Samaritan argument for abortion—most prominently associated with Judith Jarvis Thomson—similarly fail to accomplish his goal of refuting the critic of abortion on the critic's own grounds.

The "Future Like Ours" argument grounds the fetus's right to life from conception in its "having a future-like-ours that contains experiences of the sort that one now values or will later come to value (if one is not killed)."[23] Although critics and defenders of abortion differ about "whether the fetus has the same right to life as you or I," they agree "that in cases B, C, and D in the following list, the individuals in question have the same right to life as you and I do in E: (A) fetus, (B) infant, (C) suicidal teenager, (D) temporarily comatose adult, (E) you or me." Marquis "can then be understood as suggesting that the following decision procedure be used to resolve the question about the status of the fetus: Identify the property that most plausibly accounts for the wrongness of killing in cases B–E, and then determine whether that property is possessed by the individual in case A." If it is, then the fetus merits protection; if not, then it has no right to protection.[24]

21. Boonin, *Defense of Abortion*, 19. Further references will be given parenthetically.

22. Marquis's article originally appeared as "Why Abortion is Immoral," 183–202. I will quote from the text reprinted in Pojman and Beckwith, *Abortion Controversy*, cited in note 1. References will be given parenthetically. Important responses to Marquis include Cudd, "Sensationalized Philosophy," 262–64; McInerney, "Does a Fetus Already Have a Future-Like-Ours?" 264–68; Norcross, "Killing, Abortion, and Contraception," 268–77; Shirley, "Marquis's Argument Against Abortion," 79–89; Paske, "Abortion and the Neo-Natal Right to Life," 343–53. Marquis has responded to Shirley in "Fetuses, Futures and Values," 263–65, and to McInerney and Paske in "A Future Like Ours and the Concept of Person," 354–69.

23. Boonin, *Defense of Abortion*, 57, 61.

24. It should be said that the schematization of the categories as A, B, C, D, E, is

Boonin grants a good bit of intuitive rightness to Marquis's position. He believes the "future-like-ours principle that [Marquis] defends can account for the wrongness of killing in cases B–E"; that "he is also correct that the way in which this principle accounts for the wrongness of killing in these cases is intuitively plausible"; and "that an implication of this principle is that the typical human fetus has the same right to life as you or I" (62). Thus a "successful rebuttal" must "do three things": 1) "identify another property" of the individuals in B–E and thus offer "an alternative account of the wrongness of killing you or me which produces the same results in cases B–E"; 2) show that this alternative account is superior to Marquis's, that "it more convincingly identifies a feature of killing that makes it prima facie seriously wrong"; and 3) show that this alternative account has different consequences for A, the fetus (62–63).

Boonin concentrates on offering an alternative account of the kinds of desire that entitle us not to be killed. Marquis argues that D, the comatose adult, has no present desires yet surely "has the same right to life as you or I" (Boonin, 65). Thus to account for this right, we must refer to future desires that he would or will have despite his having no present desires for a future or even the present desire that his future be preserved. Boonin argues, however, that it is false that the comatose adult has no present desires. Even though he has no "occurrent" desires, he does have "dispositional" desires, despite being unaware of them. Boonin likens such dispositional desires to beliefs. I believe that triangles have three sides even though I am not consciously reflecting on that belief. My beliefs do not simply go away when I sleep, to be replaced by "a new and identical set of beliefs" when I wake up. The same seems to hold for desires. At breakfast, I am probably unaware of my desire that my "future personal life be preserved." I do not lose this "dispositional" desire when I go to sleep, and neither does the comatose adult D. Thus we do not need to invoke a future occurrent desire, as Marquis does, to account for his right not to be killed. What gives him the right not to be killed, just like you or me, is his present dispositional desire. Boonin claims the superiority of his position to Marquis's lies in its greater parsimony and moral salience (65–66).

Boonin's way of representing Marquis's argument. Marquis does, however, refer to each of Boonin's examples, but the treatment is less systematic than Boonin's characterization of the argument.

The latter claim merits brief elaboration here, as it turns on a crucial larger claim that I will later contest—that the "great merit of the future-like-ours approach in general is that it enables us to account for the prima facie wrongness of killing by understanding killing as one instance of a more general category of acts that are prima facie wrong: acts that frustrate the desires of others" (67). Now, if we consider a whole range of cases, we will find that it is frustrating dispositional rather than occurrent desires that matters most in making actions wrong. Boonin gives the example of a woman who desires her husband to be faithful yet not at the level of occurrent desire while she's playing bridge—when her desire is to be dealt a good hand. We'd find the self-defense of her husband seriously deficient if he claimed that his adultery during her bridge game was justified by her having no desire that he be faithful. Her dispositional desire matters and ought not to be frustrated. Similarly the dispositional desire of the comatose adult remains and must be respected.

Boonin again draws a distinction within the concept of desire as he considers suicidal teenager C. Here Hans, deeply depressed over rejection in love, seems to have neither the occurrent nor the dispositional desire to go on living, yet clearly he has the right to live. Marquis's "present or future occurrent desire" version seems to have "no difficulty" accounting for Hans's right not to be killed: it is based on his having future desires for a future-like-ours even if he has no such desire at present. Boonin again claims, however, that it is only partially true that Hans has no present desire for a future-like-ours. We typically distinguish, especially in cases where one is temporarily in "great emotional distress," between actual and ideal desires—the desires one "*would* have had if the actual desire had been formed under more ideal circumstances" (70). In effect, Hans's desires have been formed under a condition of partial and insufficient information: "If he were to look more objectively at what the rest of his life holds in store for him—some deep traumatic pain now but a much greater overall amount of satisfaction and happiness later on—then he would desire to persevere and get on with his life" (72). Thus, if we consider his "ideal" rather than his "actual" present desire, we do not need to point to his future desire for a "future-like-ours" in order to understand why he ought not to be killed.

Boonin claims greater parsimony and salience for his version than he finds in Marquis's. To defend his claim of greater salience, he returns to his adulterous couple. Now the wife is in therapy, occasioned by distress over the fatal illness of her only child from a previous marriage. She tells the therapist, "The only thing I care about right now is my son's health. I could care less if my husband were sleeping with every woman in town" (74). If the husband appeals to this as justification for adultery, we would surely judge his claim morally insufficient. We do so because his wife "*already* has desires about the future," even if she cannot at present reflect on them because of her circumstances. He must respect her desires: in this case, her "ideal" desire that he be faithful even if she does not currently entertain that as an "actual" desire (74).

Boonin gives relatively little attention to B, the human infant, but he believes it poses "no difficulty" for his account, which he calls ultimately the "'present ideal dispositional desire' version of the future-like-ours principle." Newborn infants do have "actual conscious desires," such as enjoying the "sensation of warmth" or being satisfied by food. Thus the infant must not be killed. Boonin makes these claims despite recognizing that the infant "does not yet possess the concept of himself as a continuing subject of experience"; that he possesses no concepts at all; and that he thus understands nothing. "But if he did understand these things," Boonin claims, "he would surely desire that his future personal life be preserved since he would understand that this is necessary in order for him to enjoy the experiences that he does already consciously desire to enjoy" (83–84). The "preconscious fetus," however, "has no actual desires," if we mean by desiring something "to be in a certain conscious state that involves caring about, valuing, wanting the object of desire." Here Boonin attempts to distinguish conscious desires that are of moral relevance from merely behavioral desires, which he grants to the "preconscious fetus." These latter include "disposition[s] to behave in certain ways or to respond to certain stimuli in certain ways"; such desires are merely "behavioral," can equally well be attributed to a thermostat, and have no moral relevance. Conscious desires "may essentially involve reference to certain propositions or sentences," but "such reference is not necessary." What does matter "is that the individual have an attraction to a given subject that is associated with certain conscious states and is not merely behavioral in nature in the way that the thermostat's desires are" (80–81). The "preconscious fetus" possesses no such "conscious desires" and thus has no right, unlike you or me, not to be killed.

There are many problems with Boonin's argument, and some of these may well be rooted in problems in Marquis's "future-like-ours" approach. For the sake of clarity, I will take up the problems in Boonin's position one by one, beginning with those that involve specific parts of the argument I have outlined and then taking up larger flaws in the whole conception. I will focus on three problems: the first involves Boonin's account of key terms like consciousness, desire, behavior, and disposition, especially as these involve his distinction between infant and fetus; the second involves his account of "ideal" as opposed to actual desire; and the third involves his treatment of C above, the suicidal teenager. In addressing the larger conceptual flaws in the overall argument, I will challenge Boonin's treatment of the prima facie wrongness of killing as one instance of the more general prima facie wrongness of frustrating desires; suggest that what he has produced is a "present-like-ours" rather than a "future-like-ours" approach; and dispute his original way of developing the categories, A–E. What I hope to show is that Boonin does not respond successfully to the abortion critic on the critic's own grounds.

I quoted Boonin on the infant's status at some length in order to suggest the strained quality of his distinction between infant and fetus, particularly on the matters of consciousness and desire. He argues that conscious desire "essentially" involves "reference to certain propositions or sentences"—language, which, of course the infant does not possess—yet "such reference is not necessary," which leaves his sense of what's "essential" quite unclear. The standard for consciousness used to disqualify the fetus also seems to involve a considerable degree of conceptual ability: "caring about, valuing, wanting the object of desire" (81). The infant passes this standard yet understands nothing, not even his own status as a subject of experience.[25] Yet to "care about" and "value" surely suggest a level of understanding, and to want something understood as an "object of desire" suggests a sense of oneself as a subject of experience. The "conscious desires" of the infant—enjoying warmth or the satisfaction of hunger—also seem insufficiently distinguishable from the mere behaviors Boonin treats so disparagingly. He overlooks, on one hand, the way fetuses, even early ones, display reactive behaviors, and, on the other,

---

25. "It is also true that the newborn infant does not yet possess the concept of himself as a continuing subject of experience, and it is true that he does not understand that death involves the annihilation of such a subject. Indeed, it seems unlikely that he has any concepts at all and so in this sense unlikely that he understands anything" (Boonin, 84). I hope the ability to understand death as "the annihilation" of the subject has not become the test of humanhood, for it seems difficult to conceive how a "continuing subject" could "understand" its own annihilation.

the way even the complex and conscious desires of adults are rooted in simple behavioral orientations. In fact, if he were not given over to such a Cartesian account of disembodied consciousness, he would not have to devise his account of ideal desire to explain why the suicidal teenager ought not to be killed. The fact that the teenager has not killed himself might simply be interpreted to mean that the whole organism that he is is disposed to—or desires to—continue living, irrespective of what he reports his conscious desires to be. To acknowledge this understanding of desire—one more parsimonious than Boonin's—would, however, commit him to recognizing that each of us is sustained and carried into our future moment to moment by the whole organism—most of it functioning quite unconsciously, or merely behaviorally. This would make "you or I" a good bit more like the fetus than we are under Boonin's mentalistic account of desire, particularly in regard to the desire that he gives supreme importance—that of continuing our present into the future, i.e., living itself. Finally, it's worth noting the near tautologies Boonin recurs to repeatedly in his account of how "preconscious fetuses" lack the features of consciousness, as he defines it. That circularity of linguistic structure—along with the fuzziness and straightforward contradictions inherent in Boonin's distinction between fetal behavior and infant consciousness—will suggest to the critic of abortion that the judgment to include infants as having a "future like you or I" may not have been taken on the grounds of their consciousness but on some other grounds—and that then a definition of consciousness has been developed in order to include the infant and disqualify the fetus.

The point I am making here can be clarified by our examining Boonin's account of "ideal" desire. Recall Boonin's example of the woman in therapy expecting the death of her child who says that, at the moment, she cares not at all whether her husband is faithful. If her husband then commits adultery, we will say that he has not adequately respected her desires. We could explain that judgment by saying that she will, in future, come again to desire her husband's faithfulness, but Boonin wants to preclude that Marquis-like interpretation because it would commit us to respecting a being now on the basis of desires it will have in the future (a position obviously aligned with a fetal right to life). Thus Boonin says she has, at present, an "ideal" desire—which she would hold under more favorable circumstances—though not an actual desire. My point is not to deny that she has a present desire for her husband's faithfulness but rather to suggest that this is better understood as an actual desire or, to use Boonin's own earlier-deployed concept, dispositional desire. Boonin's tale would seem to suggest one can have only one desire at a time, yet presumably we would not take her statement to the therapist to mean she has no desire to eat, or maintain warmth, or see her present continued into the future. Presumably her desire that her husband be faithful has been formed in the past, under a variety of circumstances, and can best be described as one of her habitual dispositions. There is no need whatever to say she would have this desire, as an ideal one, under counterfactual conditions, because she does have it now as an actual dispositional desire despite what she says at the very moment of the therapist's question. (One should add that it's also hardly unusual for one to reveal what one cares about by saying, angrily, that one does not care for it.)

What role, then, does this unparsimonious turn to a concept of "ideal" desire play in Boonin's argument? To answer this question, we need to return to case C, the suicidal teenager Hans. We're to respect Hans's life not because he will, in future, develop a desire for a "future like ours" but rather because he already has the "ideal" desire to live on—"ideal" referring to the desire he would have if he had formed his desire under more accurate and complete information about the good things life has in store for him. I have already developed the most parsimonious way to explain why Hans ought not to be killed, even given Boonin's assumption that we should understand the wrongness of killing as an instance of the wrongness of frustrating desires. Hans's *behavior*—his not having killed himself—indicates his desire to live, and we should respect that. Nevertheless we need to follow Boonin's development of Hans's ideal desire a bit further.

To develop the concept, Boonin introduces the story of Irving, a hiker nearing the end of his excursion and possessed of the primary desire to return safely and of a secondary desire to hike the easier and more scenic of two paths. He faces a fork in the road, the left path easier and more scenic, the right more difficult. He chooses the left path yet, unbeknownst to him, a land mine has been planted on this trail. Thus his actual desire is for the left path, but his ideal desire is for the right—which, of course, he would have chosen had he more complete information about the choices in question. The problem with the analogy between Irving's and Hans's case lies in the story Boonin must invent about Hans's future life. Let's say, however, that Hans has the misfortune to have a life chain like that designed by Satan for some of Eseldorf's residents in Mark Twain's *Mysterious Stranger*. Rather than enjoying the satisfactions Boonin posits for him, he will, on the way to committing suicide, attempt to rescue a young girl from a pond, contract a debilitating illness, and lay like a "paralytic log" for the next forty years.[26] In this case, if he had possessed more complete information, he might well have come to the very same desire he already has. His ideal desire, and his actual desire, might be to die. Yet still he ought not to be killed, primarily because, as I have argued, his actual desire—inferred from his behavior—indicates his desire to live. Again Boonin's own concept of dispositional desire is useful: Hans has a disposition to continue living formed in the past and which he has not lost simply because of his current depression. There is no need to invent ideal desires based on counterfactual conditions for him.

We come back, then, to asking what the role of "ideal" desire is in Boonin's account? I suggest that it is required for his defense of the infant, where he asserts a fallacious comparison between the newborn and the hiker Irving. After stating it's "unlikely that [the infant] understands anything," Boonin argues, counterfactually: "But if he did understand these things, he would surely desire that his future personal life be preserved since he would understand that this is necessary in order for him to enjoy the experiences that he does already consciously desire to enjoy. And in this sense, at least, he is no different from the hiker who would desire to turn right if he understood that this was necessary in order for him

---

26. Satan distresses Mark Twain's Theodor Fischer and Seppi Wohlmeyer by altering the life chain of their dear young friend Nikolaus. It has been "appointed" that the sleeping Nikolaus will turn over and not awaken during a rain storm, but Satan decides to alter this sequence, having Nikolaus wake up, close the window, and go back to bed. He thus "will rise in the morning two minutes later than the chain of his life had appointed him to rise. By consequence, thenceforth nothing will ever happen to him in accordance with the details of the old chain." The boys are dismayed to learn that in his new chain Nikolaus will drown in an attempt to save a young girl, Lisa, twelve days hence. Whereas in his original chain he would have arrived in time, now he will be seconds late. Lisa will "have struggled into deeper water," and both will drown. The boys plead with Satan to prevent this from happening, until Satan explains to them what was in store for Nicky in the original sequence of events: "If I had not done this, Nikolaus would save Lisa, then he would catch cold from his drenching; one of your race's fantastic and desolating scarlet fevers would follow, with pathetic after-effects; for forty-six years he would lie in his bed a paralytic log, deaf, dumb, blind, and praying night and day for the blessed relief of death. Shall I change his life back?" See *Mysterious Stranger*, 354–55.

to satisfy the strongest desires that he does in fact have"(84). But Irving's lack of understanding is utterly different from the infant's. Irving has the full capacity to understand the implications of his choices of left or right; he simply lacks full information about those choices. The infant, by Boonin's own admission, understands nothing because he does not yet have the capacity to do so. No amount of further information will modify his desires in any way. To compare the hiker and the infant is utterly misleading. We are meant to infer, I suppose, that the infant has a kind of "ideal" present desire to preserve his future even though he has only an unclear actual desire. But it's only necessary to invent this whole account of "ideal" desires based on counterfactuals if we ignore the obvious: the infant's behavior indicates quite clearly its desire to preserve itself and its future. But if we focus on organism-preserving behavior—rather than on conscious desires which the infant would have if it could understand what it cannot—then we would surely see a greater continuity between fetus and infant than Boonin will allow. The critic of abortion may very well infer that the whole account of ideal desire, with its many problems, has served only to draw a distinction, itself fallacious, between the infant and the fetus.

At this point, we should turn from the more specific problems in Boonin's argument to difficulties in his overall conception. The first concerns his claim that the wrongness of killing should be regarded "as one instance of a more general category of acts that are prima facie wrong: acts that frustrate the desires of others" (67). Boonin's language specifically diminishes the distinctiveness of the wrongness of killing. It also undermines a hierarchical ordering of the importance of duties not to frustrate desire. Such a treatment obviously overlooks the way in which life is the condition on which all other desires depend. Moreover, many desires are rightly frustrated: the desire of some to dominate others, the desire of strong peoples to conquer the weak, the desire of renegade corporate executives to fleece their shareholders. The list, of course, is endless. As we must, then, in the very nature of things, continually frustrate the desires of others and restrain our own, Boonin's way of setting the problem cannot help but undermine the force of the wrongness of killing. As desires must be frustrated, so too the right not to be killed must sometimes be abrogated.

If the prohibition against killing is to be understood as only one of many prohibitions against frustrating desire, and many desires must be frustrated, then the conditions have been set for a calculus of desires in which one's desire not to be killed is weighed against other desires. What makes such a move doubly problematic is that reducing the force of the wrongness of killing may well strengthen other desires—e.g., your country's desire for my country's territory. For desires are formed in the light of prohibitions on desire. If the wrongness of killing lies in a distinctive, exceptionless prohibition against it, we will form our desires in a way that precludes killing. Reducing the wrongness of killing to the wrongness of frustrating desire leaves us freer to form desires of sufficient intensity and value (at least to us) to override the wrongness of killing.

A second problem in Boonin's overall conception lies in his failure to recognize that what he has produced is no longer really a "future-like-ours" argument but rather a "present-like-ours" view. Boonin wants to insist that his is a "'present desire' version of the future-like-ours" principle. This enables him to keep his position within the general rubric of Marquis's "future-like-ours" argument while at the same time asserting the superiority of his version to Marquis's "present or future desire" version. But the fact that Marquis and Boonin come to directly opposing conclusions on the single matter at hand—the fetus's right to life—ought to make us wonder whether Boonin's treatment is simply a "version" of the argument being presented by Marquis. In fact it is not. In each of Boonin's modifications of Marquis's cases, what counts against killing the subject is a desire that he or she has now—the dispositional desire of the comatose patient, the ideal desire of the suicidal teenager, the conscious desire of the infant. Granted part of the desire is for the subject's future to be preserved, but this is really to say nothing that is not already implicit in the notion of desire. Desire is obviously future-directed. What matters morally in Boonin's examples is present desire.

Why, then, does Boonin want to keep his argument within the rubric provided by Marquis's "future-like-ours" position? Because only by doing so can he seem to be saying anything at all about the fetus's right to life or lack of it. If Boonin's position is—as I contend—a "present desires count" position—and desire is understood as mentalistically as Boonin does—then obviously it will disqualify at least early fetuses from having a right not to be killed. But such a position seems uninteresting and unlikely to persuade any critic of abortion to accept the permissibility of killing the fetus. In short, it must be held that the fetus has a future sufficiently like ours (typical adults) to make the argument for killing it necessary. If it has no future-like-ours, then no argument is necessary to justify its killing. On the other hand, if it has a future-like-ours, then it would seem to deserve protection. Boonin does not resolve this problem. Instead his argument remains rhetorically parasitic on Marquis's, suggesting just enough that the fetus has a future like ours to make an argument for its justified killing seem necessary. But, as I have argued, each of his case analyses reduces to a "present-desires count" model, and thus his argument is no longer a "future-like ours" position in any meaningful way. His conclusion is uncontroversial and will persuade no critic of abortion.

The most basic overall problem in Boonin's argument may derive from the way he systematizes Marquis's original conception. Here we will need to remember Boonin's categories of cases: A) fetus; B) infant; C) suicidal teenager; D) temporarily comatose patient; E) you or me. The first thing to notice here is that this is not the way the critic of abortion will distribute the categories. Critics of abortion—at least some of them—take their position because of a profoundly felt solidarity with the fetus, and thus they are likely to insist that both categories A and E should read "you, me, fetus." In fact, the critic will note the overlap between Boonin's category E and all the other categories. Each of us has been a fetus and an infant and possibly a suicidal teenager or temporarily comatose patient. If the fetus has a "future like ours," as the critic will assume, then it is either noncontroversial that the fetus has a right to life like you or me, or the right to life is a matter of controversy for the members of each of the categories. The critic of abortion will point out that Boonin's treatment suggests that the right to life for those in B, C, and D is at least controversial enough to require an argument explaining why they ought not to be killed. The only reason we will listen to the arguments in B, C, and D is that the third-person objectification and categorization induces us to forget temporarily that these are also arguments about "you" or "me." If we remembered that the argument about C, for example, is really an argument about why you or I ought not to be killed, we would inevitably and rightfully reject it out of hand. Whatever success Boonin's argument achieves depends really only on one thing: the degree to which he can induce forgetting in you and me that we were once fetuses. His first move is by far the most important one, for it puts the "fetus"—with its objectified, third-person label—in a category by itself, separate from us. But in doing this he has simply assumed what needs to be proved to the critic of abortion. The critic of abortion will not be persuaded on his own terms, for he will remember that you and I were once fetuses.

4

Abortion as Letting Die, Bad Samaritanism, or Just War

Why We Should Reject the Analogies

IN THE PROCESS OF showing "how American law and politics trivialize religious devotion," Stephen L. Carter argues, in the *Culture of Disbelief*, that religious believers must be allowed to participate in the public square without being forced to bracket their faith. On the matter of abortion, this position leads him to what might seem a counterintuitive conclusion: that the argument for abortion must be made without regard to the humanity of the fetus. Only this option avoids "derid[ing] religiously based moral judgments as inferior to secular ones," and thus Carter commends arguments that elaborate the premise of Judith Jarvis Thomson: "Even supposing that the embryo has a claim against the woman that she not end the pregnancy, it does not follow that she may not end the pregnancy."[1] One prominent class of these arguments involves the "bad Samaritan" defense, which claims that we all must have the right to be bad Samaritans. This defense appeals to our intuitions

---

1. Carter, *Culture of Disbelief*, 257–58. Laurence H. Tribe has argued similarly in *Abortion: The Clash of Absolutes*. He suggests the Court's argument in *Roe* may have "needlessly insulted and alienated those for whom the view that the fetus is a person represents a fundamental article of faith or a bedrock personal commitment." The Court should rather have said: "Even if the fetus *is* a person, our Constitution forbids compelling a woman to carry it for nine months and become a mother" (135). It is a measure of the country's division on abortion that Tribe thinks those who insist on fetal personhood will not be alienated by the language he proposes. He seems not to understand that for those for whom fetal personhood is a "fundamental article of faith," saying the fetus is a person just is a way of saying it must not be killed.

about duties to assist others. It freely grants that the fetus is a person yet argues that this does not require the mother to support it with her body. As Donald H. Regan notes, it is a "deeply rooted principle of American law that an individual is ordinarily not required to volunteer aid to another individual who is in danger or in need of assistance."[2] To require a woman to carry an unwanted fetus to term compels her to be a Good Samaritan in a way that is unjustified. Thus she must have the right to terminate the pregnancy even if we grant the personhood of the fetus.

Now surely something odd has happened to the concept of personhood here, at least to the concept as Kant conceived it. Granting herself "inclined to think . . . that we shall probably have to agree that the fetus has already become a human person well before birth," Thomson notes the way abortion opponents "commonly spend most of their time establishing that the fetus is a person, and hardly any time explaining the step from there to the impermissibility of abortion. Perhaps they think the step too simple and obvious to require much comment."[3] Not only is the step, for personhood defenders of the fetus, "simple" but unnecessary, for personhood status means precisely not being subject to being killed without consent. Whether consciously or not, those defenders follow Kant's understanding of the respect that is due to persons. Respect, as Kant defined it in the *Doctrine of Virtue*, is "to be understood as the *maxim* of limiting our self-esteem by the dignity of humanity in another person."[4] Clearly the limiting of our self-esteem before the other requires our refusal to kill. Indeed killing would seem the clearest possible violation of the second formulation of the Categorical Imperative: to kill is to regard the other, in the purest way, as simply a means to our ends, as a thing to be produced (the process of killing itself being the production, by reduction, of a thing from the living being itself).[5]

---

2. Regan, "Rewriting *Roe v. Wade*," 1569. Further citations will be given parenthetically.

3. Thomson, "A Defense of Abortion," 131–32. Further citations will be given parenthetically.

4. Respect "is not to be understood as the mere *feeling* that comes from comparing our own *worth* with another's (such as a child feels merely from habit toward his parents, a pupil toward his teacher, or any subordinate toward his superior). It is rather to be understood as the *maxim* of limiting our self-esteem by the dignity of humanity in another person, and so as respect in the practical sense." From *Doctrine of Virtue*, 244.

5. "Act so that you treat humanity, whether in your own person or in that of another, always as an end and never as a means only." In *Foundations of the Metaphysics of Morals*, 46.

If personhood has, then, meant protection against killing, how shall we understand defenses of abortion, like Thomson's, which freely grant the personhood of the fetus and yet argue for the acceptability of its killing? Or, to put this a slightly different way, how does an argument like Thomson's bring us to endorse such a seemingly impossible and paradoxical result—i.e., that the fetus is a person (in which case it can only be an innocent one) and yet that it can be justifiably killed? How is it, too, that Stephen Carter can be lead to such a paradoxical point that he claims only such abortion-despite-personhood arguments as Thomson's treat religious believers' convictions seriously?

This chapter addresses these questions through a series of interrelated arguments. It would seem to be difficult to say much that is fresh about Thomson's argument for abortion, but I hope to be able to do so. My treatment of Thomson addresses the whole of her argument, but I want to underscore three points here. First, though we might be inclined to characterize her position as an "abortion-despite-personhood" one (as I have above), it is more properly understood as an "abortion because of personhood" one—that is, her ability to make the argument *depends upon* the assumption of fetal personhood, for it depends upon invoking our whole set of responses about what is owed to persons such as her legendary violinist. One way to challenge Thomson is by making it clear that our responses to what is owed violinists will tell us little about what is owed fetuses. Second, I will argue that there is a way in which Thomson's argument actually sheds no light whatever on the question of abortions other than in the case of rape. My claim will be that "your" detaching yourself from the violinist can not meaningfully be deemed to kill him, nor can it even be considered an act of "letting him die" in a way that contributes meaningfully to the casuistry surrounding acts of "letting die," particularly in the context of abortion. In order to make this claim, I will first examine the position of James Rachels and others that letting die is actually no worse than killing. I think we should reject this position, keep a clear distinction between killing and letting die, and think harder about how the notion of letting die actually works in our moral reflection. Third, I will reject the idea that Thomson's argument be considered a defense of bad Samaritanism, at least in non-rape cases. I think we do need a secular casuistry involving our duties to anonymous others in need, though, Christianly speaking, I think we should resist gathering these under the rubric of Samaritanism, good or bad. (This is a point I make at the end of the next chapter.) My point here, though, is that Thomson does not successfully show that abortion, in non-rape cases, should be regarded as a question of good or bad Samaritanism, as this has been understood in the law.[6]

Following the discussion of Thomson, the chapter focuses on another defense of abortion as allowable bad Samaritanism. This one is described by its author, Donald H. Regan, as ultimately "an equal protection argument," for crucial to its logic is the claim that the burdens of pregnancy and childbirth are "sui generis," without parallel among the kinds of obligations we expect people to assume in assisting others (1569–1570). Regan seems no more successful than Thomson in demonstrating that abortion should be seen primarily as a problem in Samaritanism. What is most interesting about Regan's argument is his search for an analogous sacrifice to unwanted pregnancy on the part of men. His suggestion is that military conscription comes closest to providing such analogy. Evidently Regan is willing to consider forced pregnancy for women if, for instance, this could be justified as part of a campaign of national sacrifice. A careful look at Regan's logic reveals the connection between abortion and war; suggests the connection between the legitimizing of abortion and the unthinkability of American casualties in war after Vietnam (at least until Iraq)[7]; and reveals the way

---

6. Meredith W. Michaels has argued that appeals to Samaritanism are "inherently relativistic" and thus not very helpful without a "shared context for moral evaluation." She thus finds Thomson's argument unconvincing. See "Abortion and the Claims of Samaritanism," 214–15.

7. We might ask whether part of the reason we are in Iraq (and Afghanistan) is to persuade the world and ourselves that we are over the Vietnam syndrome, demonstrated by our willingness to "take casualties," as the media people put it. In short, we fight in Iraq in order to persuade ourselves that we are able to fight in Iraq, or perhaps to persuade ourselves that there is still something in the culture of consumerism worth dying for. I use the word "we" loosely, as the politicians and media do. I am fully aware that, even in our own society, we have cordoned off the work of killing and dying, assigning these to "volunteers." I do not mean to suggest that any of our leaders chose to go into Iraq or Afghanistan in order for our forces to take casualties. I only suggest that there is a kind of logic to the several military actions the United States has been in since Vietnam, the most notable before September 11, 2001, being the First Gulf War. We have been watching the post-Vietnam re-blooding of the nation, during most of which military casualties have been minor and incidental. After the demonstrations of our technological superiority in Desert Storm and Kosovo, what was left to demonstrate that we were fully "back" except the sacrifice of blood?

the "bad Samaritan" defense of abortion actually operates as a way of cordoning off violence so that it does not recoil on us.

The link between abortion and war is made quite explicit by Lloyd Steffen, whose *Life/Choice: The Theory of Just Abortion* is modeled specifically on just-war theory. Steffen's goal is to develop principles for the justification of some abortions while leaving intact a general presumption for life. Much as in Regan's case, however, the most intriguing aspects of Steffen's work lie in assumptions he does not question or perhaps even see. The most disturbing of these is his identifying questions of morality specifically with killing and membership in the "moral community" with possession of the power to kill. Unlike Thomson and Regan, Steffen does not consider fetuses liable to being killed to be "persons." Rather the fetus becomes a person when her mother extends to her the promise of bringing her to term—with twenty weeks serving as a marker at which society can reasonably assume such a promise has been extended. Thus becoming a person seems to mean little more than moving from the category of those who can be killed to that of those who are empowered to kill. The just abortion theorizing functions, then, to "construct," as Steffen puts it, a firewall between the killers and the killed. Steffen's book reveals more than the usual level of discomfort over the "fanatical" resistance to abortion of pro-lifers. That it does so may be rooted in assumptions I do not think he sees but which need to be brought to light: that abortion, like war, may be one of the ways we overcome our fear of death as power over us by exercising death itself as the moral power by which we constitute who we are.

One additional consideration, particularly of this chapter but also throughout, is with the stories philosophers tell in support of their arguments. Rachels, Thomson, et al. offer stories to test our moral intuitions or to give evidence for positions. Too often we fail to assess the kinds of narrative choices these stories embody or to recognize their rhetorical purposes. F. M. Kamm has argued that highly abstract philosophical stories allow us to bracket our emotions and thus to ponder problems rationally.[8] But I think we should recognize that stories such as those told by Rachels or Thomson are carefully constructed rhetorical devices whose purpose is to direct our attention to some features of a situation or dilemma and away from other—sometimes equally relevant—features of it. Moreover—and perhaps I mean this especially for the Christian

---

8. For Kamm's description of her "method," see *Creation and Abortion*, 7–11.

reader, who has been shaped by an alternative story—we can always ask why a particular story seems to have currency. Instead of asking what we can learn about abortion, for instance, from Thomson's famous story of the unconscious violinist, we might rather ask what has happened to sexuality and childbearing that enables Thomson's story to seem even remotely relevant.

It is often argued—as by James Childress and Tom Beauchamp in *Principles of Biomedical Ethics*—that the duties of non-maleficence and beneficence should be kept distinct, and that non-maleficence is generally, but not always, the stronger obligation.[9] Such an ordering seems in accord with common sense: surely I have a stronger obligation not to push my fishing partner into the lake than I have to rescue him should he fall into deep and treacherous water. The right to be a bad Samaritan would seem to depend on precisely this sense that we are not under equally strong obligations to do good and to refrain from harm. We might admire the one who stops to assist the stranger in peril at the side of the road: we might praise him, encourage others to do likewise, and even censure the failure to be sensitive to the one in need. But we would not require any of these forms of beneficence, or punish its failure, with the same rigor we insist on non-maleficence or punish those who act with maleficence.

A strong distinction between killing and letting die would seem to be related to this distinction between the duties of non-maleficence and beneficence. We have a very strong—to some, exceptionless—duty not to kill, killing representing perhaps the most extreme form of maleficence. On the other hand, we have a weaker obligation to prevent others from dying as a matter of beneficence. To put this in a very straightforward way, we might say it is incumbent on us—with a force approaching, at least, the absolute—to avoid killing others, whereas it is not as incumbent on us to do everything we can to save others from the possibility of dying.

James Rachels contends very directly, however, that "killing is not in itself any worse than letting die."[10] He makes this claim in a widely

---

9. Beauchamp and Childress, *Principles of Biomedical Ethics*, 107.

10. Rachels, "Active and Passive Euthanasia," 564. Further citations will be given parenthetically. The importance of the killing/letting die distinction is maintained by Foot, "The Problem of Abortion and the Doctrine of the Double Effect," 19–32, and also by Quinn in "Actions, Intentions, and Consequences," 287–312. For a critique of Foot on the double effect, one with which I substantially agree, see Anscombe, "Who Is

reprinted and influential essay arguing that the distinction between active and passive euthanasia is not as important as it was once thought to be. He points out that withholding treatment may only increase and prolong a terminal patient's agony and that, therefore, active euthanasia by lethal injection may well be "preferable to passive euthanasia" (561). He notes the inhumanity and absurdity of allowing a Down infant with intestinal obstruction to die of dehydration and starvation. The preference of passive over active euthanasia in such a case can only seem cruel. Moreover, the distinction means that the decision to allow the baby to die "is being decided on irrelevant grounds," for "it is the Down's syndrome, and not the intestines, that is the issue" (562). Rachels remains non-committal on whether the Down baby should receive corrective surgery and thus live, but this stance seems a bit disingenuous when it is placed in the middle of an argument for active euthanasia. For some of us, his case clarifies nothing at all. Down babies' lives are certainly not such a burden to them that they are insupportable. The child is simply being denied treatment that any normal infant would receive as a matter of course. Those in charge of its treatment have unfortunately not taken their duty of non-maleficence seriously enough. They are doing harm, and all that remains is a question about means. Once the decision to do harm is taken, then Rachels's logic makes sense: one ought to do that as painlessly as possible, one supposes. But this does nothing to address the reasoning for a strong distinction between killing and letting die: the prevention of harm. If the duty of non-maleficence were strongly in place, there is little doubt that the child would be treated.

Rachels's major argument that killing is no worse than letting die takes the form of a story, or rather of two stories "that are exactly alike except that one involves killing whereas the other involves letting someone die." The cases must be exactly alike except for this one difference, he argues, so that we can be "confident that it is this difference and not

---

Wronged?," 16-17. Anscombe "feel[s] a curious disagreement" about the kinds of cases in which Foot and others assume that, in situations of choice, the greater number must be saved. "If there are a lot of people stranded on a rock, and one person on another, and someone goes with a boat to rescue the single one, what cause, so far, have any of the others for complaint? They are not injured unless help that was owing to them was withheld" (17). The rescuer here does not "act badly," and it should be remembered, Anscombe adds, particularly "as the contrary may be taken for granted by some," that "when I do action A for reasons R, it is not necessary or even usual for me to have any special reason for doing-action-A-rather-than-action-B, which may also be possible."

some other that accounts for any variation in the assessments" (563). Story #1 involves Smith, who "stands to gain a large inheritance if anything should happen to his six-year-old cousin. One evening while the child is taking his bath, Smith sneaks into the bathroom and drowns the child, and then arranges things so that it will look like an accident." Story #2 involves Jones, who similarly stands to gain from the death of his six-year-old cousin. Here, then, is the somewhat different turn of Jones's story: "Like Smith, Jones sneaks in planning to drown the child in his bath. However, just as he enters the bathroom Jones sees the child slip and hit his head, and fall face down in the water. Jones is delighted; he stands by, ready to push the child's head back under if it is necessary, but it is not necessary. With only a little thrashing about, the child drowns all by himself, 'accidentally,' as Jones watches and does nothing" (563). Smith kills the child; Jones merely lets it die. Rachels asks, rhetorically, "Did either man behave better, from a moral point of view?" (563). If the killing/letting die distinction were truly significant, we should think Jones behaved somewhat better. We do not; therefore the distinction must be unimportant.

My point here is certainly not to defend Jones. What he does seems to me equally as bad as what Smith does. My contention is rather that Rachels has produced this reaction in his readers by artful elements of his storytelling and that these carefully constructed cases shed no light on the killing/letting die distinction. Three elements of the cases merit particular attention: the motives of the killers, the helplessness of the victims, and the elimination of risk from consideration. First, Jones is made to seem as bad as Smith by the attribution to him of the same selfish, instrumentalist motives; indeed Rachels goes so far as to have Jones enter the bathroom intending to kill the child. What this obscures is that the motives involved in killing and letting die—in almost every conceivable case—are utterly different. In fact, one could say that the distinction is about a distinction in motives or that it serves to condemn one kind of motive while allowing some leeway in the other because it serves freedom. The distinction serves to form us as people who do not intend killing—unlike either Smith or Jones—and who also try to avoid letting others die.[11]

11. As part of a criticism of Rachels, Kamm points out that "we would help conceal the difference between killing and letting die per se if we introduced an intention to kill into the letting die case, since that case might become as bad as a killing only because

Rachels is particularly adept at obscuring the reasons for our regarding "letting die" less seriously than killing. Part of the rhetorical trick is simply the very precise description of the process of Jones's letting the child die. Precision is exactly what is lacking in a general duty "not to let die." Would this entail my knocking cigarettes out of the mouths of everyone I meet? To fail to do so could be construed as "letting them die." Or must I go through the bars of my college town giving temperance lectures to the students? Should I advocate large increases in taxation so that people who insist on building houses in floodplains can put their dwellings up on stilts? When death comes for Willa Cather's Archbishop, Latour, he says that he will die of "having lived."[12] In a similar vein,

---

it had something in it dependent on a *definitional property* of killing. Therefore, it is a mistake to introduce the intention to kill in the letting die case." In "Killing and Letting Die," 303. For more on these issues by Kamm, see "Harming, Not Aiding, and Positive Rights," 3–32. Foot has responded to Rachels's stories by saying "the reason why it is, in ordinary circumstances, 'no worse' to leave a child drowning in a bathtub than to push it under, is that both charity and the special duty of care that we owe to children give us a positive obligation to save them, and we have no particular reason to say that it is 'less bad' to fail in this than it is to be in dereliction of the negative duty by being the agent of harm." See "Killing and Letting Die," 182. H. M. Malm presents an example very like Rachels's in "Killing, Letting Die, and Simple Conflicts," 240–41. In this case, Smith pushes a button that restarts a malfunctioning machine designed to crush a child trapped inside "solely because he is curious to see how flat a person can be." Jones discovers that a similar well-functioning machine is about to crush a child; he can stop it with the push of a button, but does not for the same reason as Smith. For Malm, "this example provides strong grounds for holding that killing is not in itself worse than letting die." Both acts are clearly wrong, and Jones "deserves as much moral disapprobation as Smith." I agree entirely with Malm's judgment about the wrongness of both acts, but I would resist the conclusion she draws. It seems to me that what they show is that cases can be drawn up that can technically be described as "letting die" but which make no meaningful contribution to casuistry about when we should turn from the otherwise justifiable actions we are pursuing because we are being insufficiently benevolent. It could be argued that Malm's cases do not contribute to moral deliberation because her two actors are clearly not moral agents, as their motives for acting/not acting make clear. Of what good would disapprobation be if directed at two men so lacking in moral imagination? Despite her judgment of this case, Malm goes on to argue that "the moral equivalence principle" regarding killing and letting die is incorrect. Malm is responding to arguments and examples put forth by Tooley, *Abortion and Infanticide*, 184–241.

12. Cather, *Death Comes for the Archbishop*, 269. After his retirement as Archbishop, Jean Latour is living on a ranch four miles north of Santa Fe. When he becomes ill with cold, he sends a young seminarian, Bernard, to Santa Fe to ask the current Archbishop if he can return to his former study in the Archbishop's house. Latour indicates he wishes to die in Santa Fe, but Bernard tells him he will not die of a cold. The old man responds, "I shall not die of a cold, my son. I shall die of having lived."

Thoreau said that as long as a man is alive, "there is always *danger* that he may die, though the danger must be allowed to be less in proportion as he is dead-and-alive to begin with."[13] If the prevention of death becomes as strenuous an obligation as not killing, will we simply prevent others from living? What are the limits on our preventing others from dying? How much freedom will we take from others, or sacrifice ourselves, in the building of comprehensive security systems designed to avoid letting die? My freedom to live, taking the risks I choose, is dependent on others' regarding the duty to avoid letting me die as considerably less binding than the duty not to kill me. Rachels's stories direct us away from the implications for freedom of the killing-letting die distinction. Moreover, his conclusion about the killing/letting die distinction seems to ignore the cardinal rule of ethics that "ought implies can." We can speak meaningfully about a duty not to kill because we can avoid killing. We cannot prescribe not letting die with the same rigor because we cannot ultimately accomplish that: people die.[14]

The third distorting aspect of Rachels' stories is his utter bracketing of risk. Jones's action is as bad as Smith's, in part, because saving the child involves absolutely no risk to him. But this is almost never the case in situations where we might have to make judgments about letting others die. If my fishing partner falls into relatively shallow water, I am a very good swimmer, and he is light and easily hauled to shore, then surely it is strongly incumbent on me to take the risks involved in saving him. If he falls into deep and turbulent water miles from shore, and I cannot swim, then it seems less obvious that I should risk my life to save him. What's involved in the casuistry is not only calculation of the risk to me but also an estimation of outcomes within an inherently uncertain world. Jones's story involves no risk and no uncertainty.[15] Rachels's stories prove only

---

13. "The amount of it is, if a man is alive, there is always *danger* that he may die, though the danger must be allowed to be less in proportion as he is dead-and-alive to begin with." *Walden*, 199.

14. "The negative duty of not killing can be discharged completely.... But the positive duty of saving can never be discharged completely." See Trammell, "Saving Life and Taking Life," 133.

15. The problems philosophers pose to get at the distinction between killing and letting die—if there is one—often obscure the fact that our moral intuitions in this area take into account calculations of risk and limitations of knowledge about outcomes. For examples of judgments based on strangely skewed degrees of knowledge and risk-calculations, see McMahan, "Killing, Letting Die, and Withdrawing Aid," 250–79. Consider McMahan's Dutch boy, who puts his finger in a cracking dike, "waits patiently" for many

that the killing/letting die distinction is very fine where one can save another from death with utter certainty, no risk to himself, and no loss of freedom to anyone. We might say that they eliminate the work made possible by retaining the difference between the two categories: a work of judgment. All of the work, interest, and moral insight made possible by the distinction of killing and letting-die involves an act of judgment by which one decides that, in a particular case, these otherwise differentiable distinctions almost warrant collapsing into one. Rachels precludes this act of judgment precisely by offering cases that are so nearly alike. His mistake lies in his assumption about the ways the stories must be told. Instead of telling identical stories dissimilar in only one particular, one must test the distinction by telling much more clearly differentiable stories in order to determine when our acts of judgment would point toward gathering these still quite different particulars under the same description.

What Rachels's stories obscure, most crucially, is the apportionment of risk under which we live. Each of us lives continually with the risk that he may lose his life—on which everything else, for him, depends. The fact I live with that risk limits my fishing friend's claim that I save him from possible drowning. On the other hand, I have the strongest possible obligation not to take from him everything he has by killing him. The strong distinction between killing and letting die emerges from this fair

---

hours for help but finally succumbs to boredom and hunger. He withdraws his finger and "within minutes the dike bursts and a flood engulfs the town, killing many" (257). The Dutch boy, in McMahan's view, lets the inhabitants die, a description I would resist because I do not see why this responsibility should be deemed the Dutch boy's alone. Why should the question, "Who let the townspeople die?" be referred to the Dutch boy alone? In fact, if the flood is only being held back by his single finger—and is so immense that it engulfs the town within minutes—then we might want to claim that the Dutch boy bears more responsibility for the drownings than "letting die" implies. What would militate against such a conclusion, it seems, is the apparent imminence of this flood, which ought surely to have moved someone else in town to have a look at the dike, move out of his or her home, or warn neighbors of the impending catastrophe. People in this town, however, are not blessed with a great deal of awareness or foresight. In McMahan's Dutch Boy 2, the boy's father, "annoyed because his son is late for dinner ... yanks the boy's finger out of the dike," again precipitating the killing flood (262). This act McMahan labels "killing," but it seems to me better described as simply a matter of accident or horrible misjudgment. Since one assumes, in both versions of Dutch Boy, that the boy and/or his father run a very great risk of being among the victims, the father in Dutch Boy 2 must surely not understand what he is doing. Or if he does, then he'd seem guilty of murder and suicide.

apportionment of risk where each of us can, at any time, lose all. To argue that the distinction is meaningless, as Rachels does, must mean that any sense of this apportionment of risk has been lost. If this is the case, it is perhaps because such a thorough denial of death has been accomplished that we have succeeded in forgetting we all bear continually the risk of dying. One might object that Rachels has set his treatment of the killing-letting die distinction within the context of euthanasia, where the risk of death is, at least in the near term, disproportionately with the one dying. But this is not an adequate defense of Rachels. He is quite clear in dismissing the general import of the distinction. His rhetorical strategy is to use euthanasia as a paradigm case for pondering and dismissing the distinction between killing and letting die. It is as if all of life is considered under the rubric of euthanasia. It is difficult to know whether this is a matter of conscious rhetorical strategy or evidence of a societal denial of death so deep and pervasive that questions regarding killing and letting die only occur in the context of euthanasia. In either case, focusing on euthanasia—where the risk of dying is temporarily quite disproportionately with the subject of the case and not with the reader—helps to accomplish that forgetting of death's ever-present threat to us all that is the source of our quite reasonable distinction between killing and letting die.

It seems to me that the practical result of Rachels's claim is likely to be the loss of "letting die" as a useful category for analyzing our actions. "Letting die" can only retain force, or even interest, if we understand "killing" as the worst thing we do. Then, when we consider whether we might, in a particular situation, be letting others die (through inattention or neglect, for instance), we will be moved to change our actions—precisely because we have been formed to believe killing the worst thing we can do. We will turn, then, from "letting die" precisely when our acts can be described as being closest to killing. Thus I contribute to relief efforts in the Sudan because my assistance there will enable some perhaps to be rescued from near certain death and at little risk to me. If I were not to do this, I could plausibly be described as letting Sudanese die. I do not, for a moment, believe that my failure to give relief—arguably to "let die"—is as bad as killing my neighbors (an absurdity Rachels's position could be construed to imply, which is why I suggest the real effect of Rachels's argument is just to blunt or defuse the force of "letting die" altogether). In fact, if I truly come to believe "letting die" is as bad as, or worse than, killing, then I'm unlikely even to raise the question whether I'm implicated in acts of letting die, for I have the strongest psychological impediments to believing myself a killer.

Rachels's argument also obscures an important difference between two senses of the phrase, "letting die." We speak of removing a patient from a ventilator in order to let her die; here we allow something to happen where we have no power to save the patient for a restoration of anything like normal functioning. Little moral evaluation is implied because there is little we could have done and there is little reason to refer the case specifically to us. A ninety-year-old patient is being killed by a variety of causes, perhaps best described, as we should hope, as having lived. Thus there is little point even in asking, in any moral sense, whether we let this person die if we choose to discontinue ventilation. At other times, however, there is a decidedly moral implication in the question whether you or I have let someone die, or are in the process of doing so. In such a case, our using the phrase suggests it makes sense to at least refer the question (and the accompanying casuistry) to me because of powers I possess to perhaps alter the outcome or my own involvement in putting events into play that have or may lead to a death. To return to my fishing example. If I have taken my friend fishing and run the boat into deep and turbulent water, where he falls out and drowns without attempted rescue on my part, it makes sense to refer the question to me: "Did I let him die?" This is true even if I can present a perfectly reasonable explanation for my making no saving effort. My prior action makes it plausible to refer the question to me.

In fact, it often seems that what's at issue in the question of "letting die" is precisely one of responsibility—that is, whether there is a question of responsibility at all and, if so, to whom it should be referred. The highway on which I drive to my university is a very treacherous one, carrying far more traffic than it was designed for and badly in need of widening. Many more people are killed on it each year than on similar stretches of road elsewhere. These problems could be remedied by funds from raised highway taxes, and many of us (especially those who use the road) argue for such an increase by saying we are unnecessarily letting people die on this unsafe stretch of road. The argument seems to be acquiring credibility slowly, and I suspect there is some body count that will cause Virginians to conclude it is no longer reasonable to let people die unnecessarily. At that point, they will have accepted implicitly the idea that it makes sense to refer the "letting die" question to them.[16] It's important to note, too, that each can accept having the question referred to him because it is not referred *exclusively* to him. Responsibility can be accepted because it can also be dispersed throughout the group. No one could bear being told that he or she is individually responsible for letting people die on Highway 81. Each would reject that indictment out of hand and probably with some anger.

I think we might say of Judith Jarvis Thomson's famous story of the unconscious violinist that it literally blinds us with anger. Its rhetorical genius lies in its so directing our emotional response into a justified an-

---

16. The literature on the killing/letting die question contains an abundance of cases involving people in particular life-saving roles: doctors, firemen, lifeguards, drivers of runaway trolleys. I believe this is the case because the obligations implicit in the roles make it possible to avoid the critical questions most of us wrestle with regarding matters of "letting die": Why is the letting die question in a particular case referred to me? Why am I obligated not to let die in this case in a way that is untrue of others? And if I am so obligated, how stringent is the obligation? Sometimes the philosophers seem to trap their role-bearers in impossible double binds. Quinn, for example, sets up a trolley problem in which the driver of the runaway is on a track where five are trapped, "but he can switch to a side-track where only one person is trapped." "The only possibly acceptable reasons for him not to switch," according to Quinn, "would be to prevent the death of the man on the side-track or to keep clean hands. But the clean-hands motive begs the question; it presupposes that the doctrine does not also speak against not switching." There's a certain cynicism about motive here, implied by the phrase "clean hands," that we should challenge. The conductor's simply letting the train go on its course could be described as a matter of his not wanting to intentionally kill another. We would probably say that that is an inaccurate description of what he does if he turns the train, and that he should bear no responsibility for the man's death. But whether *he*—having made a decision that leads to the sure death of another—can accept his "innocence" is another matter. Perhaps we begin here to get at what people sign away when they take on life-saving roles: the possibility of ever having clean hands except through a kind of general amnesty that designates such decisions as those in the trolley problems as matters of professional judgment and conduct. Clearly the numbers do count with us, and I would prefer our trolley driver to turn the train, which would then kill one instead of five. But if he does not, could any of the families of the five killed claim that they were wronged by the driver? Surely they should get damages from the trolley company and/or the trolley and track manufacturers and maintainers. But can they successfully claim they have been wronged by the driver without a showing that the life of the man "saved" is of so little value as to be unable to justify the driver's refusal to take an action that would kill him? See Quinn, "Actions, Intentions, and Consequences," 304–5. McMahan has taken up the matter of role-based obligations in relation to killing-letting die questions in "Killing, Letting Die, and Withdrawing Aid," 264–68.

ger against the violinist's imposition on us that we do not see the way in which our intuitions about what we owe the violinist actually have little to do with what is owed fetuses. Because I wish to comment specifically on its rhetoric, I give the story here:

> Let me ask you to imagine this. You wake up in the morning and find yourself back to back in bed with an unconscious violinist. A famous unconscious violinist. He has been found to have a fatal kidney ailment, and the Society of Music Lovers has canvassed all the available medical records and found that you alone have the right blood type to help. They have therefore kidnapped you, and last night the violinist's circulatory system was plugged into yours, so that your kidneys can be used to extract poisons from his blood as well as your own. The director of the hospital now tells you, "Look, we're sorry the Society of Music Lovers did this to you—we would never have permitted it if we had known. But still, they did it, and the violinist now is plugged into you. To unplug you would be to kill him. But never mind, it's only for nine months. By then he will have recovered from his ailment, and can safely be unplugged from you." (132)

Thomson asks, then, whether it is "morally incumbent on you to accede to this situation?" The answer she is counting on is, of course, "no." Being told by the director of the hospital that you cannot be unplugged—at the expense of the violinist's life—would likely seem "outrageous" (132–33). Thus she concludes that a person's right to life cannot simply outweigh the woman's right to decide what happens to her body.

Thomson's story does not elicit dispassionate response: it directs our emotional response into rage. It's worth remembering that other emotional and moral responses are possible to claims made upon us by those in need: mercy, tenderness, compassion, empathy, care. These are largely precluded by elements of Thomson's story. The kidnapping and forced attachment are very important here, of course, but also significant are the two instructions from the "director of the hospital," given as direct imperatives to the "you" who has been victimized. One of these casually tells "you" to discount nine months of your life while the other specifically overrides your right to bodily control. As it's likely we will identify the "director" of the hospital as male, his "tough luck" language effectively extends the rape metaphor implicit from the story's beginning. The story depicts a woman repeatedly violated by males, or, more appropriately, it depicts "you" repeatedly violated by males. The second person form of the story is crucial to its effects; it does not allow distance for the reader. "You" are being subjected to total determination by another. "You" are deprived of speech by the story, in which only "the director" speaks. Outrage is the inevitable and appropriate response. It is critical to the story's effects that the violinist does not speak, for if he were to appeal to the "victim," then a response different from rage would be possible (perhaps even mercy). Since he never addresses "you," the reader is prevented from imagining him in the face to face position. The violinist remains faceless. The facing position is usurped by the director, who prescribes only your complete domination by his will. One curiosity of the story, surely unintended by Thomson, is that it puts its victim in a place exactly analogous to that of the fetus being killed. The reader's rage here is caused by the sense that he or she is being totally determined by another, yet the injustice of such determination is exactly what the critic objects to in abortion.

I have assumed the "famous unconscious violinist" is male. While "famous unconscious violinist" may not connote "male" quite so automatically as "doctor," "surgeon," or "physician" once did, the phrase does seem nevertheless fairly certain to conjure up the image of a white male in a tuxedo. Thomson's pronouns reinforce the suggestion the violinist is male. This gender identification is crucial, for the genius of Thomson's story is to conflate rapist and fetus, so that the fetus becomes the violator and the appropriate object of rage. The effect of the violinist's fame is itself worth pondering. The designation suggests privilege: this is a person who has enjoyed favorable background, excellent education, extensive training in the arts. He is likely at least middle age and therefore significantly older than the woman to whom he is attached, assuming she is to represent a kind of statistical average of women seeking abortion. The dialysis-like features of the procedure also suggest the violinist is middle-aged or older. What these details do is to direct our sense of justice so that it is wholly with the woman. The life suggested by "famous violinist" has been—very likely—more advantaged than that of the woman seeking abortion. He is accomplished, distinguished, and well-known; he has already lived more years—good ones at that—than she. He has already had a life that will likely surpass hers in accomplishment. All of these factors blunt any sense we might have that there could be justice in the dependent's claim. None of the above description applies to the fetus, who has only its dependence and no history of accomplishment. All that it will ever be is dependent on its mother's carrying it to term. Thus our sense of justice, regarding the fetus, might well point to its deserving a chance from her mother. Thomson's story precludes this just reaction.

Thomson attempts to make her "famous violinist" as seemingly dependent on the woman of her story as a fetus. To unplug him is to allow him to die. But the intuition she here hopes to evoke from her reader does not apply to the fetus. Our sense that we do not owe the violinist the use of our body derives from his having access to a wide array of kinds of support provided by all of us through social means. If the Society of Music Lovers had left him in the emergency room of a public hospital, we would argue for his dialysis as a matter of what is owed him. Even if the society had plugged him in to a machine without authorization, we would surely argue that his treatment should continue, at cost to all of us. Moreover, it is precisely because we understand obligations of justice as bearing on us all that we reject the idea of his being entitled to the kind of exclusive claim he makes in Thomson's story. But we do not make similar assumptions about fetuses, precisely because they have not yet enjoyed or benefited from our systems of social protection, care, and support. What I owe the fetus is not illuminated by intuitions about what I owe a middle-aged adult because those intuitions have been shaped by the whole body of assumptions that underlie our social and institutional care for one another.

I certainly agree the violinist has no right to another's body. It is not owed him. But our sense that no particular being owes him this degree of support is surely based on larger perceptions about the support or sustenance we have received from others and the fair distribution of the risks of life. What we owe him is based on our sense of justice in ordinary arrangements: we owe him decent medical care but we do not owe him preservation from death at all costs. The constant risk of incurable illness and death is one we all must share: in fact, we show care for one another by accepting our share of that risk, which means not unjustly imposing—as the violinist does—on another for support to which we are not entitled. These intuitions do not apply to fetuses, who have no choice but to be attached to their mothers and who also have no history of benefits that enables us to say to them, as we can to the violinist: "Like us, you have benefited from the efforts and gifts of others, past and present. Like you, we bear our risks of incurable illness and death. We have benefited together and risked together: now you must not break the implicit contract by asking for more than is rightly yours." The ordinary course of things does matter. We feel the justice of rectifying things for the ailing violinist—of attempting to restore him to health—but not at the sole expense of the woman.[17] If we doubt our response to the violinist is rooted in the ordinary course of things, let's imagine a different scenario regarding attachment. If every human being needed a mid-life renewal of input from one other particular human being—involving nine months of bodily attachment—is there any doubt this would be regarded as a right? Or that our social arrangements would be designed to facilitate the procedure (paid work leave, social insurance for the poor, etc.)? Under these circumstances, need would confer the right to aid.

One curious feature of Thomson's argument is her defending the justifiability both of killing the fetus and of letting it die. If it is justifiable to kill the fetus, it would seem to follow without argument that one can let it die. The fact, then, that Thomson senses the need to argue for justifiably letting the fetus die, after she has apparently established the justifiability of its killing, may point to problems in her account of the justification for its killing. I believe this to be the case and will comment on the matter after examining first her account of abortion as justified killing.

Thomson claims that to unplug oneself from the violinist is to kill him justifiably. Reaching this conclusion depends on a prior story about justice: "Suppose a boy and his small brother are jointly given a box of chocolates for Christmas. If the older boy takes the box and refuses to give his brother any of the chocolates, he is unjust to him." But you are not being unjust to the violinist because "you gave him no right to use your kidneys." In unplugging him, "you are killing him" and thus violating his supposed "right not to be killed." Yet you do not act unjustly, a fact

---

17. Michael Davis proposes an interestingly modified version of Thomson's story to which he responds with the intuition that one ought not to unplug. You have been kidnapped just as in Thomson's story, "before you were plugged into the violinist, someone else could have been. But because you were plugged in, no one else can be. The shock of unplugging would kill him. You must stay with the violinist or he will die. He needs you in particular." Davis argues that to unplug here would be to unjustifiably pass on to an innocent "burdens it would otherwise be impermissible to impose on him." My intuitions here are different. I would hope you might respond to this evil with good, but I do not think we can insist that you do so, for you, in particular, are in no way responsible for the violinist's need of you. See Davis, "Foetuses, Famous Violinists, and the Right to Continued Aid," 267–68.

that suggests an "emendation" in the right to life, which now becomes "the right not to be killed unjustly" (138).

Two interrelated questions need particular attention here. Should we really understand the larger boy in Thomson's example to be unjust? And why does Thomson understand unplugging the violinist as killing him rather than letting him die? I suppose I agree with Thomson that her larger brother is unjust, but that is based not simply on the example she gives but rather on my sense that one who acts as he does—toward a smaller, younger sibling in a case of clear entitlement—is unlikely to be able to estimate the due claims of others in the many complex situations requiring the exercise of justice as a faculty of judgment and a virtue. In her example, he seems much more clearly a thief, one who simply steals the property of another. Proper behavior on his part requires no exercise of judgment concerning the due claims of others. The boy needs simply to be told not to steal. If Thomson's were truly a paradigm case illustrating a matter of justice, then discourse about justice would soon become vitiated or meaningless. We would soon abandon language about justice and simply teach people not to steal the property of others. For justice is about estimating the due claims of others precisely where there are no established entitlements and the necessities of life and real risks—not luxuries like Christmas chocolates—are involved. We can see, then, how Thomson's account of justice is connected to her calling the violinist's unplugging an act of killing him. Life for the violinist is an entitlement, like each boy's share of the contractually transmitted chocolates, and can only be cancelled by a counter-entitlement—in this case, that to bodily autonomy. Anything that would interfere with his, the violinist's, entitlement to life must be understood as killing him, and justice would do no more than to decide which entitlement trumps the other.

I think we can now understand something that is not said in Thomson's story, but for which we need to account. What is it that drives the violinist to attach himself to his victim? Why does he not decide he has no just claim to the kind of support he seeks? Of course Thomson explains this without explaining it by having him be unconscious. But then we can just push the question back to the Society of Music Lovers: why don't they see he has no just claim of this type? Because they are just a device. What drives him is necessity, the necessity of life itself, understood as an entitlement and without any power of being relinquished. If life is a necessity that demands what is necessary for its continuance, then it can only be met and limited by counter-necessities. How can one deny another what is a necessity for life itself?—only by insisting he has no right to it. It would seem that from Thomson's point-of-view meaningful discussion of what constitutes "letting die" would drop out altogether: after all, if there's ever a case where an action would be described as "letting die," it must surely be that of unplugging the violinist. But perhaps Thomson cannot think of the violinist as being let die because he cannot himself merely let himself die, driven as he is by the necessity of life itself.

Thus we can reject Thomson's description of the violinist's unplugging as justified killing. We can do so because we do not need to accept her understanding of justice or the apparent implicit assumption that the violinist cannot let himself die in recognition of the limits of his just claims on others. We can say that he is much more obviously killed by the disease and that he has a choice: not to impose unjustly on others by seeking access to a means of support to which he has no claim. Part of the reason he must let himself die rather than being unjust is that, by doing so, he assists the rest of us—as we have assisted him—to avoid becoming killers, even justified ones, because we recognize that it is not good to kill, even when it can be justified. Unlike the violinist, the fetus has no chance to be just; its sole dependence on another is at once both ordinary and unelected. To abort it is to kill it, in a way that is not true of unplugging the violinist.

Perhaps we can now understand why Thomson goes on to argue that we have no obligation to aid the fetus even after she has claimed—unsuccessfully, I believe—that it can be justifiably killed. Her doing so seems counterintuitive if we take it that our duty not to kill is much stronger than our duty to give aid (to prevent from dying). But if we were to accept something like Rachels's claim that "letting die" is at least as bad as "killing," then we might feel the need to make an independent argument that what can be construed as "letting die" is also not incumbent on us. In other words, if life is a necessity with a claim to whatever it needs for support and continuance (one that can only be limited by a counter claim), then any denial of a means of support is really tantamount to killing. We would need to justify any refusal to give aid—any "letting die"—with the same degree of stringency ordinarily required to justify killing.

Thomson's case for bad Samaritanism is made largely through her retelling the terrible story of Kitty Genovese's murder "while thirty-eight people watched or listened, and did nothing at all to help her."[18] She judges it "monstrous" that no one acted as a "Minimally Decent Samaritan" by calling the police, but argues "that it was not morally required of any of the thirty-eight that he rush out to give direct assistance at the risk of his own life" (142).[19] Now it seems perfectly possible to agree with Thomson's conclusion on the moral requirement to aid in this case and yet to say that it sheds no light whatever on our duty not to kill the fetus. We are not required to aid here because what we are doing cannot be even remotely compared to killing; the killing is being done by the murderers. What we must not do is to kill, in turn, in similar situations where we have the power and another is defenseless (or, in fact, in any situations). What is more interesting here is the rhetorical function of the story in Thomson's argument. In order to have abortion considered as a problem in Samaritanism, even if the fetus is a person, Thomson must, much like Rachels, induce a forgetting of death in her readers.

18. Thomson includes the story of the good Samaritan from Luke 10:30–35, commenting that the priest and the Levite "were not even Minimally Decent Samaritans, not because they were not Samaritans, but because they were not even minimally decent" (142). I prefer to think of them as not only minimally but even maximally "decent," much like all of us often ordinarily loveless people who use the seriousness of our allotted duties as justification for refusing mercy to the neighbor. It must be remembered that both priest and Levite may have become unclean—and thus unqualified for their religious duties—by contact with the wounded man's blood. Perhaps we should read the story as indicating the freedom that lies, for the Samaritan, in not being bound by "decency."

19. Noonan calls attention to a Minnesota tort case that he believes bears more resemblance to the situation of pregnancy than Thomson's "fantasy." The case involved a family of farmers who had refused the request of a cattle buyer to stay overnight at their house after he had been a guest for dinner. The family turned the cattle buyer out into the night despite his being sick and fainting. Later the court imposed liability on the farmers for the buyer's loss of his frostbitten fingers, arguing that "the law as well as humanity required that he not be exposed in his helpless condition to the merciless elements." "Although the analogy is not exact," Noonan claims the case "seems closer to the mother's situation than the case imagined by Thomson; and the emotional response of the Minnesota judges seems to be a truer reflection of what humanity requires." Noonan's judgment here seems to underestimate the burden for the mother of both the pregnancy and rearing of the child. The Minnesota case involves a very small inconvenience to the farmers whereas the woman seeking abortion may consider the burdens of pregnancy and child-rearing to be immense, even life-threatening. See Noonan, "How to Argue About Abortion," 135. The case is cited by Beckwith as evidence of legal problems with Thomson's argument. See "Arguments from Bodily Rights," 169.

Readers must be made to forget their own ever-present vulnerability to death by violence, for the reader who remembers that vulnerability will realize her first interest is in not being killed—and thus the first duty of others toward her is not to kill her. Such a reasoner will be in solidarity with the fetus, for she will see that the first question regarding it will be whether or not it can be killed (*not* whether it must be aided).

The rarity of what happened to Kitty Genovese is an unrecognized yet necessary condition for the use Thomson makes of the story. We do not, perhaps cannot, identify with Kitty Genovese. We do not really believe that what happened to Kitty Genovese will happen to us. The proof of the last two statements lies in the very fact we do not require at least "minimally decent Samaritanism." If occurrences like Kitty Genovese's murder became relatively routine, does anyone doubt that we would enact laws requiring at least minimal degrees of good Samaritanism—the required phoning of police at a very minimum? If we could truly put ourselves in the place of Kitty Genovese, would we be willing to accept being told that no one had any obligation to assist us? Here it matters greatly that it is *the story of Kitty Genovese and thus precisely not our story*. There is no second person language here, no facing of Kitty Genovese and saying, "You have no right in law to assistance from any of us, not even to our taking time to phone the police." (Interestingly, all the second person language in the violinist story is directed at the attaché; the faceless violinist is never faced and told his need confers no claim to aid.) Thomson's use of the story divides us completely from Kitty Genovese and thus from other persons who are killed, like fetuses. Her telling of the story assists us in our forgetting the possibility of violent death that hangs over us all. Violent death is something that happened to Kitty Genovese, not to me. I am induced to forget that my first right against others is that they not kill me, and I am thereby removed from solidarity with the defenseless fetus. In fact, I am most likely to identify, somewhat guiltily, with one of the thirty-eight onlookers, whose fearful inaction I can recognize to be a believable response. Thus the story induces the reader, through a subtle analogy, to think of support for the fetus as a collective matter where any of us would be in bad faith if we insisted that particular people (i.e., the parents) bear a particular responsibility for the fetus. Thus the crowd phenomenon of diffusion of responsibility is made to serve as a kind of argument excusing the non-assistance (actually destruction) of a fetus by those specifically responsible for its coming into being.

Thomson adamantly maintains that nothing is owed the fetus in justice. To make this claim, she proposes a change in her story. Suppose all the violinist needs is one hour of your life and that this hour will "not affect your health in the slightest." Or, suppose in a pregnancy resulting from rape, the woman need carry the child only one hour. In both cases, Thomson avers, one "ought" to provide the support; it "would be indecent to refuse" (140). Yet Thomson resists saying that either the violinist or the child in these emended cases has the *right* to support. Here she recurs to her story of the box of chocolates, modifying it now so that the box is not given jointly to the brothers but only to the older boy: "There he sits, stolidly eating his way through the box, his small brother watching enviously. Here we are likely to say 'You ought not to be so mean. You ought to give your brother some of those chocolates.' My own view is that it just does not follow from the truth of this that the brother has any right to any of the chocolates. If the boy refuses to give his brother any, he is greedy, stingy, callous—but not unjust." For Thomson an important distinction is at stake here, "namely the difference between the boy's refusal in this case and the boy's refusal in the earlier case, in which the box was given to both boys jointly" (140–41).[20]

Thomson seems not to imagine that the boy in the second case can be considered unjust without the differences in the cases being diminished. The boy in Chocolates #1 acts both unjustly and in violation of a right given clearly to his brother. The boy in Chocolates #2 does not violate his brother's right, but he is unjust, not only stingy and callous. I'm not sure he acts unjustly, for there may be more we need to know: perhaps the younger brother has just used his bicycle without permission, wrecked it, and refused to pay for repairs. But if no issues of restitution or retribution are involved, then the boy is unjust because he fails to understand that he has done nothing to merit this particular gift. The freedom of the gift diminishes his claim to it while the relationship to his brother increases the latter's claim. The boy should certainly reason

---

20. David S. Levin reads Thomson to mean that a late-term convenience abortion "would be unjustifiable," but this seems a misreading to me. She would find it indecent, mean-spirited, unfeeling perhaps but not unjust and therefore not unjustifiable. This seems to me an implication of her second story about the boys and the chocolates. See Levin, "Thomson and the Current State of the Abortion Controversy," 123.

to himself: "It is unfair, unjust, that I should receive all while my brother receives none." To tell him no issue of justice is involved is to urge him never to question distribution processes. We might put this another way by imagining the process of teaching this boy to be just. If justice involves developing both the disposition and the practical wisdom to properly estimate the due claims of others, then it's unlikely the boy in Chocolates #2 is ever likely to become just if he is addressed as Thomson would—for her description of his failings makes no reference to others' claims.[21]

A still more important point concerns those chocolates. Chocolates are a luxury; nothing disastrous will happen to the younger brother by his being deprived of them. He has nothing to lose. But let us modify the story a bit. Now the older brother receives a gift of grain in a time of extreme scarcity and famine. The grain is a gift to him, but, of course, he is in the position to receive the gift because of the efforts, care, nurturance, and risk-taking of his family, village, culture, nation, and so forth. If there is enough grain to sustain him and his brother but he chooses rather to hoard all the grain and allow his brother to die, would we describe him merely as "greedy, stingy, and callous," or would we want to call him unjust? Moreover, if we put ourselves in the place of the younger brother facing starvation, would we not want to appeal to our brother on the grounds of justice? Would we not want—and be entitled to—appeal to some standard outside ourselves in crying out to him? Would we not want to say that what's at stake is not just a matter of his character ("you are being greedy or callous") but rather a matter of what he owes based on all that he has received? Would we not rightly say to him, "You are being unjust to me"?

For Thomson, it is "indecent" to deny the violinist one hour of attachment if that is all that is required to preserve his life. I would probably want to call such a denial "unjust," except that, in doing so, I would want to retain the right to say his prior action of surreptitious attachment violated justice. The question should probably be regarded moot, as it is no doubt true he would not have needed to attach himself sur-

---

21. This matter may be even more complex. I suspect the child or young person is unlikely to view the issues in Chocolates #2 as ones involving justice, and it would likely only produce resentment in the older brother to tell him he's being ungrateful and unjust. Sharing the chocolates is perhaps more likely to be perceived as a matter of justice by an older person who has developed a sense of having received so much more than one could ever merit.

reptitiously if he needed only one hour's support. He could easily have negotiated it in advance. Thomson similarly labels "indecent" the request for abortion of a woman "in her seventh month" whose desire is "just to avoid the nuisance of postponing a trip abroad" (144). (Presumably this does not preclude the abortion's being allowable, under Thomson's premises.) Thomson believes, I think, that calling abortion "indecent" here precludes our calling the woman unjust, but this may not be the case. Why do we find the request for abortion here "indecent"?[22]

Let me suggest we find the seventh-month convenience abortion "indecent" because it is unjust. Surely it seems capricious, arbitrary, even cruel to allow the fetus to develop for seven months only to terminate it for purely convenience purposes. What strikes us is the apparent lack of seriousness on the part of the woman. We might ask whether she can possibly have considered the responsibilities involved in rearing a child. But, most importantly, we are struck, I believe, by a particularly gross example of what troubles pro-life people in all abortions: the utter lack of proportion between what fetus or woman will lose. The mother loses a trip that can presumably be taken at another time or compensated for in other ways. The fetus, on the other hand, stands to lose everything. What we reject in the seventh-month convenience abortion is the injustice of the mother's total determination of the fetus's prospects. No human being should have this degree of control over another. It is "indecent" for one to be so self-involved as to fail to see the utter disproportion between what one seeks for oneself and the cost to another. But our sense of the indecency is rooted in our sense of justice: it is unjust to take

---

22. Jane English argues that Thomson's judgment about "indecency" here is grounded in the "surprisingly central role" of bodies in "our attitudes toward persons." "One has only to think," she adds, "of the philosophical literature on how far physical identity suffices for personal identity or Wittgenstein's remark that the best picture of the human soul is the human body." Early abortion is thus no problem for English, but convenience abortion in the seventh month would be "wrong" because of the fetus's "resemblance" to a person. One might argue that English's position represents too restricted imagination and too little science. Part of our perception of human bodies involves a sense of their uniqueness as bearers of particular histories. Genetic identity, established at or soon after conception, is critical to that uniqueness—a point that does not imply a wide genetic determinism. Critics of abortion see what is most valuable about the human body and human soul—its uniqueness as genuinely historical being—being established at conception. See English, "Abortion: Beyond the Personhood Argument," 302. Wittgenstein's remark is in *Philosophical Investigations*, 152.

from the fetus all it will ever have for such a trivial reason as personal convenience.[23]

We are left to decide just what to call the act by which Thomson's violinist is detached. I would suggest it ought not to be called killing, for he is much more clearly killed by the disease. To call it killing is already to blur the clear distinction between detaching him and abortion, which is the intentional destruction of a human being who has no choice other than to be utterly dependent on her mother. The violinist, I insist, has another choice: to die. I am reluctant even to call the detachment an act of "letting die," at least in any sense that can contribute to the casuistry surrounding that important notion. There is nothing in Thomson's analogy (one might call this its genius) that justifies referring the "letting die" question to the person to whom the violinist attaches. It's as if Thomson has invented a Kitty Genovese case where the diffusion of responsibility can be perfectly justified. No one in particular owes the violinist what he must have in order to survive. There is no one to whom the "letting die" question can even be meaningfully referred because no one's prior actions are even possibly construable as responsible for his predicament.

Obviously this makes the case utterly unlike that of the fetus when intercourse has been voluntary. One might object to my line of reason-

---

23. Kamm would defend the woman's right to the seventh-month convenience abortion. Building on Thomson's analogy, she develops "the output cutoff principle," by which "it is permissible to end a life that is maintained by the use of your body, in order to stop that use, if the use is not required by need or special obligation, so long as the person killed is not harmed relative to the opportunities he would have had if he had never been attached, and he does not lose anything you are causally responsible for his having that he could retain without you." You have a "right not to maximize overall good consequences by suffering a loss that is less than the one that your suffering will prevent." See *Creation and Abortion*, 36. Kamm's arguments do not, in my view, escape the kinds of problems inherent in Thomson's: they are repeatedly dependent on moral intuitions developed to regulate conduct between those free-standing, non-needy beings we call persons. Thus they often have little relevance to our understanding what is owed beings who have only their need and dependence. In fact, the way the personhood of the fetus from conception actually works as an enabling feature of Kamm's argument, as I have been suggesting it does for Thomson's, is acknowledged by Kamm. See 174. Some ironies of the person-from-conception defense of the fetus emerge from Kamm's remarks. Declaring the fetus a person throughout pregnancy makes it "matter less" if the abortion is early or late, "for one will be aborting a person whenever one aborts." Moreover, if the fetus is understood as developing from a stage in which it is not a person to one in which it is, aborting it in the person stage becomes a much more serious matter than it would be otherwise, for now one must explain why it was not aborted before becoming a person.

ing here that I was earlier willing to consider cases of mass starvation in developing countries as those in which I might meaningfully raise the question whether I was letting others die. Here, as in the violinist case, no prior actions of mine are responsible for the predicaments of, say, the Sudanese. But my relationship to the Sudanese differs in two crucial ways from that of Thomson's attachee and the violinist. First, it requires almost no risk or suffering on my part to send support to an international relief agency that will prevent some Sudanese from dying (one hopes). Obviously these factors differ in Thomson's analogy of the violinist. Because I have been formed to be a person who does not want to kill, I also do not want to let others die when I can prevent that with little risk to myself. To interject a specifically Christian point here, I would say that what simultaneously nags at me and enables my response to the Sudanese is the Christian story's drawing me into community with those everywhere, the prevention of my escape into the diffused responsibility of the often irresponsible group by the story of God's choosing to die (freely and unnecessarily) for me, and the sure knowledge that I can be forgiven for not regarding myself as wholly responsible for the lives of others. God's forgiveness enables me to respond in a way I would not respond if the responsibility for letting others die were referred solely to me and without the possibility of my being forgiven. If that were the case, I would surely seek to justify myself by referring responsibility away from myself and dispersing it throughout the group.

The second crucial difference between the Sudanese and violinist cases involves judgments about the kinds of benefits one has already received and thus about the kinds of claims one is entitled to make. Our sense of what we owe the violinist is based on what he has already received: he is a member of our own society (risk pool) and has benefited from our mutual exchanges and sharing of risks. Now it is his obligation, in justice, to take his own death upon himself rather than violating those arrangements of risk and freedom that have benefited us all. As a group we owe him support, but no particular individual owes him the kind of support required in Thomson's analogy. The Sudanese, on the other hand, have not benefited from mutual exchanges and risk-sharing with us and are not dying—in the case of starvation—from anything requiring extraordinary means of alleviation. The means of alleviation can be supplied as a group, even if the call to do so comes to us primarily as individuals. We can see that by a very minimal extension of risk to our group we are able to do a great good. The disparity between what the Sudanese have received and what we in the affluent West have received is such that it should spur us to think about relief as a question of justice. The question concerning the Sudanese can be integrated into a meaningful casuistry concerning the question of "letting die" in a way that is not true of Thomson's violinist.

What, then, does Thomson's argument establish? The violinist analogy does nothing, in my view, to justify the killing of the fetus nor does it contribute meaningfully to our thinking about whether we can let fetuses die. Thomson does not succeed in making the case that abortion should be considered a matter of bad Samaritanism. Locating abortion under the rubric of Samaritanism obscures the fact that fetuses are in the predicament they're in not because they've been assaulted by thieves and left to die in the ditch. They are there, in cases of voluntary intercourse, as the result of actions taken by those who now ponder the question whether they need to be aided. Moreover, all of our intuitions about what we owe as Samaritans are based on assumptions about what justice requires of us vis-à-vis those ordinarily independent, free-standing, non-needy beings we call persons. These intuitions do not apply to fetuses, who have no choice but to be utterly dependent on their mothers. Thomson's argument is not one of justifiable abortion despite fetal personhood. Rather it is one made possible by obscuring the particular status of the fetus under the mask of personhood.

The untenability of bad Samaritan defenses of abortion is evident in the internal contradictions and omissions of Donald Regan's "Rewriting *Roe v. Wade*." Calling his position ultimately "an equal protection argument," Regan contends "that abortion should be viewed as presenting a problem in what we might call 'the law of samaritanism', that is, the law concerning obligations imposed on individuals to give aid to others" (1569). Regan argues that requiring a pregnant woman to carry an unwanted fetus to term unjustifiably compels her to be a good Samaritan. The specifically "equal protection" feature of Regan's argument lies in his contending further that "there is *no* other potential samaritan on whom burdens are imposed which are as extensive and as physically invasive as the burdens of pregnancy and childbirth" (1572). The problem with Regan's argument emerges almost immediately as he notes the difficulties with his description of unwanted pregnancy as a problem in Samaritan law. Because "the situation of the pregnant woman is *sui generis*," comparisons with specific other potential Samaritans will have difficulty establishing "the sort of unjustified inconsistency of treatment that amounts to an equal protection violation" (1570). But if unwanted pregnancy is *sui generis*, as it is, why gather it under the rubric of Samaritanism? Why should decisions we would make or endorse on other questions of Samaritanism shed any light on the matter at all? As I've argued, treating abortion as a matter of Samaritanism is neither appropriate nor helpful, especially when the intercourse leading to pregnancy has been voluntary. In addition to the problems with the analogy just noted, Regan himself identifies a further incongruity between Samaritan law's focus on omissions of assistance and the active killing of the fetus in abortion.

It seems clear, then, that Regan's gathering abortion under the heading of Samaritanism is a misstep. What is interesting to pursue is why he does this, for I believe his argument suggests, no doubt unconsciously, important things about the nature of our justification processes, the relationship between abortion and war, and the place of abortion in the life of the state. When Regan looks for examples to consider as possibly analogous to that of unwanted pregnancy, he turns to the military draft, which he finds "the most arresting statutorily created exception (or, as I think, apparent exception) to the bad-samaritan principle" (1605). The burdens imposed on draftees come closest, according to Regan, to being comparable to those imposed on pregnant women denied abortion. Among the burdens imposed on draftees, Regan mentions discomfort, pain, "considerable *physical* invasion," denial of sexual relationships, forced living "with a new group of associates" (1605). "The crucial difference between the pregnant woman denied an abortion and the military draftee is," according to Regan, "the woman is being required to aid a specific other individual (the fetus); the draftee is not. Rightly or wrongly, our tradition distinguishes between obligations to aid particular individuals and obligations to promote a more broadly based public interest" (1606).[24] (Therefore the draft presents only an "apparent," not a real case of Samaritanism and can shed no light on Samaritan questions).

What's important to note, though, is the way Regan goes about locating the possible authority to require women to carry unwanted fetuses

---

24. Michaels thinks Regan's argument here begs the question, for "the statutory enactment of a prohibition against abortion would itself create a public interest in the protection of the fetus." See "Abortion and the Claims of Samaritanism," 218.

to term. If an analogous sacrifice, on the part of men, can be found, then fairness or equal consideration could be construed as requiring women to make analogous sacrifices in childbearing. Regan's mode of argument here is highly suggestive in unintended ways. What it suggests is that perhaps part of what has underlain men's authority to forbid women abortion has been men's sacrifice in war. As long as men could be conscripted and thus compelled either to be killed or to kill for the state, they maintained the moral edge that allowed them to keep abortion illegal. Regan writes in 1979, after, as he notes, the elimination of the military draft in the United States (though the draft remains constitutional). Thomson's argument appeared originally in 1971 as the draft was in the process of being eliminated. *Roe v. Wade* was issued in 1973. One of Thomson's major claims depends on the elimination of conscription. After insisting that no one was morally required to assist Kitty Genovese "at the risk of his own life," (142) Thomson claims that no one is required to "give long stretches of his life—nine years or nine months—to sustaining the life of a person who has no special right (we were leaving open the possibility of this) to demand it." Indeed, Thomson concludes, "with one rather striking class of exceptions, no one in any country in the world is *legally* required to do anywhere near as much as this for anyone else. The class of exceptions is obvious" (142). Now the last claim only makes sense, in relation to the United States, after military conscription for Vietnam had been eliminated or discredited. As a claim about the rest of the world, it actually does not hold, as people in many nations are legally required to kill and be killed in defense of their polities or for other state reasons.

The particular ways in which abortion and war are linked can be seen more clearly by following Regan's logic a bit further. Regan grants that laws forbidding abortion "might well be constitutional if they were justified on grounds other than the right to life of the fetus":

> In particular, it seems that if there were a genuine national commitment to population growth, abortion could be prohibited in furtherance of that commitment. This will strike some readers as a curious and unacceptable conclusion, but it is a conclusion I am prepared to accept. We do sometimes require great sacrifices in the public interest. The draft is the most extreme example. If it were necessary to require women to bear children in the pursuit of a goal similar to national security, I see no reason why that sacrifice could not be required. (1607–8)

Thus the state cannot justify forbidding abortion in defense of the particular individual fetus's right not to be killed (despite Regan's granting fetal personhood) but it can do so to further a collective purpose like that of population growth required for national security. What has happened, we might ask, that the defense of life would be advocated not because it is the right of a particular person but rather a state need? The answer to that question seems, to me, to lie in Regan's account of the risks to the draftee, given previously. It curiously omits the two greatest burdens of military service, as it has historically been understood: being killed and/or being required to become one who kills. Here Regan reflects the general American policy initiative from the end of Vietnam until the present war in Iraq: to develop such technical military superiority that wars could be fought by a volunteer army virtually without the risk of violent death on our side (and with only the very limited risk that the individual soldier would have to kill, face to face, an enemy). Thus military service could be made a job like other jobs: difficult, to be sure, but fully compensable. Risk of the one loss for which one cannot be compensated was virtually eliminated. As the state ceases to need individuals to sacrifice the *irreplaceably particular*—their lives—it loses its claim and interest in protecting the lives of fetuses as irreplaceably particular.

Regan makes it clear that he regards fetuses as persons. He distinguishes his argument in this regard from Blackmun's in *Roe v. Wade*: "My argument, unlike Blackmun's, does not depend on refusing to allow the state to regard the fetus as a person. Everything I have said is consistent with the assumption that the fetus is a person" (1641). If this is true, then the state is no longer the protector of the right to life of all persons. If abortion involves killing, even justified killing, then the state would seem to be in the curious position of allowing some of its citizens to be killed. Or to describe this another way, we could say that the state extends, or parcels out, its monopoly of violence in the abortion process. As obviously none of these descriptions can be allowed, abortion is redescribed, as by Regan, as a matter of Samaritanism. The abortion decision is not primarily about whether to kill a person but rather about whether we can be required to assist one. We can see why Regan gathers abortion under the heading of Samaritanism even while admitting that it's really not like other Samaritan questions. Defining abortion as a matter of Samaritanism is not so much a matter of accurate description as it is a necessity. Killing persons suggests a violence that could recoil upon us; refusing them aid has quite different implications. The fetal person is not really killed; it dies of its own unsustainability. Regan's redescription has the additional benefit of allowing the state to maintain its benevolent posture as the sustainer and provider of good for all. What the state does in privatizing abortion is simply to allot the micro-decision regarding unmerited beneficence to the woman as most immediate provider—an allotment entirely revocable, as Regan freely admits, should state priorities change.

This is no argument for men's return to sacrifice in war in order to assure that women feel compelled to carry unwanted children to term. As a Christian, I believe, as Stanley Hauerwas has put it, "that Christ is the end of sacrifice—that is, any sacrifice that is not determined by the sacrifice of the cross."[25] With the end of sacrifice in war, men lose the moral edge required to insist with apparent justice that women be denied abortion. The sacrificial edge then shifts to women, who are able to claim, quite rightly, that making abortion unavailable causes them to sacrifice the free expression of their sexuality in a way that is not required of men. This is why Thomson's analogy of the violinist can be made to apply not only to cases of rape but also to those of voluntary intercourse. One might argue that the prior assumed risk-taking of the woman engaging in voluntary intercourse would create an obligation in her toward the fetus, and that this makes the case different from that of the violinist. But implicit in Thomson's argument is the suggestion that we cannot fairly insist that any woman carry an unwanted fetus to term because there is no equivalent sacrifice from men. This argument must perhaps remain largely implicit because it appeals to a sense of justice as fairness that is at odds with Thomson's explicit defense of a more limited libertarian notion of justice as proper acknowledgment of entitlement.

Thomson's argument should perhaps be understood as simultaneously one opposing the draft and making the case for abortion. Or, to put this another way, we might say its rhetorical force implicitly depends on the discredited status of the draft in 1971—at least to many Americans (particularly of the philosophy reading classes). Asking "what it comes to, to have a right to life," she emphatically argues "that the primary control we must place on the acceptability of an account of rights is that it should turn out in that account to be a truth that all persons have a

---

25. "Sacrificing the Sacrifices of War."

right to life." What emerges with particular clarity in the argument that follows, then, is the interrelatedness of abortion and conscription issues. Thomson asserts, "I am arguing only that having a right to life does not guarantee having either a right to be given the use of or a right to be allowed continued use of another person's body—even if one needs it for life itself" (137–38). A clear implication of this argument would seem to be the end of conscription. It is an argument that would have particular force in 1971, when the Vietnam War had simultaneously discredited the sacrifice of American soldiers (in the eyes of many) and assured Americans that they would never be in real need of the bodies of others to defend their own lives. Proof that we would never really need the bodies of conscripts for our own defense was the war itself, in which 50,000 of the nation's young could be expended for seemingly symbolic purposes. A nation really endangered could hardly afford such expenditures of life. I do not want even to seem to be accusing Thomson of bad faith: I think she fully accepts an account of rights that would both make conscription illegal and abortion legal. Her argument helps bring to light, I believe, the way sacrifice enables the gaining of a moral edge that can be used to justify kinds of coercion. This is an invaluable contribution on her part. What I do want to suggest is that her argument's reception was surely aided by the discrediting of sacrifice in Vietnam and the confidence of Americans that they would never need such sacrifice from others to preserve their own lives.

Given the linkage I've suggested between thinking about abortion and war, it seems appropriate to close this chapter with a look at Lloyd Steffen's attempt to connect them very specifically in *Life/Choice: The Theory of Just Abortion*. Steffen's concept of "just abortion" is modeled specifically on just-war theory. What he attempts is to articulate principles—themselves based on just-war thinking—by which to justify some abortions while still leaving intact a general "presumption" for life. His arguments are not successful, in my view, for reasons I will explore. Far more interesting than his specific arguments, however, are two assumptions he never questions or perhaps even sees. The first of these assumes that the "hallmark" of a "reasonable and faithful" person is a prudential self-regard that would never risk being harmed for a conviction. We might say Steffen attempts to construct a morality free of any reliance on supererogation. The effort to be free of supererogation would seem to make the conduct of war impossible: the fact it does not, for Steffen, can suggest only that he makes something like the assumption Regan does in his enumeration of the burdens to the draftee—that being killed is not a possibility. The second large, perhaps unrecognized, assumption of Steffen's is his identifying questions of morality specifically with killing, and membership in the "moral community" with possession of the power to kill.

Many treatments of the abortion topic begin with concern that differences over abortion threaten national unity. Steffen, however, is unusually fearful about this matter: "Abortion has fractured a nation, threatened the rule of law, disrupted religious communities, divided families, decided elections, spurred violence, and presented women—and couples—facing unwanted pregnancies with difficult personal decisions."[26] He attributes this "distressing polarization" to those who hold extremist and absolutist views on the issue. Here he means "pro-lifers," for the "just abortion" theory he advances is explicitly pro-choice: "Just abortion steers clear of extremism and absolutism in favor of a morally moderate position; and moral moderation on the abortion issue means one thing: that some abortions are morally justifiable and others are not" (4). That pro-choice people are right to be concerned about pro-lifers' violence against abortion providers and seekers is beyond question, particularly to those of us who confess Jesus as Messiah. Arguments such as Steffen's, however, seem less concerned with this particular matter than with some general amorphous threat to national unity. In Steffen's case, in fact, it's difficult to understand whom he is addressing. Presumably most pro-choice people already agree with him. As he often casts pro-life people as "extremists," "absolutists," and "fanatics," it seems unlikely he considers them really able to be persuaded of his position. How, then, are we to understand what he is doing? If, as he has told us, "moral moderation" on abortion means only "one thing," then everyone who does not subscribe to this position is, by definition, an extremist and thus presumably incapable of being persuaded. What must be recognized is that equating abortion and war dramatically isolates fetuses and those who speak for them. They are positioned as the enemy.

Steffen argues repeatedly that one of his purposes is to reclaim abortion as a moral problem. Steffen believes it has ceased to be a moral problem for most people, who have aligned themselves with one or another social policy alternative (this oversimplification of the issue itself

---

26. Steffen, *Life/Choice*, 2. Further citations will be given parenthetically.

being driven by the extremism of the drive for prohibition) (3). What makes a problem specifically a moral one, for Steffen, seems to be its involving killing: "Because life is universally regarded as a basic good of life, the act of extinguishing a life requires moral reflection" (15). Elsewhere Steffen is even more explicit about the meaning of "moral": "If abortion is a moral problem, it is so because abortion involves a killing" (50). Because our presumption is for life, it requires a moral argument to set it aside. This would seem to suggest that moral people are specifically those willing, under some circumstances, to kill. To be unwilling to kill human beings under any circumstances is, thus, to be amoral, if not perhaps immoral. To be unwilling to kill is surely also, in Steffen's terms, to be a "fanatic," for he defines fanatics as "persons who hold to positions with such inflexibility that they would allow themselves to be harmed and destroyed by so doing" (152–53). Being reasonable, then, seems to mean never holding a conviction at the risk of being harmed. One might respond to Steffen here by saying that a conviction one is not willing to be harmed for is not much of a conviction. "To allow oneself to be sacrificed to a moral superior, represented by the fetus," Steffen argues, is to love the fetus more than oneself and oneself-as-neighbor. So much does this offend against prudential and practical reason, and fundamental commitments to self-regard that are the hallmarks of reasonable and faithful people, that one who held to such an absolutist perspective would be termed not only a moral absolutist but a fanatic as well (152–53)

It's not clear why being harmed or even dying for another must represent "sacrifice to a moral superior." Perhaps such actions could simply be seen as evidence of that great love by which one lays down his or her life for a friend. One bothersome feature of Steffen's definition of the fanatic, from a Christian point-of-view, is its identification of prudential self-regard with faithfulness. If I'm so reasonably self-regarding as to risk no conviction that could harm me, how will I ever discover the self God wants me to be? Given his attitude toward fanaticism, Steffen would surely have little use for the martyrs, whose blood, one remembers, was once considered the seed of the church.

It seems clear, then, that the Christian pacifist could never be assimilated into the moral state, as Steffen defines it, for the "moral" state is just that populated by those willing to kill rather than take the fanatical risk of being harmed for their convictions. To be so fearful of risk as to define as "fanatical" anyone willing to be harmed for her convictions would seem to necessitate the building of an extraordinarily secure state. Perhaps this concern for security explains why Steffen seems so alarmed at divisions in the nation caused by defenders of the fetus. The more we become devoted to ensuring security, the greater the apparent threat posed by even the seemingly weakest of foes.

Problems with Steffen's analogy between war and abortion should now be apparent. If we are never to ask anyone to risk being harmed for a conviction, or to act from anything other than prudential self-regard, then war would surely cease to exist, as these standards are utterly inconsistent with the kinds of risks and behaviors perennially expected of soldiers. Yet Steffen is not in the business of making a pacifist argument; he clearly believes that some killing can be justified, as in abortion. If the abortion–war analogy is to hold, then, for the purpose of his "just abortion" position, the conduct of war must be entirely consistent, in his view, with prudential self-regard. The intriguing question is how such an assumption, so inconsistent with nearly the entire history of warfare, could come to be. Again I would suggest the answer lies in American policy between Vietnam and the current Iraq war: that is, to establish such military and technological superiority that war could be conducted with very low risks of casualties by free market soldiers. This professionalization of war also had the effect of isolating it from the ongoing life of the American people; it became a kind of technical function of the state, carried out by a highly specialized group, and thus nothing that one had to consider in reflection about all the other political matters that concern our daily lives. Steffen's assumptions also reflect an extraordinarily nationalistic, or at least Americano-centric, view of war. For people nearly everywhere else on earth continued throughout the period of seemingly impenetrable American security—roughly 1975 to September 11, 2001—to conduct war in the usual ways, with the usual risks and required sacrifices.

Thus one reason for rejecting Steffen's notion of just abortion is that it relies on assumptions about war that are untenable. It also seems to make any real debate about "just cause" meaningless, for that must, in some way, depend upon an assessment that the "enemy" has acted unjustly. The "enemy" here is the fetus, and it has "acted" in the only way possible to it, neither justly nor unjustly. Proportionality of response seems also a standard hardly applicable to abortion, except perhaps in the case of danger to the life of the mother—and even, in this case, there is no warrant for the analogy to just war. Nor does it really clarify the problem of legitimation to establish the mother as legitimate authority in a way analogous to the legitimate authority necessary in the declaration of a just war. Surely what makes for the legitimate authority to declare a just war is a larger political process, operating to empower, to criticize, and, if need be, to check the exercise of authority. Judgments about legitimacy will involve also the degree to which the authority has attempted to negotiate with the enemy, to pursue all political measures short of war. None of this applies to abortion, where the woman's "authority" derives simply from her possession of the power to terminate the fetus and no possibility of negotiation exists. Obviously, for Steffen, war—if it can serve as an analogy to abortion—has been completely sundered from the political process. The important distinction between combatant and non-combatant in *jus in bello* seems also inapplicable to abortion, where the only casualty is surely not a combatant but one whose existence is solely dependent upon the health and well-being of the one contemplating killing it.

Steffen's picture of moral conflict would effectively make traditional just-war thinking impossible. Abortion, and presumably war, present simple conflicts of will in which there are only two alternatives—the free exercise of moral will or subjection. One is either an end in oneself or a thing; remaining an end in oneself means reducing the other to a thing. Possession of full moral standing becomes effectively equated with the power to kill. The "abortion conflict" centers not on a conflict of rights, Steffen maintains, but rather "on whether the fetus possesses sufficient moral status to withstand a challenge the effect of which would be to allow the fetus to be killed" (51). Possessing moral status means being able to resist being killed; it means to move from the category of those who can be killed—the unjustified—to those who can kill. In "framing the theory" of just abortion, Steffen argues "the moral question [of abortion] is whether or under what circumstances" the "direct and willful killing of a developing form of human life" can be justified. "Just abortion" is "unique in doggedly holding to the idea that abortion always presents itself to reflection as a moral problem"—again precisely because the character of specifically moral problems lies in their concerning the distinction between those empowered to kill and those who can be killed (70). Steffen repeatedly asserts the presumption of just war is in favor of life, but this presumption seems ultimately not to possess much actual force in limiting the decision for abortion. Regarding the "last resort" criterion, for example—that drawn by analogy from just war's insistence that war be the "last resort" of policy—Steffen argues that "the assumption that abortion must be a last resort in the sense that any possible way of preserving fetal life is preferable to killing a fetus actually positions the mother as a moral inferior to the fetus. This is, as previously argued, a morally reprehensible and unjustifiable move to make" (96).

Thus the "presumption for life," together with the "last resort" criterion, does not point to carrying the child to term and putting it up for adoption. To do so might seem the best way to clearly serve a presumption for life. But as Steffen's description makes clear, the concern here is not really with life but with moral superiority and inferiority: the mother must have the freedom not to bring a pregnancy to term "against her will" (97). She must be free to enact her will, even to killing the fetus. To deprive her of her will is to render her a moral inferior, a less than fully endowed moral subject.

To be a fully endowed moral subject is to be a person. Steffen recognizes that personhood is a moral category, not grounded in facts about fetal life or development. For him the fetus becomes a person through its mother's extending the promise to bring it to term. At twenty weeks, he proposes, we should judge that "an implicit promise to bring the fetus to term has been made, and that aborting it beyond that point, unless the woman's life is in danger, is not morally appropriate" (118). Steffen regards this twenty-week "cut-off" point as an "extreme limit" and asserts that "clearly any justified abortion ought to be performed earlier rather than later" (119). Since personhood depends on a purely moral determination, however, it's not clear why Steffen should regard abortion at eight weeks as preferable to that at twenty weeks. In neither case is the fetus a person presumably, as what determines its status as person is simply its mother's promise not to kill it. In fact, Steffen would seem to have difficulty giving reasons for opposing abortion of fetuses even much farther along than twenty weeks. The fetus's status in the moral community, its personhood, is made to depend on the mother's promise not to kill it. But if the mother decides to kill it, at say thirty-five weeks, what is to prevent its being killed? She has retracted the promise and thus the fetus has presumably lost its status. Steffen argues that the "moral community" has an obligation to "infer" that the mother's not killing her fetus in twenty weeks means she has made a tacit promise to bring it to term.

Thus the community "can claim a right to enforce that promise even if the pregnant woman should change her mind" (119).

Steffen's attempt to establish a twenty-week cut-off date seems somewhat inconsistent with his first criterion for just abortion: the establishment of the mother as legitimate authority for the abortion decision. If the mother is to be judged the "legitimate and just authority" before twenty weeks, why not later as well? Steffen seems to recognize this apparent problem, as he will not designate even a very late-term abortion "murder," arguing that "murder" implies the kind of "morally absolutist" judgment that he wishes to eschew. Late-term abortions might be impermissible or even "despicable," but this would be "for reasons that take into account the moral relation of the mother (and the moral community) to the unborn fetus—and not for reasons that are morally absolutist and unconditional, which is what murder implies" (121).

What prevents Steffen, one might ask, from declaring that "murder" inappropriately describes the morally relational matter of infanticide—or even the killing of older children? He claims these are matters about which the "moral community" shows no equivocation: "The moral community does not seek to justify a willful killing of babies, even under difficult circumstances. Infanticide does not present problems of moral perplexity. Membership in the moral community is granted once a baby is born, so that the killing of an infant, which is defenseless, strikes persons of goodwill as morally abhorrent" (61). This claim ignores the defenses of infanticide by Tooley, Singer, Rachels, et al., as well as those defenses of abortion that freely grant the personhood of fetuses—whose importance is surely to suggest that a being's simply being regarded one of the moral community is insufficient reason to prevent its being killed. Steffen's claim seems also at odds with his drawing the analogy between abortion and war. Just war theory offers reasons and conditions under which members of the moral community can be killed. If abortion does not kill members of the moral community, there's no particular reason to look for an analogy to war. If abortion does kill members of the moral community, then criteria established for just abortion might also be made to fit infanticide.

Steffen himself works out principles for "just non-treatment of neonates." This section of his argument is meant to undermine absolutist opposition to abortion by showing that the "good of life is not an absolute good" (65). Once that has been shown, a much more permissive definition of just abortion can be established. But, in fact, Steffen's argument for "just non-treatment" establishes nothing relevant to his later defense of just abortion. His criteria for "just non-treatment" are unequivocally *patient-centered*, dependent above all on the judgment that "the life of the neonatal patient is clearly a burden to the infant itself" (67). But this is just what is not at stake in the defenses of abortion he later offers. "Just abortion" develops criteria by which women may abort their fetuses without regard to the later interests of those fetuses.

Steffen depends on a "presumption for life" to limit the frequency of abortions. His "just abortion" criteria include the specification that "one do no harm to, or in any way subvert, the value of the good of life that is protected by the moral presumption against abortion" (100). Yet "just cause" for terminating pregnancy can be as ill-defined and vague, for Steffen, as the need to "preserve [the woman's] well-being and relational integrity" (91). Moreover, as the woman is herself the appropriate and legitimate authority in the decision, "just abortion" effectively functions as abortion on demand. What Steffen's treatment of the pro-life presumption reveals, in fact, is the impossibility of our believing we can simultaneously establish presumptions and yet set them aside without undermining them. In the process of "framing the theory," Steffen argues that "constructing a theory of just abortion cannot proceed unless the common moral presumption at stake in the abortion debate has been adequately articulated" (71). But when we know so clearly in advance that there are reasons for the lifting of a presumption, can the presumption really be said to possess any force? We establish the presumption; we decide when it can be set aside; we aver that there are circumstances in which we act directly contrary to the presumption and yet the presumption is not damaged. To treat a presumption in this way risks rendering it meaningless.

It seems, in fact, that Steffen's analogy of abortion and war would tend to weaken the very presumption for life required for just-war discipline. If abortion can be as routinely justified as it can be under Steffen's standard—and as it currently is in practice—then his analogy seems unwittingly to encourage similar routinization of justified killing in war. It is unclear just how strong the presumption for life is in Steffen's work. He repeatedly sounds the note of a Niebuhrian moral realism in which taking responsibility in an imperfect world means deciding when to dirty one's hands by justified killing. To understand God's commandment not to kill as an exceptionless prohibition is thus to have no place in the moral community, defined, as we have seen, as those empowered to kill under appropriate circumstances. Opponents of abortion present a threat to national unity: they must come to see that accepting "moral responsibility" in a flawed world means exercising violence in justified ways against external enemies and granting to women the power to kill their fetuses when such killing can be justified.

Steffen's attempt is to render abortion uncontroversial by constructing a "firewall," as he puts it, between those justified in killing and the killed. Those who oppose abortion thus precipitate a crisis of difference, a challenge to the distinction. Their opposition suggests that our attempts to erect such firewalls are grounded less in justice than simply in power. The problematizing of the distinction suggests that perhaps we should understand the killing of abortion as simply something we do because we can, an exercise of the power to kill necessary to constitute the moral community. A just abortion is one that can be described in such a way that no one ever need fear its undermining the presumption for life— our life, that is. Remembering Hobbes's claim that our first fear is that of violent death, we can see what is most dangerous about pro-life fanatics.[27] They prevent us from converting death as power over us into power to kill and threaten us doubly by refusing to endorse the justifications by which we diminish our fear of being killed by distinguishing ourselves from those justifiably killed. They would leave us, in other words, in the intolerable position of being under the dominion of death without the compensating power to kill.

---

27. Hobbes, *Leviathan*, 65.

5

Why David Boonin's Defense of Thomson Fails to Persuade the Abortion Critic

JUDITH JARVIS THOMSON's "GOOD SAMARITAN ARGUMENT" for the permissibility of abortion has recently been defended at length by David Boonin. Boonin breaks out the objections to the argument in sixteen categories, answering each of the objections—as in the case of the "future like ours" argument—in what he believes to be the abortion critic's own terms. A full response to Boonin is beyond the scope of the present argument, but the seriousness and weight of his defense of Thomson require at least some attention and answer. What I offer here, then, is an engagement with four of his most important refutations of objections to Thomson. None of these succeeds in accomplishing Boonin's aim of answering the critic of abortion on grounds he or she already accepts.

One of the disturbing consequences of the Good Samaritan defense of abortion is evident from Boonin's way of defining the position. "From the moral point of view," he writes, "a woman who carries a pregnancy to term is like a person who generously offers at some considerable cost to herself to provide what another needs but does not have the right to, while a woman who declines to carry a pregnancy to term is like a person who declines to offer such assistance. It is not the case that abortion violates the requirements of morality, on this account, but rather that continuing to incur the burdens involved in a typical pregnancy goes beyond them, even if the fetus does have the same right to life that you or I have."[1]

---

1. Boonin, *Defense of Abortion*, 133–34. Further references will be given parenthetically.

Boonin's description matches closely the distinction between supererogatory and ordinary behavior. As to carry to term becomes supererogatory, on his account, the killing of the fetus becomes ordinary. Neither Thomson nor Boonin shies away from the language of killing. Their accounts grant (indeed depend upon, in my view) the personhood of the fetus and make arguments for its justifiable killing. Thus the ordinary level of conduct that we can expect from pregnant women is the justified killing of persons.

Several odd and disturbing conclusions follow from Boonin's way of linking carrying to term with Good Samaritanism or supererogation. First, it seems odd to define what the majority of women still do—carry to term—as supererogatory. Surely we know what is supererogatory or exceptional in part by distinguishing it from the ordinary or typical. Second, if abortion is the justified killing of persons, then we have put the power to kill in women's hands on a scale unprecedented in history. We should ask whether it can be good for any of our souls to engage in killing—*even if completely justifiable*—on this scale. The belief that killing can be so often and routinely justified seems likely to undermine the prohibition against killing—which must depend on killing's being only very infrequently justifiable. Finally, it should be noted how Boonin's distinction of the supererogatory and the ordinary may have the rhetorical effect of encouraging abortion. To call something ordinary or typical is not simply neutral description but rather a way of giving permission. Societies do not require heroic behavior; they require and expect ordinary or typical behavior.

One ancillary result of Boonin's understanding of child-bearing as supererogation must surely be to undermine public support for care, nurturance, and education of children. Doing the heroic in the absence of a clear societal requirement is perhaps praiseworthy, but it hardly obligates the rest of us to support one's choices. One thing I'm suggesting is that the context for good Samaritan style arguments like those of Thomson or Boonin is the increasing privatization of childbearing and rearing. A consequence of this privatization is the increased understanding of children as resources for public consumption. As childbearing ceases to be a norm, it becomes necessary rhetorically to present children as resources in order to make claims on public funding necessary for education and social welfare. Self-interested maximizers who see childbearing as extraordinary will quite appropriately expect their support for other people's children to yield a return. It seems inevitable that children will come to seem private commodities at home—where they must satisfy parents convinced of their own heroism in even venturing to have children—and resources available for others' use in their public lives.[2]

2. I might as well declare myself as one who despises hearing children spoken of as "our most important resource for the future." I felt this way long before reading Wendell Berry, but his analyses of economic or market totalitarianism have confirmed it. The mind concerned with particulars, as he puts it, "feels threatened and sickened when it hears people and creatures and places spoken of as labor, management, capital, and raw material." See "The Whole Horse," 239. Nevertheless having children in the United States or Canada is perhaps approaching the status of supererogation, at least in an economic sense. Economist Shirley Burggraf estimates the transfer of wealth "out of the family and into the Social Security System" at $16 trillion. She asks where politicians got the idea that this could be done "without affecting family behavior" (51). For her our public discourse on the family verges on schizophrenia, with one side "chanting 'family values'" and the other hoping that "with enough parental leave and enough child care, everyone can have a career and a family" (55). Neither is paying any attention to the economic influences operating on the family, not the least of which is women's now understanding fully the opportunity costs of rearing children. "It violates every principle of economic rationality," she writes, "to think that we can collectivize a major portion of the social wealth produced by families, and still continue to privatize the costs" (55). Rolf George has shown just what a bad investment children are through an economic parable of the Crusoes and Fridays. Robinson and Mrs. Crusoe have four children, the Fridays have none. All four adults are 29 years old and the Crusoe children are quadruplets. The Crusoes will care for their children until age 18 and then work another 18 years before retiring at 65; the Fridays will work and save until 65 as well. The men can then expect to live another 15 years, the women 19. (Canadian figures for life expectancy). During that period the Fridays will purchase goods and services from the Crusoe children. If "the Fridays save at the rate at which the Crusoes spend on their children, and if the Crusoes do the same after they have raised them, then, at an interest rate of about 4%," the Fridays will have three times more money than the Crusoes at age 65. One could say they could "obtain the services of three of the Crusoe children, leaving the Crusoes to be supported by only one of their offspring" (1). George concludes that the "sole reason for this lamentable turn of events is that the Crusoes have invested their money in the very children that now maintain all of them." Moreover, as the "percentage of childless persons grows, it becomes more and more irrational, in a capitalist economy, to have children" (3). For Burggraf, see "How Should the Costs of Child Rearing Be Distributed?," 48–55; and for George, "Who Should Bear the Cost of Children?," 1–42, especially 1–3. See also George, "On the External Benefits of Children," 209–17. Paula Casal rejects George's arguments for parental subsidies on the grounds that these will encourage population growth among those in the developed nations who are the world's greatest overconsumers of resources. See "Environmentalism, Procreation, and the Principle of Fairness," 363–76.

I

But my primary purpose here is to address Boonin's "refutations" of the objections to Thomson's good Samaritan argument. One such objection concerns the matter of "tacit consent." As summarized by Bonnie Steinbock, this objection holds that "by engaging in intercourse, knowing that this may result in the creation of a person inside her body, [the pregnant woman] implicitly gives the resulting person a right to remain."[3] Boonin's challenge to this position begins with a distinction between "a) voluntarily bringing about a certain state of affairs, and b) voluntarily doing an action foreseeing that this may lead to a certain state of affairs." His claim is that "only a) is a plausible candidate for grounding tacit consent," but that plausible attempts to "apply tacit consent to nonrape cases of pregnancy must appeal to b)" (154). In short, the woman engaging in voluntary intercourse without contraception only "foresees" but does not "bring about" an unintended pregnancy. Thus the case for her giving a kind of tacit consent fails.

To clarify the distinction of bringing about and foreseeing on which his refutation depends, Boonin introduces the cases of Bill and Ted. Bill goes to a restaurant, eats, removes money from his wallet, places it on the table, and walks out. Obviously he brings it about that some of his money, according to the conventions, goes for a tip to the waiter and staff. Ted enters and sits down, but finds that a "crumpled wad of dollar bills in his pants pocket made him uncomfortable." Thus he puts these on the table while he is eating, "intending to put most of them back in his pocket when it was time to leave." A friend warns him to put the money back in his pocket but Ted refuses. He again refuses when the friend suggests he tie a piece of string around his finger to remind him. Ted claims he does not like the way the string "made him feel" as he's eating. Unfortunately Ted becomes "so lost in the rapture of his meal" that he does forget to put the money back in his pocket. Later, after he "left the restaurant, he suddenly realized his mistake and headed back to clear things up" (156). Boonin's argument is that the woman seeking abortion is like Ted rather than Bill. Since "Ted's relation to the unwanted state of affairs he has foreseeably produced is not sufficient to warrant the claim that he has consented to bear the burdens it imposes on him, the same is true of her" (159).

---

3. Steinbock, *Life Before Birth*, 78.

Why David Boonin's Defense of Thomson Fails to Persuade ⁜ 149

Boonin's strong distinction between "bringing about" and "foreseeing" should strike us as immediately suspect. Clearly "foreseeing" is an integral part of acts "bringing about" states of affairs. We bring about desirable consequences that we foresee and take action to avoid bringing about undesirable consequences that can be foreseen. Ted's failure is actually a failure to foresee. He does not foresee that he will leave the restaurant with his money still on the table. If he had actually foreseen this, he would surely have put the money back in his pocket or even asked his friend to hold it for him. Boonin uses the word "foreseeable" in the sense of possibility, and surely it is possible that Ted could foresee he might leave his money unintentionally. In the same sense, I could, at fourteen years old, foresee that I might some day be a major league shortstop. That was a possibility within my ability to foresee. But I did not make any plans on it, because I did not really foresee its happening. No one would hold me responsible for not developing my abilities as a shortstop, and we'd be unlikely to hold Ted responsible for leaving his money. Certainly good restaurant practice would dictate returning it to him when he came to claim it.

But the whole concept of negligence depends on an assessment that some states of affairs can be reasonably foreseen. We can be held responsible for foreseeing consequences with a certain likelihood of happening. Our foreseeing depends on the structure of acts themselves leading to certain kinds of typical, expectable consequences. There is no real comparison between Ted's action and that of the woman voluntarily having unprotected intercourse. This is because inadvertently leaving one's money on the table has no regular, typical, expectable relationship to eating dinner in a restaurant in the same way that pregnancy has to sexual intercourse. Intercourse is the kind of act that leads to pregnancy; eating in a restaurant is not the kind of act that leads to losing one's money. We might well consider whether Ted might be less likely to lose his money if he had similarly lost it on ten previous occasions (or even if he had heard of ten others who had done so). Were that the case, he would truly *foresee* that this will happen to him again and put away his cash. Boonin does not successfully respond to the advocate of the tacit consent position on the advocate's own terms. The holder of that position can insist that the woman engaging in voluntary unprotected intercourse not only foresees but brings about her pregnancy—and she can be said to bring it about because it is a reasonably foreseeable result.

Ted's leaving his money, on the other hand, is possibly but not reasonably foreseeable. He does not really foresee it. If he did, he would have taken the simple expedient of putting his money back in his pocket.[4]

II

A second argument Boonin addresses is what he calls the "responsibility objection." In its simplest form, this objection to the good Samaritan argument consists of saying that the woman acquires a responsibility to support the fetus because her "voluntary act foreseeably brought about the state of affairs in which [the fetus] is in need" of "assistance." It is perhaps worth a reminder here that the responsibility critic shares Thomson's and Boonin's view that you may detach yourself from the violinist. The responsibility critic argues that Thomson's violinist case is relevantly similar to pregnancy resulting from rape but that pregnancy resulting from voluntary intercourse is different.

Boonin's refutation of the responsibility objection depends upon a distinction he draws between one's being responsible for another's existence and another's neediness. He puts the distinction like this:

4. In a note Boonin explains that he does not want to suggest that the woman's right to abort follows from "Ted's right to reclaim his money." He claims rather that his purpose is only to respond "to an argument that claims to show that she lacks the right to abort because she has consented to refrain from doing so. That argument turns on the claim that the voluntariness of the action which produced the state of affairs justifies the attribution of consent, not on the claim that she is obligated to sustain the fetus because its very life is at stake. And the example of Bill and Ted demonstrates that this foundational claim about consent is untenable" (158). But this last claim is unsustainable. Bill and Ted's examples tell us nothing meaningful about the kind of consent involved in a woman's engaging in sex that she knows to have a reasonably expectable, though uncertain, outcome. Bill's case involves a certainty; the conventions of tipping are such that if he leaves an amount of money roughly 20% of his bill on the table, it will certainly be understood by all as a tip. Ted's case involves no issues of consent at all and actually no consequences, as no restaurant is going to refuse to return his money (perhaps minus what might be regarded an appropriate tip). Boonin has announced that his overall purpose is to answer the critic of abortion on the critic's own terms, but his examples here will certainly not persuade the holder of the tacit consent objection. Moreover, the critic will not endorse the separation Boonin insists on between the issue of consent and the obligation to support the fetus whose "very life is at stake." The importance of the issue of consent is grounded in the fact that what results here is not losing one's money but rather the creation of another and utterly vulnerable human being. Criticism of abortion, in short, is meant to insist on the seriousness of the consequences so that people will foresee the utterly predictable results of their actions and approach sex with somewhat more care than Ted evinces with his money.

Responsibility (1): You are responsible for the fact that the other person now exists.

Responsibility (2): You are responsible for the fact that, given that the other person now exists, he stands in need of your assistance. (169)

Boonin's strategy is to grant that the pregnant woman is responsible in sense 1) but not in sense 2), and that she is therefore not responsible for allowing the fetus to remain. To make this argument, he characterizes the critic as maintaining that the voluntary intercourse case is "relevantly similar" to cases "in which a voluntary act of yours foreseeably (but not intentionally) causes an accident that leads an innocent bystander to be in need of your assistance to survive" (170). Thus the kind of case Boonin chooses to represent the critic is one involving a hunter who accidentally injures an innocent bystander or another in which one's engaging in a pleasurable activity has "the unfortunate side effect of destroying someone's food supply" (167).[5] In these cases, we would conclude that one is responsible in sense 2), as through a voluntary activity one has caused another's neediness and thus incurred the obligation of assistance. Boonin argues, however, that the woman's case is different from these, for "there was no option available to her on which the fetus would now exist and not be in need of her assistance." Thus "there is no voluntary action that she did such that had she not done it the fetus would now exist and not be in need of her assistance." Boonin then concludes that, "in the sense in which I defined these terms above, a woman whose pregnancy arises from voluntary intercourse is responsible for the fetus's existence, but she is not responsible for its neediness, given that it exists" (171).

We can begin answering Boonin by questioning his division of responsibility into that for 1) existence and 2) neediness. Such a distinction would seem to make sense only for beings whose existence can meaningfully be distinguished from their neediness, and this is, of course, not the case for fetuses. Surely Boonin is right that the creation of neediness in another is central to our attribution of responsibility. If, like the hunter or a bad driver, I injure another and thus create a need for assistance, then I have the responsibility to supply such assistance. But this understanding of responsibility is predicated on the assumption that we are ordinar-

---

5. Boonin borrows the case involving destruction of food supply from Tooley, *Abortion and Infanticide*, 45.

ily non-needy beings. Clearly it is important to organize our notions of responsibility in this fashion in order to limit people's claims against one another. The wounded person must be able to show that he has been injured by the hunter in order to establish the hunter's responsibility to assist him. The presumption is that the hunter has no responsibility to assist him—apart from a specific showing of harm—because we are ordinarily non-needy. None of this applies to the fetus. It makes no sense to judge the pregnant woman free of responsibility based on standards of responsibility grounded in assessments of harm measured against a baseline of non-neediness. A revision of the food supply example above will help to make my point. In the revised case, we knowingly engage in an optional activity that has a very great likelihood of creating people in a place where the food supply is inadequate. We have brought about their existence as people who are in need of assistance. Would we not be responsible for assisting them? Surely it could plausibly be argued that we assumed that responsibility when we engaged in the optional activity that we knew might lead to their being created as the needy beings they have no choice but to be.

I conclude, then, that neither Boonin's Responsibility 1 nor Responsibility 2 provides an accurate description of the responsibility incurred when creating a being who is, by definition, needy. A more accurate description of the sense in which one is responsible for bringing a fetus into existence is 3: You are responsible for the fact that the other person now exists as one who needs your assistance. Boonin may successfully answer the responsibility objection as it is presented in the kinds of examples he chooses (i.e., those by Tooley, Beckwith, Carrier et al.) but he does not successfully answer one who would push the question of responsibility back to the act of intercourse. This is where it must be addressed, the critic might insist, if we are to consider the fetus as the kind of needy being it cannot help but be. Again we see how the Thomson–Boonin position is not merely an abortion-despite-fetal-personhood argument but rather one that *depends upon* the fetus's being a person. The notions of responsibility Boonin works with are derived from the ordinary experience of those free-standing, non-needy beings we call persons. These he then applies to the fetus, which, because it has only its need, apparently cannot qualify for responsible treatment from others (since this depends on demonstrating that one has become needy against a baseline of non-neediness). I am struck, too, by how differences about abortion are deeply embedded in the very language we use to describe what is going on. For Boonin procreative intercourse brings about a "state of affairs in which" one may require "assistance." For the critic of abortion, procreative intercourse brings about a unique and particular fetus for whom the question is not "assistance"—a kind of help directed to one already separate and independent—but rather "sustenance," support that is in no way optional but instead essential to this new being's developing life. Such deeply imbedded differences in the very grammar of abortion make Boonin's attempt to refute the critic on the critic's own terms a great deal more problematic than Boonin allows.

III

The significant differences in moral description between critics of abortion and Boonin become especially evident in his handling of the "killing versus letting die objection." The holder of this objection to the good Samaritan argument maintains "that there is a morally relevant difference between killing a person and letting a person die, and that abortion kills the fetus while unplugging yourself merely allows the violinist to die" (188). Here again Boonin's strategy is to grant the critic's assumption—that killing is indeed worse than letting die—and yet to show that it does not undermine the analogy between unplugging the violinist and aborting the fetus. Boonin's argument depends upon a highly contestable description of abortion by hysterotomy—in which the living fetus is removed "through an abdominal incision of the uterus and then allow[ed] ... to die"—as "more plausibly" a "case of letting die" than "a case of killing." In this case, as also in abortion by hysterectomy, the woman is effectively discontinuing support, "and when an agent discontinues providing another with needed life support, this seems clearly to be a case of letting die rather than of killing" (193). Boonin's language here should be contested on several counts. First we should notice the inapplicability to the relationship of woman and fetus of his phrase concerning the "agent discontinu[ing] providing another with needed life support." The missing word here is "agent," which should follow "another," and indeed it is plausible that we would consider one agent's discontinuation of support to another agent to be "letting die" rather than killing. But we would do so because implicit in the word "agent" is the assumption that the agent has both some measure of ability and responsibility to sustain him or herself. This is not true of the fetus.

Let us suppose a large group of young potential parents in the developed world suddenly become converted to the conviction that we must radically reduce population. They thus expose thousands of their own young infants to death by starvation. Would we not more reasonably describe this as mass killing than as an act of letting die? There is some evidence Boonin might see this as letting die rather than killing, for he argues elsewhere that "surely a person who fails to feed a hungry infant allows it to die and does not kill it" (199). Or let us suppose that a powerful and wealthy nation, rich in resources, made a small and ethnically different country entirely dependent upon it. After the small country lost all ability to survive independently, the large nation suddenly discontinued all support. The people of the small country, predictably, died. Would we not plausibly describe the large country's actions as genocide? Indeed, we would, I believe, be inclined to describe the actions as genocide in direct proportion to our ability to show the large nation to be responsible for the small country's dependence and the small country unable to support itself and thus not responsible for doing so. The critic of abortion, already unpersuaded by Boonin's refutation of the responsibility objection, will similarly argue that abortion by hysterotomy is more properly described as killing than as letting die. In the non-rape case, the woman bears at least some responsibility for the fetus's existence and the fetus has no choice but to exist as a being who is totally dependent. In such circumstances, to initiate a process that can only lead to the certain death of the fetus seems appropriately described as killing rather than letting die.

If we characterize hysterotomy as killing, Boonin argues further, we must "by parity of reasoning" also "say that unplugging yourself from the violinist kills him and does not merely let him die, since it is equally true that unplugging yourself from him actively disconnects the violinist from the support that he needs in order to survive" (195). But this line of argument ignores two very important differences between the violinist and the fetus. The first is that the fetus has no choice but to remain connected to her mother until aborted or born. The violinist does have the choice to be disconnected, and this is true even if he is comatose and must rely on a proxy to exercise the choice. Thomson and Boonin think they have rendered him choiceless by making his continued living contingent on the attachment. But this reveals only that survival has become an idol. Emily Dickinson is only partly right when she concludes one famous poem with the claim that we have "the power to kill without the power to die."[6] We are without the power to die, for our dying happens to us, comes to us, without exertion of power on our part. But we are able to allow ourselves to die without making unjust claims on others, and this the violinist can and should do. He should disconnect himself (or provide that a proxy will do so) in order to keep faith with the general bargain of risk-sharing under which all live and from which he has benefited in the past. Part of the reason he should do so is to enable distinctions to be made between unjustifiable claims to total support from another—as in his own case—and fully justified claims to such support by beings who have no ability to choose otherwise, fetuses.

A second very important difference between violinist and fetus involves who is responsible for each's dependence. In the non-rape abortion case, the person who terminates support to the dependent fetus is the very same person who is, at least partially, responsible for the fetus's existence in the first place (and responsible for its existence as the only kind of being it can be, a dependent one). But this is not true of the violinist, who has been made dependent on one unique other only through the vagaries of the natural lottery. Boonin may fail to see this distinction because of the way he has so systematically divided the abortion critic's arguments off from one another. He has dealt with the responsibility objection earlier—inadequately, as I hope to have shown—and thus does not see how the matter of responsibility is involved here also in the question of how to describe discontinuation of support. To discontinue supporting a being for whose existence one is responsible will seem, to the critic of abortion, like killing (not only in abortion but in failing to feed one's infant). Unplugging the violinist—for whose condition one is in no way responsible—will seem much more appropriately described as allowing disease to take its course.

Part of Boonin's argument in this section depends upon Phillipa Foot's attempts to capture the difference between killing and letting die through her well-known trolley problems.[7] My concern here is not so much with the trolley problems as such or with Boonin's modifications of Foot's examples but rather with the argument Boonin makes against Foot's conclusions concerning the relevance of the trolley problems to

---

6. "My Life had stood—a Loaded Gun" ends "For I have but the power to kill, / Without—the power to die."*Complete Poems of Emily Dickinson*, 369–70.

7. Foot, "Killing and Letting Die," 280–89.

abortion. Boonin's slightly adapted version of Foot's basic trolley problem sets up two rescue situations. In both cases, one is driving a trolley north along a track that one knows well. The track divides into right and left forks but then these come back together into a single track, at whose end is a hospital. In Rescue 1, one learns that there is a single dying person on the right hand fork and five dying people on the left hand one. If one chooses to save the single person on the right hand fork, one cannot return in time to save the five. Similarly, if one chooses to turn left and save the five, then one does not have sufficient time to rescue the one person on the right fork. Choosing to turn left means, obviously, letting one die in order to save five. In Rescue 2, no one is on the right hand fork. Instead, there is a "healthy (but temporarily unconscious) person stuck to the track near the beginning of the left-hand branch" (191) and the same five dying people further on down the left hand fork. One does have time to rescue the person stuck to the track, but doing so will prevent one from getting the other five to the hospital in time to save them. Running over the person stuck to the track, however, will allow one to get to the five in time to save them. In short, Rescue 2 involves killing one to save five. Foot argues that our sense of the difference between Rescues 1 and 2 involves that between initiating and merely allowing the events in question. She concludes that this distinction undermines the violinist analogy, which is best understood, in her view, as involving allowing a sequence of fatal events to continue. Abortion, on the other hand, is "completely different," for it "originates the sequence which ends in the death of the fetus."[8]

Boonin responds by claiming that Foot "fails to establish that the act of removing the fetus from the womb is the act that originates the fatal sequence of events in the case of procedures such as hysterotomy" (196). He begins by attempting to discredit Foot's distinction between the violinist and the fetus. Simply because the fetus is "not in jeopardy" in the womb "does not suffice to establish that the act of removing it from the womb is the act that originates the fatal sequence" (196). "After all," Boonin continues, "the violinist while plugged into you is not in jeopardy either, and the act of unplugging yourself is not the act that originates the fatal sequence in that case: It merely allows a preexisting sequence to continue. Unplugging yourself results in the violinist's death only because his condition is such that he cannot survive on his

---

8. Foot, "Killing and Letting Die," 288–89.

own" (196). Here Boonin is misled by the false certainty possible in philosophical examples such as the trolley problems. It is untrue that the violinist is not in jeopardy when plugged into you. Both he and the fetus are in some measure of jeopardy, as we all are, at all times. Because we are ordinarily in some measure of jeopardy, it becomes necessary to distinguish ordinary from extraordinary kinds of jeopardy. The fetus in the womb is subject only to the ordinary degree of jeopardy; thus to actively impose on it a much greater degree of jeopardy can reasonably be considered initiating the sequence that leads to its death—or, to put this simply, to kill it. The violinist is exposed to a quite extraordinary degree of jeopardy caused by the disease. Unquestionably this degree of jeopardy entitles him to a claim against the rest of us for care. What it does not entitle him to is complete bodily support from one other particular human being. He cannot reasonably say that any other has intervened in his life in order to subject him to an extraordinary degree of jeopardy. He cannot claim that he is killed, only that he has been justifiably let die. Foot's distinction between the fetus and the violinist stands, and Boonin's refutation of her position fails.

Boonin's claim that abortion allows an already fatal sequence to continue might well undermine opposition to killing of all sorts. In order to insist that abortion is similar to unplugging the violinist, he is forced to argue that we should understand the fetus's death in hysterotomy as being attributable to its insufficient lung functioning at this point in its development. Thus the act that originates the fatal sequence for the fetus is its conception: "Whatever caused the fetus to have such poorly developed lungs at this point in time is what initiated the fatal sequence. And since it is presumably part of the normal course of things that a fetus at an early stage of gestation has lungs of this level of development, the act which causally led to this state of affairs was simply the act of conceiving it in the first place" (196). John Paul II might well point to this argument as evidence for his claim that demands for total autonomy lead to a culture of death, for it seems here that the fetus has been made eligible for death by its being conceived as the only kind of being it can be, a dependent one. One wonders if Boonin's logic would lead one to defend Susan Smith by saying that what originated the fatal sequence of events for her children was their being conceived as beings whose lungs would not sustain them underwater.[9] Or if X shoots and kills Y, can X

9. Susan Smith of South Carolina was convicted in 1995 of murdering her two small sons by strapping them into a vehicle which she let roll into John D. Long lake.

be defended by our saying that the fatal sequence for Y began when he was conceived as the kind of being who could not sustain being shot? Of course, in neither of these cases would we, or Boonin, want to make these arguments. We'd rightly say Susan Smith is responsible for killing her children, and X is responsible for killing Y. Similarly, abortion intervenes in the ordinary course of things for the fetus, thus initiating the fatal sequence of events leading to its death. For the violinist, disease—not the unplugging—initiates that sequence. Foot's distinction stands, and, for the critic of abortion, killing the fetus remains substantially worse than allowing the violinist to die.

IV

One last argument of Boonin's deserves attention, for it suggests he does not understand the way the presumption against killing works for the Christian critic of abortion.[10] At issue is what Boonin terms the "intending versus foreseeing objection," which depends upon a distinction often made in discussions of the principle of double effect. In some cases, "such as those in which a woman's cancerous uterus must be removed in order to save her life, it can be permissible to do an action that foreseeably brings about the death of the fetus (since the fetus will surely die if the uterus is removed), even though it would not be permissible intentionally to kill the fetus" (212). Boonin points out that this distinction seems also applicable to the violinist example. When you unplug the violinist, you do so foreseeing his death, but that death is not what you intend. Abortion, on the other hand, involves not just foreseeing but intending the death of the fetus. As there "is a morally relevant difference between intending death and foreseeing it, it does not follow from the fact that unplugging yourself from the violinist is permissible that abortion is also permissible" (212–13). Thus Boonin characterizes the objection to the Good Samaritan argument that he proceeds to address. Once again his task is to grant the force of the distinction—intending versus foreseeing—and yet to argue that it does not undermine the Good Samaritan argument.

Boonin's argument begins with a hypothetical involving two bombers fighting in a just war for Nation A against Nation B, which is "starting

---

10. On the way just-war thinking shares pacifism's strong presumption against doing harm, against violence, see Childress, "Just-War Criteria," 40-58.

to run low on ammunition and on morale, but is continuing to inflict severe casualties nonetheless, resulting in retaliation and heavy losses on both sides." The bombers' target is "a large ammunitions plant closely surrounded by buildings that house athletes training to compete for Nation B in the Olympics." The two bombers of Nation A "each decide to drop a bomb on the center of the ammunitions plant and each do so because this will hasten the end of the war saving many lives on both sides." But the "values that underlie their reasoning" differ. Bomber I wants to "force the enemy to surrender by reducing its already low ammunition supply." Arguing that "the most efficient way to do that" is to bomb the ammunitions plant, he does so, recognizing that "the explosion will also kill some innocent civilians, and this is a very bad thing, but their deaths are not a part of my plan or intention; I merely foresee that they will occur. And the good of ending the war suffices to outweigh the evil of their deaths." Bomber II, on the other hand, wants to force Nation B to surrender by reducing its morale directly. "The most efficient way to do that is to kill all the Olympic athletes living around the ammunitions plant," thus crippling support for the war in Nation B and "saving countless lives on both sides." Bomber II closes by saying, "I recognize, of course, that killing innocent civilians is in itself a very bad thing, but I intend to kill them nonetheless, since the good of ending the war suffices to outweigh the evil of killing them" (213–14).

Boonin's next move is to argue that what Bomber I does is permissible whereas Bomber II's action is not. Bomber I, in his view, merely foresees the deaths of the athletes whereas Bomber II clearly intends to kill them. If we doubt this characterization of their motives, Boonin adds, we need merely to imagine a counterfactual in which the athletes are no longer living near the munitions plant.[11] Bomber I would go ahead to the

---

11. Boonin's treatment of Bomber I's intention here seems similar to Oliver O'Donovan's suggested way of testing "for the intention to harm non-combatants." O'Donovan proposes the following hypothetical as a way of discerning whether appropriate discrimination has been exercised (*Just War Revisited*, 44–45): "If it were to chance that by some unexpected intervention of Providence the predicted harm to non-combatants did not ensue, would the point of the attack have been frustrated?" (45). By this standard Boonin's Bomber I might seem to exhibit appropriate discrimination. But Boonin's case gives us no way to judge whether Bomber I's actions meet an "important corollary" of O'Donovan's regarding "what intention means": "The foresight that *disproportionate* non-combatant damage will be done, combined with a *failure to intend to avoid* that disproportionate damage, presumes an intention to do that damage." Gratuitous foreseen damage can be "presumed to be intended"; thus "discrimina-

target whereas Bomber II would not, as his intention is precisely to kill the athletes to lower their nation's morale. This may be true of Bomber I, but it does nothing to change the fact that what he does in the original hypothetical is not consistent with just war. Regarding the original hypothetical, one must begin by noting how little Boonin's language takes note of the way judgments about justice in war involve decisions taken by legitimate authority. In short, it's at least inconsistent with the spirit of just-war thinking to imagine individual bombers making decisions about the legitimacy of their targets and then offering up accounts of their own motives as justifications. Secondly, standards of *jus in bello* would not allow for Bomber I's actions to be regarded as just. The prudential portion of his reasoning is much too general to justify a violation of the distinction between combatants and non-combatants. The "good of ending the war" might be used to justify just about any conceivable action against enemy civilians.

If Bomber I is to be in conformity with *jus in bello*, he must also ask other preliminary questions, such as whether the bombs can be delivered from a lower altitude that will make for more precise targeting and reduce the casualties.[12] As he can clearly foresee that his action will

---

tion is not solely a matter of selecting a military object for attack, or simple 'targeting'. It is also a matter of attacking the target discriminatingly, i.e., proportioning the means to the object." The very vagueness of Bomber I's "object"—bringing an end to the war and thus saving countless lives—gives us little reason to believe he has exercised this kind of discrimination regarding the proportioning of means to ends in this particular case. In fact, we should ask whether Bomber I is not attempting to circumvent the requirement of discrimination by describing his ends in such a way as to justify the widest possible range of means.

In relation to O'Donovan's revisiting of the just war, the fact that Boonin's Bomber's civilian victims are Olympic trainees might also need to be considered more specifically. O'Donovan's is a "radically evangelical proposal for reinterpreting armed conflict in terms of judgment," one that "takes issue from the outset with the generally antagonistic shape of our natural intuitions about war" (27). The killing of non-combatants is wrong, of course, irrespective of whether they are Olympic athletes or not. As an act of political judgment, however, killing those training for participation in games often considered a witness to the possibility of peace might seem extraordinarily antagonistic. Killing Olympic athletes seems to reinforce precisely the opposition of "we" and "they"—the "antagonistic conception"—that O'Donovan wants to break with decisively by revisiting just war as an evangelical proposal with judgment as its center (32).

12. On this point, see Walzer, *Arguing About War*, 17. In assessing the justice and injustice of the Gulf War, Walzer offers an account of the kind of procedures (unlike those hypothesized by Boonin) required for targeting consistent with *jus in bello*: "This effort to limit civilian casualties was embodied in clear-cut orders. Pilots were instructed to

cause non-combatant casualties, he must not drop his bomb on the munitions plant. We might well say, in fact, that his doing so, with the clear foreknowledge of civilian casualties, is tantamount to intending those casualties—though, of course, his case is less clear than that of Bomber II. It is easy to see, in fact, how *jus in bello* standards could never be maintained if we did not condemn the actions of Bomber I. For it would be a short step from Bomber I's rationale to developing strategy and targeting in such a way as to concentrate on military targets where damage to civilians could be maximized—all in the name, of course, of reducing total casualties on both sides.

If we reject the justifiability of Bomber I's actions, then Boonin's argument fails, for his further strategy is to identify unplugging the violinist with the, to him, justifiable actions of Bomber I. In his view, both Bomber I and you, as you unplug the violinist, foresee but do not intend death. On the view I am developing, Bomber I and you are relevantly different. Unplugging the violinist simply refuses him a claim he cannot justifiably make. You act justly in unplugging him. Bomber I unjustifiably kills civilians. Whether he intends or merely foresees doing so is perhaps a moot point, but a strong case can be made, as I have shown, for describing his action as intentional. Thus we do not need to follow Boonin's argument further, but I believe it would be helpful to look briefly at two further Bomber scenarios he proposes in order to understand how he construes abortion in relation to the intending versus foreseeing distinction.[13]

---

return to base with their bombs and missiles intact whenever they were unable to get a clear 'fix' on their assigned targets. They were not to drop their bombs in the general vicinity of the targets; nor were they to aim freely at 'targets of opportunity' (except in specified battle zones). In their bombing runs, they were to accept risks for themselves in order to reduce the risk of causing 'collateral damage' to civilians. So we were told, and so, presumably, the pilots were told. The first studies of the bombing, after the war, suggest that those orders were often not followed—that bombs were commonly dropped from altitudes much too high for anything like confident aiming. But the policy, if it was the actual policy, was the right one" (95).

13. One reason Bomber I's action must be impermissible according to *jus in bello* standards is to prevent Bomber II from describing his intentions in exactly the same way as Boonin ascribes to Bomber I. If what Bomber I does were acceptable, no Bomber II would ever describe his actions in the way Boonin attributes to him. He would simply say, as Bomber I does, that he dropped the bomb on the ammunitions plant foreseeing but not intending that a certain number of noncombatants living near to the plant would be killed. The distinction between combatants and noncombatants has been one of the most-debated features of just-war thinking. It is certainly by no means clear even

Boonin argues next that there is a "third alternative" to conceiving of consequences as either intended or foreseen. Sometimes an act can produce two effects, and one can reasonably be said to intend both. We'd say this of a dieter, for instance, whose intention in losing weight is to improve his health but who also foresees that he will gain in attractiveness. Boonin claims further that we must distinguish two possible construals here. On one, dieting to improve health is a sufficient inten-

---

that the workers in the ammunitions plant would qualify as combatants, something Boonin seems to take for granted. Under the kinds of definitions suggested by Michael Walzer or Jeffrie Murphy, they would be assimilated into the ranks of combatants. Walzer argues that the crucial differentiating characteristic is whether one makes what soldiers need to fight or simply what they need to live. For Murphy the distinction turns on whether one has a "necessary" or a merely "contingent" relationship to the war effort. Daniel Zupan, however, advocates a very strong version of noncombatant immunity based on a principle of "autonomy" grounded in a Kantian understanding of the human being as a rational end in himself. Zupan contends "that munitions factory workers are not combatants. The relevant principle to consult here is whether they have adopted the sort of maxim that justifies our use of force against them. Since they are not involved in direct harming, have not adopted this sort of maxim, they are not legitimate targets" (87). For Zupan, the factory itself might qualify as a legitimate target for bombing, but proper respect for the war convention and the workers' autonomy requires our issuing a warning before the bombing. See Walzer, *Just and Unjust Wars*, 146; Murphy, "Killing of the Innocent," 349–51; and Zupan, *War, Morality, and Autonomy*, 81–102.

But my judgment that the actions of Bomber I are inconsistent with *jus in bello* is based primarily on his going to the target despite knowing that the Olympic athletes will be killed. He might defend his action by pointing out, as Richard B. Miller has, that while "it is a common assumption of popular discourse about war that non-combatant immunity prohibits any and all killing of innocent parties," such "an interpretation of *in bello* criteria is wrong" (151). Paul Ramsey was one who was very concerned to retrieve the tradition's ability to make precise discriminations between "acts of war which directly intend and directly effect the death of non-combatants" and those in which noncombatants were killed as an indirect effect of action against combatants. Indeed Bomber I might use Ramsey to defend his action: "A desired and desirable victory may, however, justify conduct in warfare that causes the death, and is foreknown to cause the death, of non-combatants *indirectly*. This would *not* be directly to do evil that good may come of it" (Ramsey 154). But as Miller points out, Ramsey "argues that consequentialist calculations are appropriate only after our duties have been met. Within our discourse about war, judgments about moral means (i.e. noncombatant immunity) must precede judgments about whether consequences can be 'prudentially balanced.' Anything less would weaken the strict demands of noncombatant immunity, placing the morality of means on a slippery slope" (151). War is, for Ramsey, "not a 'boundary' case for morality" but "yet another sphere in which care is obligatory" (Miller, 150). There is no evidence in the example of Bomber I that the requirements of care or judgments about means have preceded the consequentialist reasoning, which is itself far too vague and general to allow for any precision of decision-making. See Miller, *Interpretations of Conflict*, 150–51; and Ramsey, "The Case for Making 'Just War' Possible," 154.

tion in itself to cause the action, with increased attractiveness simply a foreseen secondary effect. On the second, neither of the above effects is sufficient in itself to motivate the action, but the combination of them is enough to persuade the dieter "that the diet is justified" (217). Boonin then introduces what he conceives to be Bomber scenarios analogous to the pair of dieters. Bomber III wants "to force the enemy to surrender by reducing its already low ammunition supply *and* by reducing its already low morale." "The best way to satisfy this combination of desires" is to bomb the ammunitions plant, destroying weapons and "killing some of their Olympic athletes." Bomber III reasons further: "If dropping the bomb only destroyed the ammunitions plant and didn't kill any innocent civilians, then dropping the bomb would still be justified. Destroying the plant would be a sufficient reason to drop the bomb. But since the bomb will also kill the Olympic athletes, and since I view that as another legitimate goal, I drop the bomb with the intention of causing both effects" (217). Thus Bomber III is, for Boonin, relevantly like the dieter who would lose weight in order to improve his health even if he did not also gain in attractiveness.

Bomber IV, however, is more like the dieter who must be assured both that he will improve in health and attractiveness. He insists the bomb must both destroy the ammunitions plant and kill the Olympic athletes: "If it only killed the civilians and didn't destroy the ammunitions plant, then the bomb would be better used elsewhere where it could do more damage." And he concludes likewise if it only "destroyed the ammunitions plant and didn't kill any innocent civilians." As "things stand," however, in the hypothetical, "dropping the bomb will have both effects, and for that reason I view the decision to drop the bomb as justified" (217).

Boonin makes two assertions about this pair of bomber scenarios. First, he argues that what Bomber III does is permissible whereas the action of Bomber IV is not. Second, he claims "the intention of a woman who has an abortion is relevantly like the intention of Bomber III rather than that of Bomber IV" (218). Boonin does disapprove of the intention of Bomber III but claims "the mere presence of this intention is not enough to render such acts impermissible." What matters for Boonin, in the case of Bomber III, is that when he "drops the bomb, unlike when Bomber IV does, the presence of this intention [that of killing civilians] is not essential to the act he is performing" (218). Boonin says we are thus entitled to criticize "the kind of person Bomber III is" but not what he does. The most relevant analogy, for Boonin, is between Bomber III and the woman who has abortion by hysterotomy. There the essential act, the sufficient intention, is to rid oneself of bodily encumberment. The death of the fetus is also not simply foreseen but intended, as Boonin grants most women who abort would not be willing to see their child reared by someone else. (In other words, the death of the fetus is something intended.) Yet freeing oneself of bodily encumberment is sufficient intention in itself—like bombing the ammunitions plant even if no civilians would be killed. To prove this, Boonin turns to another counterfactual. If women seeking abortions were told that their fetuses would survive "no matter what happens," they would still undoubtedly have the procedures. Thus "most women who seek abortions" are relevantly "like the dieter for whom an improvement in appearance is a sufficient reason to stick with his diet even if it is not the only reason he acts on"—and, "more importantly, they are thus like Bomber III, who, like Bomber I, would still drop the bomb on the ammunitions plant even if it would not cause the death of any innocent civilians." Thus, in Boonin's view, if we accept the permissibility of Bomber III's action, "we can accept the claim that there is a morally relevant difference between intending death and foreseeing it without abandoning the good samaritan argument, at least as it applies to abortion by hysterotomy" (221) He regards his argument, then, as fulfilling his standard of responding to the abortion critic on the critic's own grounds.

To begin with, it seems reasonable to make two observations regarding Boonin's hypotheticals and the possibility of continued just-war thinking. Stanley Hauerwas has argued that perhaps only a people whose first commitment is to pacifism can maintain the rigorous presumption against killing needed for classical Christian just war thinking.[14] Boonin's hypotheticals suggest Hauerwas may be right. All four of the bomber scenarios are inconsistent with *jus in bello*, as I demonstrated above with Bomber I, the one Boonin considers the most clearly justifiable. What is striking about the scenarios, moreover, is that the reasoning about "justifiability" never turns on anything more than considerations of expediency. Bomber III's decision that dropping the bomb on the plant is "justified" even if doing so "only destroyed the ammunitions plant and didn't kill any innocent civilians" is not really a matter of justice at all. It

---

14. Hauerwas, "Epilogue," 152, and *Against the Nations*, 132–40.

is simply a self-interested judgment about the "best way"—which here means only the "most efficient way"—to go about satisfying one's "combination of desires" (217). The language of *jus in bello* would insist that Bomber III is justified in bombing the plant "if and only if" no civilians were killed, and if the war were justified according to the criteria of *jus ad bellum*. That the hypotheticals of Bomber III and IV never approach questions of justice is apparent, too, from Boonin's dieter analogy. The dieter never has to justify his intentions or his actions to anyone but himself. His "sufficient" reason is not a reason capable of being demonstrated to others as justifying a course of action; it's merely a judgment about the level of motivation required to move him to a completely self-interested pursuit.

Boonin's hypotheticals also suggest how completely principles like justice have ceased, for him, to operate as action-guiding or intention-forming qualities or virtues. What's wrong with the intentions of Bomber III—and, of course, Bomber IV—is that intending the killing of civilians as a legitimate goal is inconsistent with just war discipline—and this is true irrespective of the immediate consequences of a particular bombing (i.e., that the Olympic athletes just happen to have moved away temporarily from their training site next to the plant). There is every reason to believe that Bomber III will next time seek a target that allows him to maximize the destruction of military resources and innocent civilians. In short, what Bomber III does is inconsistent with justice, as is not the case with your decision to unplug yourself from the violinist. The critic of abortion has not been answered, for he can easily maintain that you justly unplug yourself from the violinist in a way that is not true of the woman who, in a non-rape case, has abortion by hysterotomy—particularly if she is to be understood as being like Bomber III.

At this point, it seems necessary to say something about Boonin's and Thomson's use of counterfactuals. Boonin's counterfactuals obscure the way people form their intentions and explain their actions in light of the real consequences of those actions. If many women confronting abortion indicate that the death of the fetus is part of what they want, this is because abortion does result in the death of fetuses. Claiming to want the death of the fetus is important to maintaining the resolution to undertake an action that can only result in the death of the fetus. To ask women whether they would still abort if the fetus could survive and be reared by someone else is not likely to shed much light on their intentions. The question can only suggest the process of carrying the baby to term and putting it up for adoption, and this is precisely what the woman seeking abortion has already decided against doing. If it were really the case that aborted fetuses would stay alive, then women would probably, as Boonin speculates, have the abortions they desire. Yet it seems specious to use this as an argument to prove that women abort primarily to relieve themselves of burden. For if fetuses could live on their own, then presumably they would not be very burdensome. Let's imagine that seventy-five day old fetuses could be removed from the womb and remain necessarily alive (Boonin's condition). I would guess a high percentage of women would choose the procedure and that pregnancy would also quickly come to seem much less a burden. (I use the term "procedure" because, under such circumstances, it would also soon cease being called "abortion"). In short, Boonin's use of counterfactuals to characterize intentions formed in the light of quite contradictory real consequences seems to me highly dubious at best. Worth noting, in fact, is that guaranteeing the survival of fetuses that are aborted would likely eliminate the moral question of abortion.

The value of Thomson's story as counterfactual should also be challenged. Throughout his defenses of Thomson, Boonin relies on our intuition that unplugging the violinist is "permissible." Yet this seems curiously paradoxical, as surely one would only frame the issue in terms of "permissibility" if there were at least some sentiment that unplugging should not be permissible. In that case, it would be necessary to argue for its permissibility. But, as Boonin grants, almost no one ever challenges Thomson on the grounds that it is impermissible to unplug the violinist. Thus we are asked for an intuition about permissibility in a context where it is not really a question. One could say we are asked for an irresponsible response, for we all know it will never again be necessary for us to depend on one unique other in quite the same way as the violinist. I have argued earlier that if each of us did need to be attached, in adulthood, to a unique other for nine months, that it would be understood as a matter of just claim. Various kinds of social support and compensation would undoubtedly be available. If, to modify the counterfactual, it were highly unlikely yet statistically possible that we could find ourselves with a need similar to the violinist's, then social debate might emerge regarding ways to accommodate the special need of "violinists." If the chance were 1 in 10,000, the church might appeal to those needed for the support to look on this as supererogatory service. If 1 in 1000, it's likely that insurance schemes would be devised to cover and compensate the liabilities. It's difficult to say, with any precision, how likely the need of such support would have to be before its refusal began to be discussed as a matter of what is "permissible" or "unpermissible." One thing is certain. The question of unplugging oneself from the violinist would never be discussed in terms of "permissibility" by people who know they will never be in the position of the violinist. Whatever insights we have, then, about unplugging ourselves from violinists are not insights about "permissibility." This seems to me a problem neither Thomson nor Boonin confronts adequately.

V

I will close by registering a specifically Christian reservation about Thomson's and Boonin's situating the story of the violinist under the rubric of good Samaritanism. In doing so, they place their accounts, of course, in relation to the American legal tradition's use of the good Samaritan label to refer to cases involving duties to aid or assist those in need. But it is crucial to note a difference between the way Thomson or the legal tradition understands being a good Samaritan and the gloss Jesus provides for his parable. Thomson's story gives one person the power to determine the fate of another. It is a story about power. "You" have the power to save the life of another; the question is whether you are obligated to do so and at what sacrifice to yourself.

Jesus's story, however, is not about the Samaritan's saving the man at the side of the road from death. The story is not premised on the efficacy or inefficacy of the Samaritan's efforts. "Who acted as neighbor to the man?" the lawyer asks, and Jesus responds, "The one who showed mercy." As we are all continually in response to our neighbors and equally capable of mercy, being a good Samaritan is something that involves the constant exercise of mercifulness. Christians should resist the appropriation of the good Samaritan to name situations contrived in order to make us uniquely powerful over others. Such examples can hardly fail to produce resentment on our part. We need to say with Kierkegaard, "Let journalists and tax-collectors and parish clerks talk about charity and calculate and calculate; but let us never fail to hear that Christianity speaks *essentially* of mercifulness."[15] Commenting on Jesus's story, Kierkegaard asks, "If the Samaritan [horseless and penniless] had gone away carrying the unfortunate man, had sought a softer resting-place for the wounded man, had sat by his side, had done everything in his power to halt the loss of blood—but the unfortunate man died in his arms: would he not have been just as merciful, equally as merciful as that merciful Samaritan[?]" (294). The exercise of mercy is independent of the power to save from death. The world, in Kierkegaard's view, has forgotten this. The world wants charity, lots of it, and forgets mercifulness. This is because "money is the world's god," and "therefore it thinks that everything which has to do with money or has a relationship to money is earnestness" (296). It cannot conceive the value of mercifulness, for "*mercifulness is able to do nothing*" (299).

"But the main thing is still this, that need be met in every way, and that everything possible be done to remedy every need." Here Kierkegaard perfectly anticipates the premise of Thomson's story of the violinist. He attributes this way of speaking to "temporality," grants it is "well-intentioned," and notes that temporality "cannot very well speak otherwise" (301). "Temporal existence" has a "temporal and to that degree an activist conception of need and also has a materialistic conception of the greatness of a gift and of the ability to do something to meet need" (302). Yet this well-intentioned temporality presents the greatest danger, for it makes mercifulness unintelligible. Kierkegaard is not insensitive to the importance of meeting human needs. If preaching is "solely and only about mercifulness," as it should be, "charity will follow of itself and come by itself to the degree to which the individual is capable" (292). But mercifulness is the true ground of our equality before God precisely because it does not depend on anything but obedience to Christ. To "preach ecclesiastically-worldly and worldly-ecclesiastically about charity [and] well-doing" is, "Christianly understood, indecent" (292). It leaves the "poor man" to "groan against" the preacher, in the Biblical sense, for he has been done the "greatest injustice." The poor man lacks the means to be as charitable as the rich, but he is equally able to exercise the qualitatively different virtue of mercy. To Kierkegaard's paradoxical sense of things, it would be truly "terrible" of us to "constrain the poor and wretched to 'hinder our prayers,' as Scriptures say (1 Peter 3:7) by

---

15. Kierkegaard, *Works of Love*, 292. Further references will be given parenthetically.

their groaning against us to God, because we insultingly rebuffed the poor and the wretched by not speaking about how *they* can practise mercy" (293).

If Kierkegaard is right, then something very important is at stake in the insistence that Thomson's famous story is not—Christianly speaking—a matter of good Samaritanism. This is not to deny the need for careful moral reasoning about the extent of our obligation to others. It is, however, to insist that the exercise of mercy marks the good Samaritan, not the generous offering of resources with the power and efficacy to save from death—however well-intentioned and important such action is. Temporality teaches us we are self-interested individuals with the right to expend our time and resources as we wish. The need of another cannot help, then, but be a problem, and we develop accounts of obligation to help us define and limit the amounts we owe. But the good Samaritan, seeking always to act as neighbor in the exercise of mercy, is unlikely to see need either in the other or himself as a threat. Rather he is likely to rest in his need and to seek, as Kierkegaard puts it, to remain in the "debt of love."[16] How the exercise of mercy is likely to play out in concrete circumstances is difficult to say. What must be insisted on, however, is that, Christianly speaking, it is inappropriate to use good Samaritanism to frame issues in such a way that our response can hardly be anything but the practical exercise of mercilessness.

---

16. "We shall not, then, speak about *one's coming into debt by receiving love*. No, it is the one who loves who is in debt; because he is aware of being gripped by love, he perceives this as being in infinite debt. Remarkable! To give a person one's love is, as has been said, certainly the highest a human being can give—and yet, precisely when he gives his love and precisely by giving it he comes into infinite debt. One can therefore say that this is the *essential characteristic of love: that the lover by giving infinitely comes into—infinite debt*. But this is the relationship of infinitude, and love is infinite." *Works of Love*, 172.

6

The Ethics of Genetic Enhancement
A Test of Pragmatism as Democratic Tradition

In *Democracy and Tradition*, Jeffrey Stout makes a wide-ranging case for pragmatism as the philosophical style best suited for ethical discussion in a democracy. The major heroes of Stout's account are Emerson, Whitman, and Dewey; its lesser ones, Thoreau, Rorty, Hegel. Those whom Stout sets himself in opposition to he styles the "new traditionalists": these include John Milbank, Alasdair MacIntyre, and Stanley Hauerwas. The work of the new traditionalists—with its emphasis on the need for communities of virtue and highly self-conscious rearticulation of tradition, particularly the Christian one—has done much, in Stout's view, to undermine democracy. Stout treats Milbank's "radical orthodoxy" as essentially an expression of resentment against the secular whose worst consequence is to encourage formation of a "refuge of aggressive like-mindedness" reinforced by ritualistic denunciations of the "secular 'other' and the unmasking of liberal theological error."[1] Stout suspects MacIntyre's return to Aristotelian virtue cannot help but reinforce hierarchical habits of mind and social arrangements that are deeply in conflict with democracy. Perhaps Stout's most trenchant and sustained criticism is directed at Hauerwas, about whom he remarks, "No theologian has done more to inflame Christian resentment of secular political culture" (140). Many things about Hauerwas rankle Stout, but perhaps nothing more seriously than Hauerwas's insistence that Christians distance themselves from the accounts of justice offered by

---

1. *Democracy and Tradition*, 115. Further citations will be given in the text.

liberal democracy. Hauerwas has, of course, argued that the first task of Christians is to be the church, a community of character shaped ultimately by the narrative of Scripture. This has involved him in stringent criticism of liberalism, understood as a political philosophy that both tries to get along without any sustaining story and which, then, cannot help but undermine every other sustaining story. "There is no doubt," Stout argues, that "the main effect of [Hauerwas's] antiliberal rhetoric, aside from significantly widening his audience, is to undercut Christian identification with democracy" (140).

Stout rejects the new traditionalists' tendency to oppose modernity to tradition. He acknowledges that many early Enlightenment thinkers did regard "themselves as the heralds of a complete break from the past," as champions of modernity and reason over against tradition. But, in retrospect, it is possible to see how much even these figures shared with the past, and, by now, democracy must itself be regarded as a tradition. Democracy "has an ethical life of its own," Stout contends, "which philosophers would do well to articulate," as he, of course, seeks to do. Pragmatism, then, is "best viewed as an attempt to bring the notions of democratic deliberation and tradition together in a single philosophical vision." "*Pragmatism is democratic traditionalism*," Stout argues, a claim best understood as meaning "that pragmatism is the philosophical space in which democratic rebellion against hierarchy combines with traditionalist love of virtue to form a new intellectual tradition that is indebted to both" (13). What Stout cherishes in Emerson and Whitman is a combination of natural piety—rooted in gratitude for what they have received from the past—with strong, anti-hierarchical emphasis on self-reliance. What he derives from Dewey is the "pragmatic insistence that democratic ideals and principles depend for their conceptual content and justification on contingent social practices" (247). "Ethical deliberation and political debate" are the "social practices that matter most directly to democracy," according to Stout, and such essential "discursive exchange" is "likely to thrive only where individuals identify to some significant extent with a community of reason-givers" (293)—hence some of his fears not only of the new traditionalists but of a "business elite" whose involvement in global capitalism causes it to have "some need for the American state" but also allows it to "get along without attending very carefully to the needs of the nation, the people who constitute the community of American citizens."² The model of ethical deliberation and political discussion envisioned by Stout involves the public exchange of intelligible reasons, a holding of one another accountable, and cooperation "in crafting political arrangements that promote justice and decency" (298) in our relations with one another. This is to be done without compromising the integrity necessary to the democratic citizen's crucial self-respect.

Perhaps this may seem a greater foray into political philosophy than the reader of a book on bioethics cares to follow, but I hope that is not the case. One of my purposes throughout has been to place the issues of bioethics in larger ethical, theological, social, and political contexts. It seems critical to do this if crucial decisions about developing bioethical practices are not to be left simply to an ever-more-professionalized cadre of experts. In short, with Stout, I am committed to the public exchange of reasons and the process by which individuals and groups hold one another accountable through reasoned discourse. My contention here is that bioethics may provide a test of pragmatism as democratic traditionalism. A significant group of bioethicists has argued that pragmatism is particularly well-suited to ethical discussion in the field. Jonathan D. Moreno defines bioethics as a naturalism rooted in strongly pragmatic tendencies: rejection of foundationalism, insistence on the experimental character of experience, the "contexted" or "embedded" quality of actual moral problems, the social character of knowing, the intelligent "use of the best available information to craft improved living conditions."³ Joseph J. Fins, Matthew D. Bacchetta, and Franklin G. Miller have stressed the efficacy of "clinical pragmatism" in finding workable solutions to moral problems encountered in clinical settings. For these authors, pragmatism primarily provides a method for conflict resolution between clinicians and patients, one whose goal is to "reach consensus on good outcomes" by a "thorough process of inquiry, discussion, negotiation, and reflective evaluation." Such an approach "embraces principles" but "understands them as tools for guiding conduct, not as absolute fixed moral laws."⁴ Noting pragmatic thought's "basic nonideological but moral tone," Herman J. Saatkamp Jr. describes pragmatism as

---

2. Stout here quotes Hollinger, *Postethnic America*, 15ff. See Stout, *Democracy and Tradition*, 291.

3. Moreno, "Bioethics Is a Naturalism," 16.

4. Fins et al., "Clinical Pragmatism," 30.

"maintaining the priority of the good over truth and as strongly favoring some form of individualism." Saatkamp believes these qualities make pragmatism useful in assessing the innovations of the "new genetics," although he worries that, among other things, pragmatism's too-great insistence on the constant improvement of life may alienate us from "the aesthetic delight of being alive."[5] Summarizing the contributions of the twenty writers for *Pragmatic Bioethics*—where the work of the above writers appears—editor Glenn McGee identifies pragmatism unabashedly with America: "Rooted in American culture, tied to American ideas about social and scientific progress and about health and disease, in many ways pragmatism is America's philosophy." "Its obvious strength," McGee argues, "is its relevance to real life," and with this in mind, he suggests pragmatism's ability "to form a community of inquiry to debate, reform, and finally reconstruct aspects of personal, institutional, and social health care and science."[6]

McGee has given an extended example of a kind of pragmatist ethical argument in *The Perfect Baby: Parenthood in the New World of Cloning and Genetics*. My purpose here is to engage McGee's arguments on the question of genetic enhancement specifically, giving reasons for modifying them or rejecting them outright. A further purpose is to suggest how McGee's practice of pragmatism suggests that pragmatism may not be able to fulfill the function Stout claims for it as the language of democratic traditionalism. In fact, we can see how pragmatism gives rise to the kinds of challenges offered by MacIntyre, Hauerwas, and other advocates of ethics whose primary terms are narrative, community, character, and the virtues. For McGee's pragmatic rhetoric—with its seemingly neutral descriptions of social practices like "reproduction," child rearing, and education—tends to mask important, substantive assumptions about the ends of life, about the kinds of people we should be. In short, one soon finds that engaging McGee in the exchange of reason-giving leads to articulating differences that "go all the way down." If Stout is right that American pragmatism has become a tradition, then perhaps it should be challenged as a tradition, one that—in search of a common faith—insufficiently recognizes differences in practices among groups.[7]

5. Saatkamp, "Genetics and Pragmatism," 155, 167.
6. McGee, introduction to *Pragmatic Bioethics*, xv.
7. One might say that neither Stout nor McGee adequately understands the way technological artifacts become, as Joel Shuman argues, "normal and even 'natural'

McGee's pragmatism is evident in the kind of commonsense reasonableness he brings to the matter of genetic enhancement of children. He begins by defining what he regards to be more extreme positions on biotechnology, positions grounded in metaphysics or, at the very least, in large abstractions like nature and culture. The rhetorical stance is akin to the "just folks" appeal favored by American politicians, media figures, movie stars, and other elites. The opponents McGee needs in order to define his own position include the radical critic of technology, Jeremy Rifkin, feminist Robyn Rowland, phenomenologist Hans Jonas, and to a lesser extent, Leon Kass and Paul Ramsey. McGee treats Rifkin as a Luddite gadfly whose insistence on our "participating with" rather than "dominating" nature reflects a false dichotomy between nature, on the one hand, and human technology on the other.[8] Rowland's fears that bioengineering represents a patriarchal attempt to usurp women's control over the power of reproduction are presented in such a way as to seem extreme or even unreal to any readers unaccustomed to academic feminist discourse.[9] The position of Jonas's that interests McGee most is his claim that genetic engineering posed "ethical questions of a wholly new kind" because it broke down the past "distinction between human beings and the subject of their experiments." In directly contrary fashion, McGee argues that questions like those of genetic enhancement can be resolved pragmatically precisely because they do not pose radically dif-

---

aspects of a way of life that" is consequently deprived of any permanent standards by which to judge the fabricating process. We might see the new traditionalists as rearticulating standards by which the "infinite policing of life and of the body" in the name of technology can be challenged. See Shuman, "Desperately Seeking Perfection," 146. Shuman is following the analysis of technology of Hannah Arendt, particularly that of *The Human Condition*. Shuman's essay is part of an issue of *Christian Bioethics* devoted to considerations of enhancement from various Christian understandings. These include McKenny, "Enhancements and the Quest for Perfection," 99–103; Keenan., "Whose Perfection is it Anyway?," 104–20; Hanson, "Indulging Anxiety," 121–38; Khushf, "Thinking Theologically About Reproductive and Genetic Enhancements," 154–82; Taboada, "Human Genetic Enhancement," 183–96; Engelhardt, "Genetic Enhancement and Theosis," 197–99.

8. McGee, *Perfect Baby*, 52. Further citations will be given parenthetically. McGee quotes from Rifkin's *Algeny*, 251.

9. See *Perfect Baby*, 52–55. The book McGee cites is Rowland, *Living Laboratories*. For a helpful consideration of feminist understandings of women and the reproductive technologies, see Deane-Drummond, *Genetics and Christian Ethics*, 191–219. Deane-Drummond's own positions combine feminist commitments with virtue ethics, with particular emphasis on prudence, justice, charity, and temperance.

ferent issues than other social practices. Contra Jonas, he argues that genetic enhancement poses very similar questions to those posed by other kinds of enhancement—education, for example.[10] Leon Kass and Paul Ramsey figure similarly as foils for McGee. Kass seems too fearful of the hope generated by innovations in biotechnology, too concerned with "big questions" at the expense of modest pragmatic advances.[11] Ramsey is invoked for his comment that "Men ought not to play God before they learn to be men, and after they learn to be men they will not play God." Ramsey is thus made to stand for an attitude of prohibition against delving into the secrets of human biology. Theologians like Ramsey "caution against the coming interference in the restricted territory of hereditary information."[12] This sentence is nicely calculated to at once conjure up images of the Church persecuting Galileo and to appeal to the general American resentment of being interfered with or restricted in any way.

Immediately following McGee's chapter on the thinkers mentioned above is one entitled "Debunking the Myths." Part of such debunking is to score academia for being too distanced from the practical concerns of American citizens, including those regarding bioethics. "Why," McGee asks, "has scholarship concerning genetic technologies failed to produce proactive public hearings, sensible commentary, and nationwide public policy debate?" The answer, he believes, "is fairly simple," and it lies in the failure of American bioethics "to consider what William James, among the last philosophers to play an active role in American political life, termed the *cash value* of our scholarship." "Philosophical discussions of ethical issues in genetics" have too often been written in "jargon-ridden dense" prose suited only for scholars and specialists; such work represents a betrayal of the "universities' promises to be of service to the community at large." Having invoked one founding father of pragmatism, James, McGee now goes on to summon another, Dewey:

> American philosophers have developed ways to measure rigor and success, rankings and professional protocols that have little to do with the life of ideas in the community. Philosophical scholarship thus tends to settle for truths that work within what

---

10. On Jonas, see *Perfect Baby*, 55–58. McGee engages Jonas's *Philosophical Essays*.

11. For McGee on Kass, see *Perfect Baby*, 59–61. McGee has in mind Kass's *Toward a More Natural Science*.

12. On Ramsey, see *Perfect Baby*, 58–60. The quote from Ramsey is from *Fabricated Man*, 138.

> John Dewey called "hermetically sealed systems" of philosophical thinking. Our systems claim to be grounded in religion or "pure reason," and we too often fail to descend from our lofty and elegant ideals into the mundane world of everyday experiences, where we live and make all of our important choices. (64)

Surely there is much that is valid in this assessment of American university scholarship. Alasdair MacIntyre has made a similar point in *Three Rival Versions of Moral Enquiry*, where he argues that the contemporary liberal university is almost completely unable to give an account to the public of what it is doing in such fields as philosophy or literary study.[13]

Where McGee wants to take the argument, though, is quite different from where MacIntyre takes it, and the difference is worth considering for what it suggests about problems with McGee's pragmatism (as well as that of Dewey and Stout). MacIntyre argues, of course, for the university's being revivified by a conscious recapturing and rearticulation of a tradition rooted in practices shared by a wider community. He understands the university's life and the larger social life as being rooted in practices oriented toward particular ends. Ultimately it is possible, then, to ask about university work: What kinds of ends has it historically served? What kinds of ends does it serve best? Under this understanding, it is more possible to sustain the life of the university in some independence from larger social practices than seems possible under McGee's pragmatism. We must note how McGee's description sets the philosophically sealed systems and pure reason of university work over against the social practices of ordinary people, which he argues must form the grounding for real reflection in bioethics and presumably other fields. Rifkin, Rowland, Jonas, Ramsey, Kass represent one kind of discourse rooted in ideology and abstraction whereas a saving pragmatism is instead rooted in the ordinary questions and practices of people as they make real decisions about reproductive choices. But this ignores the fact that university scholarship like that done by any of the five people named above is also rooted in practices. Moreover, it ignores the fact that all five of them are fulfilling one of the traditional ends of the university: that of looking at practices from somewhat greater distance than that of the self-interested participants faced with immediate ethical decisions. The differences between Rifkin et al. and McGee are not differences between abstraction, ideology, and pure reason, on the one hand, and practice on the other.

---

13. MacIntyre, *Three Rival Versions of Moral Enquiry*, 225–28.

Rather they are differences about what practices count, what they mean, how they are to be understood, what sorts of ramifications they have. To take just one example: Jonas and Kass have been particularly concerned about reproductive cloning precisely because they think it will change our whole practice of child-rearing. In setting up his grand opposition of nature and technology, Rifkin may have enlarged the contexts of the practices he is considering beyond the place where his insights are useful or clarifying. But they are nevertheless insights rooted in understanding the practices of technology and how it is changing the world.

McGee's understanding of pragmatism cannot help but have the effect of undermining the university as a place in which specific kinds of disciplined reflection are carried out. If academic philosophic discourse has become too removed from the concerns of ordinary citizens, it is, at least in part, due to the triumph, not the weakness, of pragmatism. The contemporary multiversity is ever more exclusively focused on precisely the kinds of questions McGee, following Dewey, foregrounds: how to find the best possible adjustments between the means made available by current science and the ends of self-interested consumers. If philosophers are out of touch with this—an hypothesis I'm not sure will hold generally—it is because there is still some rearguard action by traditionalists and embattled university departments to maintain an identity distinguishable from generalized sociological reflection on technology—its benefits, liabilities, distribution, and so forth. Philosophical, not to mention theological, reflection may seem removed, too, from the concerns of ordinary citizens because it is no longer deemed necessary for those citizens to be educated in philosophy or theology. Without any larger categories with which to think, citizens will increasingly consider themselves simply self-interested participants in the market.

Offering his work as an alternative to that of Rifkin, Jonas et al., McGee proposes to look at "Commonsense Reproduction and the Idea of the Perfect Baby," to cite the subtitle of one of his chapters. He begins, in pragmatic fashion, by observing that "parenthood is the principal social institution concerned with reproduction" and that "*Hope* defines the journey of parenthood" (81). "Central to preparation for birth and parenthood" is "hope for a parent's 'perfect baby'": "Just as our society celebrates the marrying woman as 'perfect bride,' so too there is emphasis, as an intimate relationship with baby is undertaken, on the perfection of the child" (81).[14] But even "more than hope," "responsible parenting," according to McGee, involves "*choices*," for "choosing to *make* a baby involves a commitment to work to make life better for that baby." Parents make a whole set of choices, from prenatal care onward, which, together with their hopes, "create a moral atmosphere in which our children dwell" (81). McGee does acknowledge that there can be a "dark side" to such hopes: "baby may be forced to attain rigid or foreign ideals," pushed to become the "first doctor in the family" even though such a role does not fit. But McGee never relinquishes the language of perfection: the loss to "baby" in having "foreign ideals" foisted on it is that it will fail "to enjoy perfection of its own sort" (82).

This description of McGee's starting-point makes clear how difficult it can be to engage in intellectual dialogue with pragmatism, for the philosophical style hides highly contestable judgments under the apparently neutral descriptive language of "our" practices. Some of what McGee says seems innocent enough: of course parents have hopes for their children, and responsible parenting means doing what one can to ensure children's health and welfare. But much of McGee's language is not so innocent. Take, for instance, the infatuation with the "perfect baby." I would dispute, as a matter of description, that most people hope for a "perfect baby." If they do, then it would be wise—as a matter of prescription—to urge them to relinquish such hopes, for they can only be disappointed. What McGee is really offering is a description of the way some affluent Western elites have come to think of parenting. These are people affluent and secure enough that having children has become a highly self-conscious process rather than something simply natural

---

14. In an excellent article by an M.D., Taboada has asked whether the issue at stake in genetic enhancement really should be framed as "perfection." McGee's rhetoric certainly suggests that it has been or will be, however unrealistic or damaging to children this will be. Taboada points out that "in medicine, the expression *gene therapy* is used to designate any gene transfer carried out for medical purposes" (190). What she fears is that anti-enhancement arguments may lead to the "undifferentiated rejection" of a whole class of procedures that perhaps do not pose the ethical problems ordinarily associated with enhancements. Among the research lines "that may fall under the general category of *human genetic enhancement*" are "genetic engineering to bolster immune function, to improve the efficiency of DNA repair, to add cellular receptors to capture and process cholesterol, and to enable the patient's bone marrow cells to resist the non-intended effects of chemotherapy" (191). It's worth noting that none of these is obviously intended to confer positional advantage. Each seems classifiable as therapeutic. See "Human Genetic Enhancement," 183–96.

or expected of them by tradition and culture. The welfare democracies provide such elites enough protection against the ravages of life that they no longer need children as providers of security in their own old age. Having children thus becomes a matter of choice, and intelligent consumer behavior dictates, of course, that one should make the best choices possible—thus perfection as an "idea."

The comparison of "baby" to "perfect bride" is telling. It suggests why feminists are right to attack the enterprise of genetic engineering as male usurpation of reproduction. The "perfect bride" is a product of male fantasy, conjurable by a Pygmalion creating Galatea or Hawthorne's Aylmer obsessed with Georgiana's apparent single imperfection in "The Birthmark." Moreover, "perfect bride" or "perfect baby" can exist only as "idea"—as in McGee's language—and thus represent the products of a particularly male kind of objectifying language. The matter is especially critical here—epistemologically, one might say—because McGee's objectifying idealism is being applied to what might be the paradigmatic practices underlying realism: that is, childbirth and child-rearing. We need to think about how child-bearing and rearing might be the underpinnings of a distinctive way of looking at the world. The child is formed in the woman's body, in a kind of continuity with her body, and yet emerges as a being in its own right who nevertheless combines features of both parents and even other ancestors. As the child grows and develops, she or he is present to the parents (and to a lesser degree, the larger group) as a constant continuity in otherness, and otherness in continuity. And this continuity/otherness is always present as embodied human being, not as "idea." Surely this kind of intimate connection with what is "other" must lead to a sense of one's embeddedness in the world that would militate against philosophic idealism. It will lead parents to resist any such attempt as that of an idealist like Emerson to divide the universe into "Nature and the Soul," where nature includes all that is "NOT ME, that is, both nature and art, all other men and my own body"—the lack of gender inclusive language here being, in my view, highly significant.[15] People who tend children's bodies, worry about their survival in the face of earthquake, epidemic, and starvation, and who risk themselves for and in their children seem quite likely to see nature as the real surrounding, sustaining, and potentially killing context of life. Such a nature is the partly knowable yet ultimately mysterious ground of existence, not

---

15. Emerson, *Nature*, 4.

simply an other that functions either for us to construct through our ideas or to elicit ideas from us, as William James would have it.[16]

My point is that McGee's language describes and attempts to normalize childbearing and rearing only as they have come to be understood by people with sufficient technological resources and control to conceive of what they are doing as baby "making" within a process of "reproduction." The bioethical literature on reproduction is filled with hand-wringing over the "commodification" of children that is supposedly a danger, for example, of surrogacy.[17] But what McGee's language reveals is the degree to which children have already become commodified: that babies have become commodities is obvious in descriptions of them as perfect objects capable of being "re-produced" within the social institution of parenthood. McGee's language simultaneously privatizes parenthood, so that the child's "moral atmosphere" results from parental hopes and choices, and reconstitutes it as a problem in "public health." An alternative description would describe parenthood as the form in which people give birth to, rear, and love unique, unrepeatable, imperfect human beings. In the process parents learn how to rear and love and how to accept and rejoice in both their children's and their own inevitable failures to conform to any preconceived idea of what is going on. The effect can be, then, to turn the parents to traditioned sources of wisdom about the parenting and generational process. Parenthood certainly plays a role in social life but it is not primarily a matter of "reproduction," as there are no reproducible commodities involved in it. It is not even primarily a matter of "mak[ing] life better" for baby. Even that seemingly innocuous phrase of McGee's needs to be challenged for the way it inevitably leads to a focus on quantitative measures of the good life. This is not to say we should be unconcerned about making life conditions better for all people. But it is to insist that there is wisdom in Thoreau's saying that one comes "into this world, not chiefly to make this

---

16. I have in mind James's pondering whether "previous reality" is not itself "there, far less for the purpose of reappearing unaltered in our knowledge, than for the very purpose of stimulating our minds to such additions as shall enhance the universe's total value." See *Pragmatism*, 123. In a copy of the *Logic* of Rudolph Hermann Lotze, James wrote in the following terse summary of the matter: "Things for the sake of knowledge not knowledge for that of things." Quoted in James, *Pragmatism*, 172.

17. For an example from a theological point-of-view, see Peters, *For the Love of Children*, 33–34.

a good place to live in, but to live in it, be it good or bad."[18] I want my children to live in it and to learn to serve. If we become too focused on "making life better" for our children—or for each successive generation of Americans, as the current wisdom has it—we will be inclined to focus on quantitative measures because these lend themselves more easily to judgments of comparative success and improvement. There are, in my view, already far too many families in which the absenteeism of working parents is explained always as part of what's required to ensure a "better life" for the children.

McGee's reasons for unpacking the thought of Hans Jonas become especially apparent when he turns to the matter of genetic enhancement of children. With his insistence that genetic technology raises fundamentally new questions for ethics, Jonas serves as the perfect foil for McGee's pragmatist claim that genetic enhancement be seen "within a wider range of other, more mundane parental decisions" (121). For McGee, parents are continually in the process of making enhancement decisions: "The question is not whether but how to enhance the lives and character of our children" (121). At this point in his argument, McGee turns very explicitly to a social constructionist view of the language of medicine. Rejecting our culture's "naïve reliance on a hypostatized idea of what counts as medicine," he offers a loose definition rooted in our practices: "The fact is that our culture happens to choose to deal with certain kinds of problems in buildings called hospitals, where we locate people whom we have trained to do things that we see as desirable to our bodies" (126). When "new interventions are proposed," then, we should not ask "Is this medicine or enhancement? But rather 'Will this approach to this issue work better than others?'" (126).

Norman Daniels's "species-typical functioning" comes in for particular criticism from McGee. The "species-typical account of normalcy posits without justification that members of the species are born with largely determined sets of capacities." Such capacities cannot be understood "without reference to human social norms." "According to this account," McGee continues, "we first unearth data about what counts as an impairment, then round up everyone who is affected, and finally make sure that those with the most impairment receive the most treatment, while those who are unimpaired are entitled to no treatment. But who

---

18. "Civil Disobedience," 396.

decides what to measure in the first place, or how to draw the line between impairment and enhancement in the raw data?" (125).[19]

Open to question here is McGee's assumption that defining species-typical function depends on assuming "largely determined sets of capacities." The language of "capacities" itself pictures human beings as so much force or power to do, to work, to produce output. An alternative description might stress our vulnerability to pain, suffering, and death. Such a description would lead to the conclusion that our accounts of disease do have a grounding in the natural experience of the body. The major childhood illnesses, AIDS, polio, typhoid, malaria, cancer, heart disease; these produce pain and premature death—"premature" by species-typical standards. Bodily experience provides the norms by which these conditions can be judged diseases. I would suggest that it is only our relative security against these diseases in the Western bourgeois democracies—where most bioethics is done—that gives credence to a purely pragmatic definition of medicine. If the Western democracies still suffered from the great childhood epidemics, it would be more difficult to argue credibly that "disease" and "health" name only "cultural evaluations of what kinds of traits are problematic or desirable in our lives" (125).

Christians might well want to endorse the very notion of treatment caricatured by McGee as a round-up of all the impaired (I'd prefer "afflicted") for triage. Such a picture of care might well lead us to fund broad programs of vaccination or drug distribution in developing countries before we support cosmetic plastic surgery, therapy for shyness, or genetically enhanced intelligence for Americans.[20]

Contra McGee, it is not question-begging to insist "that plastic surgery or designer drugs are 'not medical'" (126). "We get much more mileage," he reasons, out of judgments about "whether a particular method works well in clinical settings or is the most effective option in our social or personal quiver than judgments based on whether an intervention is properly classed as natural or medical" (126). McGee himself simply begs the question of who "we" are here; he assumes an agreement about ends that he has not demonstrated to exist. His pragmatism seems typically managerial: questions about ends are made to disappear through

---

19. McGee is responding to Daniels, *Just Health Care*.

20. For ways to begin thinking about national and international health care reform, see Cahill, *Theological Bioethics*, 131–68.

concentration on adopting the right means, which, in practice, means the most efficient ones—the ones that give us the most mileage, the most bang for our buck, the most Jamesian "cash value." When some of us insist, then, that procedures like cosmetic surgery be regarded as "non-medical," we do so as a way to resist the omnicompetent managers. The rhetorical choice appeals to our common experience of bodily suffering and invokes an implicit agreement about the sorts of burdens one must bear without assistance from others. Of course the language is value-laden, but it is not simply "constructed," for it responds to the lived bodily experience of pain, suffering, and limitation.

McGee makes the issue of genetic enhancement go away by placing it within the context of other things we do to "improve" our children. The pragmatic focus on means forecloses all discussion of ends, and "we" are enlisted for action in causes whose worth we are not to question. First he assures us that the power of genetic manipulation is unlikely to "revamp the human species" or "destroy our human natures." It seems we should have greater fear of "conventional social institutions, such as schools and churches," for these "have a much more immediate effect on who we become" (127). Yet later we're told, quite without qualification, that we ought not to see a difference in kind between genetic improvement of human beings and "public education," in which "we invest billions of dollars in the attempt to make people more intelligent and less aggressive" (127–28). The possibility that our skepticism about genetic enhancement might carry over into reservations about public education—when it understands itself as an attempt to "improve" our children—is not examined.

A tendency to foreclose assumptions is evident, again, in the way McGee frames the issue of eugenics. Here there is plenty to fear, McGee grants, but "the fear is not of genetic control, it is of socially prescribed blueprints of perfection, enforced by intolerant scientists-cum-bureaucrats" (127). I'd like to be able to choose my own fears. Some of us do fear "genetic control"—particularly that resulting in what we regard as "enhancement"—and especially because we think intolerant bureaucrats are unlikely to recognize their own intolerance. Commenting further on eugenics, McGee can find no harsher word than "misadventures" to describe "the results in our century." I should add that I fear the inability to imagine evil represented by such a pallid description.

The displacement of moral by practical language is an important part of pragmatism's mystification of power. McGee argues that "a scientifically styled 'perfect society,' stratified by genes, makes little sense in a world where genetic variability turns out to be a virtue—and in which specialization and rigidity spell extinction" (127). Arguing the policy "makes little sense" precludes consideration of its rightness; the question becomes an empirical one, whose answer could presumably be different if a way could be found to make it "make sense." Moreover, it obscures the way in which different groups might be impacted by such a policy; wealthy elites with a relatively short time-horizon might well be benefited by the ability to encourage genetic design of masses of workers, consumers, taxpayers, and soldiers. McGee then closes his account of legitimate fears of eugenics by observing that "there are also plenty of practical examples of the danger of replacing parental responsibility with overarching social control" (127). Again parental and social control raise only practical questions, not moral ones about the degree of power one person should exercise over another. These questions simply disappear as the pragmatist concentrates on the practical questions.

The guiding assumption of McGee's defense of genetic enhancement is that it represents only an extension of ways parents currently seek to enhance their children. In a descriptive sense, what he argues is probably accurate: many parents do seem to think of what they're doing as enhancement or improvement of their children. And stated in general terms, the goal seems unexceptionable. Who could oppose enhancing children? Or, to paraphrase the authors of *From Chance to Choice*, why shouldn't parents "be free to use genetic intervention techniques to produce the best offspring they can"?[21] One answer to this question may seem improbable here, but I will defend it from a Christian point-of-view. Parents ought not to seek to produce "the best offspring," because, in doing so, they will fail to recognize what they already have.

This is to say that Christians should challenge the first assumption of McGee's. How to do this is very difficult, as pragmatism, in its very assumptions, tends to preclude moral questioning. McGee, for instance, begins with a description of how people parent (that is, how affluent Western elites parent), then shows that genetic enhancement is basically continuous with practices already in place, and concludes there's no very good reason to prevent parents from genetically enhancing children as

---

21. Buchanan et al., *From Chance to Choice*, 156.

long as they do so within certain practical limits. The method of foreclosing moral challenge is evident in a concluding remark of McGee's on the specific matter of cloning and individuality: "No child has an open future, and even a cursory examination of the changing history of parenthood makes clear that it is not individuality but rather correct forms of responsible relation that is the goal" (152). I would call this a too easy move from fact to value, the kind Hume warned against long ago, except I suspect that pragmatism simply gradually squeezes out questions of value. McGee argues that from parenthood's history we can know its goal. How does one challenge this morally? How does one say that parenting should not involve certain practices, no matter what is true historically? Guided by the history of what parents have done, we know the goal of parenting and something of what the best means to achieve parental preferences has been. The question becomes simply one of finding the best match between means and ends as we go about enhancing our children.

One way to respond to McGee's claims is by offering a different description of parenting. The beginning of McGee's account of ordinary enhancements provides a place to begin differentiating Christian parenting from enhancement. "Parenthood," McGee asserts, "sometimes feels like a laboratory in enhancement" (126–27). The laboratory metaphor is revealing in its implicit objectification of the child and the distancing it suggests between the experimenter and the one subjected to experimentation. The living bond between parent and child seems excluded by the metaphor. Children appear rather as resources "to develop": "All of us with children experience the pressure to develop the life of an infant, a young person, a young adult." It is difficult to see how the performer of experiments aimed at developing the child can experience anything like wonder at the child's presence, wonder that would be the first sign of a reality transcending his own will. Making his case further for continuity of genetic enhancement with enhancements already sanctioned, McGee refers to education:

> We invest billions of dollars in the attempt to make people more intelligent and less aggressive. We call this attempt public education. As with eugenics, the goal of education is to design and inculcate skills and norms in the behaviors of offspring, from sexual mores through beliefs about history to respect for the law. Athletic activity and school lunches are designed so that children

grow up to be stronger, more capable, and smarter. Those who do not perform well in school are "failed," and miss out on college, better-paying work, or social success. (127–28)

I have quoted McGee at length here in order to examine the ideas closely. First, I have a good bit of anecdotal evidence that suggests public education does not make people "less aggressive." Each year I teach a considerable number of recent graduates of public education, and if there's one conviction they share, it is that life is a kind of ruthless Darwinian struggle endlessly working to separate winners from losers. They are made more aggressive, not less, by education as it is now conducted. The reason for this is evident in McGee's own language with its heavy use of comparative judgments. He would provide athletic programs and school lunches to make children "stronger, more capable, and smarter" rather than healthy, able to learn, well-nourished, and perhaps even trusting of adults who care for them. But it's critical to be "strong, capable, and smart" in McGee's school world, for there one must "perform" and the judgment of the school seems as either-or as the thumbs up or down of performances in other empires: to fail is to "miss out on college, better paying work or social success." To cite the language of one of my students, to fail to go to college is to become "disposable." One hopes the division of the failed from the successful is not as absolute in our society as this suggests. If it is, one might suggest the divide is due less to the enhanced skills of the successful than to the success of the credentialed in getting a bachelor's degree established as the entrance requirement for all kinds of jobs that really require almost nothing learned in one's formal education beyond grade school. The psychological and economic value of such credentialing ought not to be ignored: it allows masses of the educated to feel themselves justified in earning incomes hundreds or even thousands of times greater than the world's poor—and consuming commensurately.

Perhaps even more disturbing is McGee's straightforward connection of eugenics to public education. He wants, of course, to sanitize eugenics by comparing it to something we all grant to be necessary, if not entirely desirable. But perhaps one should simply reverse the comparison and use it to raise the deepest kinds of questions about public education in mass society. The "misadventures" of eugenics (to use McGee's words) sought straightforwardly to improve populations by killing or sterilizing those deemed undesirable. We might say, in Deweyan terms, that the eugenicists of the twentieth century found the perfect adjustment between means and ends. To think that public education could even conceivably be compared to eugenics, as McGee does, ought perhaps to be seen as reason to close all the schools tomorrow. One might ask what happened to the conception of the school as a specifically educational institution, one entrusted with teaching academic subjects such as mathematics, physical and biological sciences, philosophy, history, and literature. Clearly one thing that has happened under pragmatism is the triumph of behaviorism, which undermines basic assumptions about mind, choice, will, and judgment: note that, for McGee, even "beliefs about history" are simply one form of "the behaviors of offspring." Rarely has there been a clearer echo of Plato's *Republic*, with its insistence that social order depends on the elite's carefully designing the kinds of stories to be told (and, of course, censoring those unconducive to socially-desired behaviors).

Perhaps it has been necessary to identify education with the "improvement of children" in order to ensure its support by a utilitarian public. Perhaps it is only possible to garner support for mass education by designing the schools to produce a particular product: the "strong, capable, smart" winner-worker (white collar), consumer, taxpayer, and supporter of the nation. In any case, conceiving of students as tools to be designed serves the functionalist conception of mass society identified by Gabriel Marcel fifty years ago.[22] It hardly matters whether this pragmatic, top-down model of education as management preceded and caused the development of mass societies or is a consequence of it. What should be observed is how neatly the reduction of children to tools dovetails with the total organization of societies required by the mass wars of the twentieth century and the welfare states' systematic movement of resources from the young to old. Capitalism's need for a highly mobile work force also is served by reduction of the parent-child relationship to that between detached scientist-experimenter and object of experiment. Large corporate structures—private and state—put enormous demands on workers' time and energy, both directly and through taxation. How convenient, then, to conceive of parenting as management; it's difficult to see how parents who spend only a few minutes a day interacting with the child could conceive of it otherwise. Efficiency must rule in the home, as elsewhere. One particularly troubling feature of the new eugenics is its

---

22. See Marcel's wonderful and underappreciated *Man Against Mass Society*.

conversion of the home into simply another institution devoted to manipulating the child. There is no longer room, or time, for unconditional love even in the home. The total mobilization of social effort requires every child to be improved—by education now, by eugenics as soon as possible.

To be committed to ceaseless improvement is to believe, necessarily, that nothing is ever good enough. Parents committed to improving their children communicate the conviction that their children are not good enough. One need hardly point out the connection between parental expectations of this kind and our children's lack of self-esteem. To argue against improving our children is not to diminish the importance of education. All children, by birthright, ought to be introduced to as much as possible of the accumulated wisdom of human beings; they should be given the knowledge, tools, and methods needed to explore the physical and natural sciences; and they should be assisted in acquiring the learning and skills necessary for them to find satisfying ways of serving others through their knowledge. But there is every difference between enabling our children to know and to serve and making better children. The first implies greater respect for our children's integrity, the design of institutions to fit the particulars of individuals, and reduced emphasis on competition; the latter ensures that all children will be inadequate yet some, the winners, will be less so than others, and they will design social practices and institutions to perpetuate and strengthen their advantages. Once one can produce a better tool, it would be irrational not to alter systems and environments in such a way as to maximize its utility.

One wonders whether the obsession with improving children doesn't derive from a deep conviction that we ourselves are unworthy. Perhaps we fear that our children will not be good enough, that they will not represent us in the way we would like. The desire to have one's identity perpetuated is a powerful motive in parents; we should ask seriously whether arguments for enhancing children are based on concern for children or on the parental desire to reduce the risk of producing children inadequate to our self-conceptions (delusions). Genetic enhancement would ensure in advance that parental "investment" would be adequately compensated. (Although the increasing of control and thus of expectation may very well, in practice, leave parents less satisfied with their children than previously).

Conceiving of children as products or objects to be fashioned may help parents limit the psychological cost of losing them. Conceiving of children as objects of our fashioning seems clearly to limit or reduce emotional attachment on the part of parents. "Making" itself implies an objectification; the language of "baby making" and even of "re-production" involve a forgetting or suppression of the mother's bodily connection to the child. The language of objectification reflects and encourages thinking of children as replaceable. Of course the standard response of many geneticists, at this point, is to say that increased genetic control, even cloning, poses no threat to human uniqueness as every person is largely the product of his or her own experiences. There is truth to this claim, although it seems just a little disingenuous as a defense of cloning, which is, after all, an attempt to replicate. But perhaps it's a mistake to think of replaceability in simple binary fashion. We sometimes speak of finding near-replacements for objects that we lose, or even for beloved pets. The objectifying language of baby-making moves children further toward this category of the nearly replaceable. The controlled shaping of genetic inheritance can be replicated: whatever we learn to shape and control can be repeated. Moreover, to stress parental enhancement of children is to encourage parents to see their own images of their children rather than the children themselves. And parental images are replicable, infinitely.

In recommending the single life for the man who would seek great accomplishments, Francis Bacon anticipated the attitude toward marriage and children of today's affluent idolaters of work: "He that hath wife and children hath given hostages to fortune; for they are impediments to great enterprises, either of virtue or mischief."[23] Under the guise of encouraging greatness, Bacon advocates an eminently safe doctrine, one that provides justification for avoiding exposure to "fortune." For children are "hostages" to fortune, and, as Bacon understands, parents become hostages themselves in having children. A central part of the experience of parenthood and parental love is to realize that one is now more exposed to hostile fortune in the person of another, the child, than in oneself. Parenthood is an experience of learning to live "out of control"; it is to take the radical risk of loving another "as oneself," and, because of that very love, to allow and even encourage that other to become him or herself—thus exposing the parent to maximum risk. One Christian

---

23. Bacon, "Of Marriage and Single Life," 22.

objection to the pragmatist model of "parent as scientist-enhancer" is that the model precludes change and transformation in the parents as they rear their children. Parents too often think of rearing as a one-way process, ignoring the way children rear their parents. One learns to parent by doing it and by the child's showing the parent how to do it. What one learns from rearing one child often has nothing to tell one about rearing the next; in fact it often must be forgotten or unlearned. Thus parenthood is one of the experiences by which we learn to see human beings, lovingly, as individuals. Jesus illumined our own experience of parenthood when he spoke of his Father's knowing the very number of hairs on our heads, his ability to differentiate infinitely among his children, all held in love.

Why should Christian parents avoid using genetic techniques for purely enhancement purposes?[24] Because ultimately to become the omnipotent administrator of the child's future is to refuse the discipline of the Trinity as guide to one's parenting. The parent as laboratory scientist suggests the self-enclosed isolation specifically rejected by God. As Karl Barth writes, "God could also be a God enthroned high above man," omnipotently running everything in the human world like some perfect manager or technician who never needed even to consult with those he manipulates. And "it might be asked whether it would not be better for all concerned if God were to act in this manner." But he has not done so. He has willed to honor human beings as our commander and partner, and in his grace he wills to need us "truly and seriously," though this need must be construed as part of his freedom and not as a lack or imperfection.[25] The Trinitarian love is continually being offered by the Father to the Son and freely offered back by the Son. Rather than seeing this relationship as somehow the "product of a sublimation of strictly human relationships," Gabriel Marcel has suggested we should recognize how much our human "relationships themselves, in the course of history, have been deepened and renewed under the action of a transcendental idea, without which what we call our nature would never have been able to evolve fully."[26] The Trinitarian love, freely given and freely returned,

---

24. By "purely" enhancement purposes here I mean those not designed to restore or establish ordinary functioning. I have in mind the kinds of examples usually cited in the literature: improvement of intelligence, height, memory beyond species-typical norms.

25. Barth, *Church Dogmatics*, 4/3, 649.

26. Marcel, *Homo Viator*, 101.

should, and does, discipline our parenting. That love—which takes the form of kenosis, the self-emptying in ultimate risk that trusts in God's infinite love—seems utterly inconsistent with designing the child as an artifact.

This chapter has, I hope, suggested both the limitations of pragmatism as a philosophic framework for bioethics, at least regarding genetic enhancement, and the reasons one must articulate a broad, traditioned understanding of practices like childrearing in order to challenge pragmatism. McGee's version of pragmatism simply assumes too much in its description of "our" social practices: that genetic enhancement is like education is not, to some of us, obvious; that education itself be understood as enhancement is, to some of us, odious; that species-typical functioning should be disregarded in defining what constitutes enhancement depends upon a bracketing of justice considerations that some of us resist. In order to challenge McGee's assumptions, I have had to develop something like a mini-narrative of Christian parenting. This way of proceeding sheds light, I think, on the much larger project of the new traditionalists whose work Stout finds so unfriendly to democracy. In order to challenge the reigning paradigms of American pragmatic-scientific progressivism, writers like MacIntyre and Hauerwas have found it necessary to rearticulate whole traditioned ways of life rooted in narratives, practices, and virtues related to particular ends of life. That such a thoroughgoing challenge has arisen at this moment of history may well reflect the near hegemony of the American progressivism called into question by the new traditionalists. There is, in my view, nothing anti-democratic about the work of either MacIntyre or Hauerwas unless it has become anti-democratic to locate descriptions of the good life within narratives sufficiently authoritative to challenge the pretensions of consumerism, scientism, and American power. Indeed Hauerwas has, in my judgment, performed a real, if unintended, service to American democracy through his insistence that the first task of the church is to be the church. For only if the church understands itself in this way can the world understand itself as world—that is, as a realm of limited powers whose ultimate dependence on violence to ensure security has been brought under judgment in the cross of Christ.

This is not the place for a full-scale assessment of pragmatism, but before closing, I do want to highlight three things that concern me in the way McGee's pragmatism functions. I'll pose them, in the spirit of pragmatic inquiry that guides my own analysis, as questions for Jeff Stout.

The first springs from McGee's observation that pragmatism is "America's philosophy." It is difficult to assess just what such a statement means or implies, and I am not one to engage in simplistic America bashing. Nevertheless, if this is the case, should it give us pause? Should it make us wary of pragmatism as part and parcel of the American transformation of the globe? I think we can see in McGee's work some cause to be wary of pragmatism precisely for this reason. I have in mind McGee's argument that we should ignore species-typical accounts of functioning in distinguishing therapies from enhancements. He claims we get "more mileage" if we focus on the effectiveness of a particular intervention and abandon concern about whether it's "properly classed as natural or medical" (126). The approach seems typically American, even to the driving metaphor, and it's no doubt true that effectiveness or efficiency can be maximized by declaring contrary considerations irrelevant. The argument brackets considerations of justice implicit in species-typical language, as I pointed out earlier. The justice of health-care distribution has apparently ceased to matter, which, if we remember Hume's analysis of justice, might make us conclude that a condition of such abundance has been reached as to make justice no longer necessary.[27] McGee's pragmatic way of defining medicine, then, may simply reflect the condition of abundant resources available, at least until very recently, in America's wealthiest HMOs and hospitals. To continue thinking of medicine pragmatically—that is, in terms of finding the most effective means to get what we want—would seem to require an economy of ceaseless growth. The implications of one nation's committing itself to a policy of limitless economic expansion in a world of very unequal powers are, to say the least, ominous. This nation would be required, at a minimum, to ensure the dependable, steady flow of inexpensive energy sources; to encourage vast concentrations of corporate power in the name of efficiency (efficiencies they could then deliver, at least in the short term, by using their power to dictate market and labor conditions); to convert every available

---

27. See *An Enquiry Concerning the Principles of Morals*, 39. Hume writes, "Thus, the rules of equity or justice depend entirely on the particular state and condition in which men are placed, and owe their origin and existence to that utility, which results to the public from their strict and regular observance. Reverse, in any considerable circumstance, the condition of men: Produce extreme abundance or extreme necessity: Implant in the human breast perfect moderation and humanity, or perfect rapaciousness and malice: By rendering justice totally *useless*, you thereby totally destroy its essence, and suspend its obligation upon mankind."

citizen into an economic subject first, at whatever cost to their other roles or identities; and to displace a whole variety of costs—monetary, human, natural—from present to future—i.e., to incur great levels of debt because the imperative of growth is *now*. To what degree, we should ask, is pragmatism implicated in these problems? Does its apparent claim that the only meaningful questions of ethics or policy are those that can be resolved consequentially tend to undermine traditional sources of wisdom that would enable people to live within limits? Does the focus on "cash value" encourage the dangerous illusion that we have greater predictive power than we do? Do we protect ourselves from recognizing this illusion by exerting ever greater social control (now by education, perhaps later by genetic design) in order to guarantee consequences we've predicted? Are we required—by the demands of prediction—to persuade everyone that no matter what else they may be, they are—in something like *essence*—self-interested economic maximizers, rational consumers? What, then, are the consequences for citizenship and democracy of these trends in which pragmatism is, at least arguably, implicated?

My second question for pragmatism is closely related to the first. Does pragmatism inevitably foster short-term thinking, perhaps through the very substitution of what Dewey called "intelligent method" for more traditional kinds of wisdom? Consider the following from Dewey, quoted by McGee: "If intelligent method is lacking, prejudice, the pressure of immediate circumstance, self-interest and class-interest, traditional customs, institutions of accidental historical origin, are *not* lacking, and they tend to take the place of intelligence" (138). This quote poses a whole nest of problems, only a couple of which I'll point out here. Surely intelligent method has been, and can be, successfully and happily employed against prejudice and the too great pressure of immediate circumstance. But Dewey seems too willing to deny that traditions, institutions, and even class consciousness carry forms of wisdom unavailable to the "intelligence" of the isolated individual—forms of wisdom rooted, specifically, in the experience of communities through time.

Jeff Stout has shown some willingness to admire the criticism of our contemporary culture by Wendell Berry, and Berry seems precisely the necessary contrast to Dewey here.[28] Dewey sounds like no one so much as the advocates of industrial farming against whom Berry inveighs. These largely academic and government advocates of agribusi-

---

28. On Berry, see Stout, *Democracy and Tradition*, 134–35.

ness tend to consider agricultural problems always as those involving production and distribution within the world food system. These can be approached—they confidently aver—through the systematic application of intelligent method. But Berry would argue that any intelligent method worth its salt will have to begin by learning the intimate particularities of all the innumerable fields, orchards, and pastures where food is grown, not produced, by farmers. That kind of intimate learning will soon discover that "intelligent method" can hardly discount the wisdom preserved in traditions, in people's character, in institutions that have arisen in response to historical conditions, in local custom and memory. A wise regard for these minutely particularized kinds of knowing will caution us against a too-great reliance on the abstractions of method, which, in their focus on finding the appropriate means to solve current problems, cannot help but be somewhat shortsighted. We might well ask pragmatists, then, whether they ought not to seek correction and discipline from traditionalists, old and new, who carry kinds of knowledge unavailable to the intelligent expert isolated in his own moment in time.

What makes this question particularly significant in the context of genetic enhancement and design is that we are here proposing to alter the relationship between parent and child that is surely central to our whole sense of time frames—of what counts as short-term and long-term. What, in my view, stands the best chance of causing us to take long-term views of the consequences of our actions is a sense of the adequacy of what we have received from the past. As we discover the adequacy of the past to sustain us over a whole lifetime, we learn to trust our children to become the people they will be without excessive intervention from us. Actually the process works in both directions; we learn to trust that what sustains us is good as we see it coming to good in our children—sometimes in ways we could hardly anticipate. Like Jacob, when he discovers Joseph alive in Egypt, we learn over the course of a whole life that it is "enough" (Gen 45:28). And because it is enough we want to pass the sustaining contexts of life on to future generations. We come to this knowledge of the way generations sustain one another only through full lives understood in narrative terms. This is not, of course, to say we should never intervene in the conditions of life from fear of breaking the generational bond. It is to say, however, that we should be extremely wary of processes like genetic enhancement that threaten to change altogether the relations between one generation and another.

My last question for pragmatism concerns the effect on the imagination caused by a too exclusive focus on means-end rationality. It is prompted by a comment of McGee's offered as illustration of the truth of Dewey's comments on intelligent method quoted above. As an example of the kinds of influences that operate where "intelligent method is lacking," McGee notes, "the few fetal diagnoses available now are so expensive that only the wealthy can use them. As a consequence, a disproportionate number of children with Down's syndome are 'almost certainly born to the less affluent'" (138). The passage offers a clear illustration of why Hauerwas has insisted that Christians should be wary of committing themselves to programs of Rawlsian justice. Social policy is unintelligent, for McGee, where the poor lack equal access to the means to identify and abort Down fetuses. The problem is basically one of society's failure to realize Rawlsian justice as fairness. And, given McGee's assumptions about the kind of life that counts, it would be difficult to argue with him. Who could be opposed to egalitarian access to the means of genetic control and enhancement? Moreover, is there any real doubt that care of a Down child will tend to cause a "less affluent" American family to remain "less affluent," thereby missing out on the sacred promise of our national life? Part of what I want to say is that McGee, despite the best intentions, has said nothing of relevance to Down children (I resist here saying "to the *issue* or *problem* of Down children"). But to say that McGee's comments about Down children (or poverty) are not exhaustive requires an alternative imagination, one nurtured by other sources than pragmatism's account of intelligence as problem-solving rationality or our culture's standard accounts of justice, whether egalitarian or libertarian. One of the sources capable of nurturing an imagination receptive to all children, however imperfect, is the gospel, as Hauerwas has faithfully reminded us. If pragmatism undermines this kind of imagination, as McGee's practice of it arguably does, then it surely cannot be a sustaining philosophy for democracy.

7

Why Designing the Subjects of Justice Is Likely to Be Unjust

In *From Chance to Choice: Genetics and Justice*, Allen Buchanan, Dan Brock, Norman Daniels, and Daniel Wikler pose a series of knotty problems for the theory of justice in an "age of genetic intervention."[1] The book's central conclusions are sometimes a bit difficult to discern precisely, perhaps because of its multiple authorship, its method of seeking wide reflective equilibrium, and the inherently speculative quality of some of the possibilities addressed. The authors' statement of intention seems modest enough. They begin by noting that the sorry history of eugenics has largely discredited public health approaches to genetic intervention, and, as a result, the "personal service model"—with necessary moral firebreaks—has dominated ethical reflection on the issues. Finding this approach arbitrary and unsystematic, Buchanan et al. "argue that although respect for individual autonomy requires an extensive sphere of protected reproductive freedoms and hence a broad range of personal discretion in decisions to use genetic interventions, both the need to prevent harm to offspring and the demands of justice, especially those regarding equal opportunity, place systematic limits on individuals' freedom to use or not use genetic interventions" (13–14). That one might be limited in one's freedom to refuse genetic intervention seems chilling, but otherwise the aim seems modest, especially as the authors insist that health care, "so far as it is a concern of justice, has to do only with the treatment and prevention of disease" (17).

1. Buchanan et al., *From Chance to Choice*, 3. Further references will be given parenthetically.

Despite these apparently limited purposes, at times the authors seem to be laying the groundwork for a vast expansion of social control over human genetics based on appeals to justice. Immediately following the passage cited above, for instance, they argue "that some versions of the level playing field conception extend the requirements of equal opportunity, at least in principle, to interventions to counteract natural inequalities that do not constitute diseases" (17). Traditionally, the authors note, natural inequalities have not been regarded to be within the scope of justice. The unequal distribution of talents and capacities has not, in itself, been seen as something justice requires us to correct. Some recent theorists, however, have proposed that "justice requires redistributing social goods in order to compensate those with less desirable natural assets." Yet these theorists "have not considered the possibility that justice might sometimes require altering the natural assets themselves, perhaps for the simple reason that until very recently this has been unthinkable" (63–64). Now, of course, the possibility of altering natural assets has at least become "thinkable," and thus, according to the authors, the theory of justice must engage the issue. If "precise and safe control over the distribution of natural assets becomes feasible," then justice may require compensating for bad luck "by attacking natural inequalities directly" rather than through intervention in the social lottery alone (64).

Numerous areas of the authors' discussion of genetics and justice demand a widening of the reflection and a disturbing of the equilibrium. In order to keep my treatment limited here, I will focus on four specifically. I begin by raising some questions about the equal opportunities rationale for treatment of disease and then about the authors' "ethical autopsy" of eugenics—specifically about the claim that the "greatest single flaw of eugenics was its failure to take justice seriously" (100). The third area I want to address involves the authors' treatment of the distinction between enhancement and therapy. Although they set out to defend the distinction as reasonable, some of their argument seems to discount the distinction in favor of a much more expansive role for genetic intervention. I will defend the distinction and suggest the authors' problematic test cases are perhaps not as problematic as they seem to be. The final area of my analysis concerns the conception of justice itself under which the authors believe themselves to be operating. They draw a sharp distinction between two broad approaches to justice: one they call justice as "self-interested reciprocity," the other, "subject-centered justice." Basically justice as self-interested reciprocity holds that justice is obligatory among members of a community who are capable of engaging in productive exchanges. Subject-centered theories, on the other hand, constitute communities based on some quality such as sentience and then insist that we have obligations of justice to all quite apart from their "capacity to make a net contribution to social cooperation" (295).[2] The authors identify themselves with a subject-centered theory, but it is my contention that their work is better understood as the expression of justice as self-interested reciprocity. By reflecting on the way they correlate each of these theories with issues of genetic intervention, we can see how each captures something of our fundamental intuitions about justice and yet how each needs to be supplemented by insights captured better by the other.

I

The authors of *From Chance to Choice* ground their arguments in an equal-opportunity rationale for the treatment of disease. Aligning themselves with a "level playing field" construal of equal opportunity, they distinguish between a "social-structural view," associated with Rawls, and the "much more expansive" brute-luck view (66–68). The first requires efforts to counter the effects of "past institutional injustice, including the unjust distribution of wealth," but it focuses on "limitations on opportunity that originate in unjust institutions, not in natural differences between persons." The brute-luck view, on the other hand, insists that equal opportunity "requires efforts to counteract the effects of all factors beyond an individual's control," including how she "fares in the natural lottery" (67). Obviously the brute-luck view would seem more supportive of genetic interventions, but the authors ultimately contend that even their preferred social-structural view may do so.

The argument for an apparent extension of the social-structural view begins with the assumption that "the significance of disease is that it limits opportunity in the most serious cases, at least, by preventing persons from developing the threshold of abilities necessary for being 'normal competitors' in social cooperation" (74). This description ought

---

2. The authors find "variants" of justice as self-interested reciprocity in "Epicurus, Hobbes, Hume, and, with the greatest sophistication, in the work of David Gauthier"; "subject-centered" theories are those of Kant and utilitarianism (295). For Gauthier, see especially *Morals By Agreement*.

not to go unquestioned. First, it gives inadequate attention to the ill person's own bodily experience, to the pain, suffering, isolation, fear and threat of death that illness brings. Some people also will probably never develop the abilities necessary for the kind of "competition" seemingly implicit in the authors' description. Others have no desire to engage in such competition, and still others have retired from it. In short, there is no prospect of "bringing these people up" to levels of normal competition, and yet surely we do not want to use this fact to limit their claims to be treated.[3]

One of the authors' examples should help us to think about the reasons we support something so fundamental as care of the sick. The authors note, quite appropriately, that "if a baby is born with a hip deformity . . . an effort will be made to marshal social resources to pay for surgical repair of this condition if the parents lack health insurance and cannot afford to pay the surgical bill" (70). They go on to argue that "one obvious and compelling justification for subsidizing this procedure is that it is necessary in order to remove a serious obstacle to opportunity" (70–71). But if this is the case, would there be less obvious justification for subsidizing the hip repair if the child showed evidence of mental limitation sufficient to prevent his ever being a normal social competitor? I would argue we ought to subsidize the hip repair without regard to the child's ability ever to become a future competitor because prevention or correction of undue harm, not provision of equal opportunity, is the goal of medical treatment. One might object that prevention of harm and provision of equal opportunity are so closely related as to be inextricable: that we prevent harm from a concern for equal opportunity. But I would contend the two motives are indeed very different and that it is important to keep this clear, for quite different understandings of polity and power flow from the way we construe the relation between these descriptions of motive.

Prevention of harm keeps the focus on the sufferer herself rather than on some imagined capacity for social contribution she may later make. It is a subject-centered description rather than one that erases the subject in reconceiving her illness as a matter of social policy. Treatment of illness to prevent or correct harm affirms an equality that already exists.[4] I would suggest its roots lie in an understanding of our equal

    3. "Bringing up" is the authors' language; see, e.g., 74.
    4. The difficulties involved in defining such terms as "disease," "health," "needs," and "opportunity" are helpfully addressed in Daniels, *Just Health Care*, 19–35. One major

vulnerability to disease and death. As long as we think of ourselves as standing continually under that "power of deduction," to adapt Foucault, we will see the justice of remedying that which threatens to take away from the way we normally are—in short, we will focus on preventing harm.[5] But as medicine has diminished the ever-present threat of death, at least in the affluent West, and become the enterprise of bio-power claiming to be able to improve all aspects of life, a different kind of rationale for health care will seem necessary. The equal opportunity approach is an attempt at such a rationale, and a relatively good one. Now the appeal is to the fairness implicit in enabling all to participate in social cooperation. What needs to be noted, however (and this is to get ahead of the argument a bit), is that the rationale is not "subject-centered" but rather one appealing to reciprocal self-interest. The very significance of disease is now made to depend not on its experience by the subject but rather on its preventing people from participating in schemes of cooperation whose ultimate justification lies in their furthering the interests of all.[6]

Arguing for health care on grounds of "equal opportunity" seems also paradoxically to make possible the justification of even greater stratification in health care than we now already have. The normal

---

problem for Daniels's concept of "species-typical functioning" is caused by the kinds of genetic revision advocated by *From Chance to Choice*. "A fact central to [his] approach," Daniels states, is that "impairment of normal functioning through disease and disability restricts an individual's opportunity *relative to that portion of the normal range his skills and talents would have made available to him were he healthy.*" He insists "there is no presumption that we should eliminate or level individual differences: *these act as a baseline constraint on the degree to which individuals enjoy the normal range.* Only where differences in talents and skills are the results of disease and disability, not merely normal variation, is some effort required to correct for the effects of the 'natural lottery'"(33–34). The program of *From Chance to Choice* is to argue that justice may demand genetic revision of normal variation, thus eliminating the "baseline constraint" necessary for the definition of disease or disability. The result can be well described in the language Daniels himself uses to criticize the World Health Organization's definition of health as "complete physical, mental, and social well-being." This definition leads to an "over-medicaliz[ing]" of "social philosophy," something that might equally be said of the genetic interventions contemplated by Buchanan et al.

5. Foucault, *History of Sexuality*, 135–45.

6. "All" should be read here to mean all those included within the particular scheme of reciprocal exchanges; it is unlikely that "social resources" will be marshaled in the United States to assist a child with a broken hip in Malawi. We need to imagine ever larger schemes of reciprocity but without diminishing differences in the process: in short, love is needed to extend and discipline justice.

competition of social cooperation operates at several different levels of complexity in today's information economies, as the authors' accounts frequently emphasize. If equal opportunity involves preventing disease that "hinders people from developing the abilities that would allow them to compete," (74) will it not be necessary to correlate the potential of the sufferer with some particular level of the game of social competition/cooperation? Suppose, for explanatory purposes, we can describe a particular society's system of cooperation as operating at five levels: A, B, C, D, and E. If a C- child is born with a need for genetic interventions, is he/she to be revised to a C or to a higher level, B or A—revisions that seem likely to be more complex and expensive? How would we balance the interests of the various groups involved? C's interest might seem clearly to lie in being revised to A, but this might well be counter to the interests of those in the A, B, and C categories—particularly if some A- could be revised to A much more cheaply and/or some process like cloning could guarantee more than the adequate number of beings with at least A potential genes. Indeed, cloning might ultimately become the means of reproduction included in standard health care packages precisely to avoid situations like the one above. Cloning C's would guarantee equal opportunity at that level of cooperation and minimize the need for costly interventions to revise naturally produced C-s to Cs.[7]

7. Obviously my scheme here is meant to suggest Aldous Huxley's *Brave New World*, in which the Bokhanovsky process produces Alphas, Betas, and so on who are designed to function perfectly and satisfyingly in the kinds of social roles allotted to them. Huxley's conception provides an elegant solution to problems caused by differences in human abilities and in the requirements of various kinds of work. The Bokhanovsky process could be described as providing a technological solution to the problem of justice, the kind a society might turn to, for instance, if it loses confidence in social-structural means to reconcile the ends of justice with the outcomes of the natural and social lotteries. The process ensures social peace by producing the perfect match between the ends of life for each cadre of functioners and the means available to them. It solves problems articulated by Plato in *The Republic*, namely that while "all of you in this land are brothers . . . the god who fashioned you mixed gold in the composition of those among you who are fit to rule, so that they are of the most precious quality; and he put silver in the Auxiliaries, and iron and brass in the farmers and craftsmen." Most of the time parents whose constitution includes gold produce offspring of gold, but this is not invariable. When parents of a more valuable metal produce children of a lesser, they must unpityingly see that the children are assigned to "station[s] proper" to their "nature." We should, of course, reject both Plato and Huxley's ways of grappling with these problems of human differentiation, but both have taken the issues at least as seriously as the authors of *From Chance to Choice*. Their rhetoric suggests a clear sense that the game of social competition will remain hierarchical; they allude continually

Nothing in this argument should be conceived as restricting efforts to ensure equality of opportunity achieved through social means. Indeed one of the reasons to eschew attempts to promote equality of opportunity through genetic intervention is that it will undermine efforts to do so through social means. If it becomes possible to move toward a level playing field by manipulation of genes for mathematical ability or improved memory (two of the authors' repeatedly introduced examples), then political efforts are likely to focus on such measures to assist the disadvantaged. But whether such interventions can succeed apart from extensive social change seems doubtful: children with genetically improved mathematics ability are unlikely to realize much benefit from the improvement if they still must go to failing schools. More important, the degree of hidden social coercion in a program of genetic intervention for enhancement seems enormous. Buchanan et al. aver that parents will freely choose to have their children "improved" if given the choice. But how free will such a choice be? If a competitive ratcheting up of genetic endowments becomes the norm, will parents really have the choice not to "improve" their children? If parents choose not to do so, will this not undermine their claim to other kinds of social assistance?[8]

---

to "the most desirable offices and positions" and so forth. Thus they do not envision "genetic maximization," to coin a phrase, for everyone, and surely it's difficult to believe that significant genetic enhancement will ever be inexpensive enough to be broadly distributed. Thus it seems they are implicitly committed to a scheme in which elites would be able to ensure that their children have the qualities necessary to remain Alphas. The golden would no longer have to reckon even with the possibility of giving birth to a child of iron. Whether any redistributive notions of justice could survive that change is worth considering. See *Republic*, 106–9.

8. This is perhaps a good place to insist on the unlikelihood that eugenics can remain "liberal," to use Nicholas Agar's term. Agar advocates a eugenics in which "the state would not presume to make any eugenic choices" but rather "foster the development of a wide range of technologies of enhancement ensuring that prospective parents were fully informed about what kinds of people these technologies would make." If it becomes possible, however, to increase genetically children's mathematical ability, is there any doubt that state funding of schools will be directed toward forcing parents to use the genetic technology? It's easy to see how this would be done. Full funding could be awarded those schools where 100 percent of the students are mathematically-improved, 60% to those where only 60 percent are genetically enhanced, and so forth. Parental behavior is also easy to predict. Parents of improved children would seek to place their children with others similarly improved, relocating to areas with genetically approved schools if necessary. Unimproved children and their parents would likely meet with hostility from the enhanced as they would, of course, be seen to be holding back their improved classmates. It's difficult to imagine how one would frame a public argument

The argument for genetic intervention put forth by Buchanan et al. masks powerful assumptions about the good life, the life worth living, despite their acknowledgment of "value pluralism" and the "moral individualism" they identify as a major emphasis of their understanding of liberalism. First, it places far too much emphasis on economic activity as the defining, even salvific, aspect of life. "Who is and who is not 'disabled,'" for example, is not determined by reference to judgment about a person's ability or inability to participate in and enjoy the wide range of things most of us like to do and believe worth doing. Rather disability is determined by "the most basic cooperative framework in a society": "in other words, what the most basic institutions for production and exchange are like will determine the capacities an individual must have in order to be an effective participant in social cooperation" (20). To be disabled, on this definition, is to fall below some threshold of value as a worker, consumer, and taxpayer.

That the authors' assumed norm for the good life is high-level participation in the symbolic economy is evident throughout the text. Even in the middle of a discussion of how genetic policy-making must include "safeguards against exclusion," the authors reveal their biases in their comments on enhancement: "Although we do not rule out the usefulness of these techniques even to the highest-functioning, most-able members of the population, the (perhaps unintended) risk of 'disabling' already-vulnerable fellow-citizens by raising the ante on abilities needed to participate fully in society can be avoided by steps adopted toward that end" (332). But to be "most-able" involves ability in a certain practice, to be "most able" at something. To be the "highest functioner" can similarly only be gauged in relation to some practice or activity. Yet to be among the most-abled highest functioners here is equated with participating "fully" in society. Other "less-able functioners" apparently participate less fully. The language suggests very strongly that a particular kind of life is more worth living than other kinds of lives. Elsewhere in the text, it's clear that the life most worth living is one of competing "for desirable social positions" (74). The authors uncritically assert that "those with

---

against such state coercion. One suspects the state policy I outline here would be met with resounding endorsement, as it provides a pragmatic solution to making the best use of social resources, monetary and human. This is particularly true under the positive view of freedom—with its stress on capabilities—advocated by Agar. If improved mathematics ability for all assists all to realize the positive freedom of enhanced capabilities, then who could be against it? See *Liberal Eugenics*, 5, 103.

the least marketable capabilities will have lower prospects in life than those with more marketable capabilities" (132). To argue that "those with the least marketable" skills will, on average, enjoy less economic success than those with more marketable skills would be one thing: the logic of the market itself undergirds the conclusion. But the authors' language, here and throughout the text, goes much too far toward conflating the goodness of a life with ability to secure "desirable jobs and offices" in the market. Such conflation is particularly apparent in a chapter that addresses the question "whether parents should be free to use genetic intervention techniques to produce the best offspring they can" (156). The authors favor at least some parental discretion in genetic design of the "best children," and part of their argument depends on diminishing the distinction between social or environmental ways of producing the "best" and genetic ones.[9]

The larger argument is not my concern here. Rather I wish to call attention to the attitudes toward children evident in their language. Children here are "human capital" (158) in whom parents "invest." Thus we are told—in language that reveals much about the authors' conception of the good life—that "parents who have the means often invest in the development of capabilities other than athletic ones: They give their children violin or piano or ballet lessons, enroll them in chess clubs and tournaments, or encourage their computer skills or interest in math teams or science fairs." And, in the same vein, some parents' "strategy is to spot special skills or talents and to invest heavily in developing these strengths" (158). Perhaps one comment on the larger argument is appropriate here. The authors seem to believe that genetic design of children by parents is consistent with children retaining an "open future," but the ubiquitous language of capital and investment undermines their contention in ways they fail to recognize.[10] People invest in order to receive a

---

9. The comparison of genetic enhancement to education is a favorite one of those arguing for enhancement. See Agar, *Liberal Eugenics*, 11–12; McGee, *The Perfect Baby*, 122–24; Robertson, *Children of Choice*, 167; and Harris, *Clones, Genes, and Immortality*, 171–72. If schools do conceive of what they're doing as fashioning the "best people," it seems little wonder that they alienate many as badly as they do. For how is one to react if he understands this to be the message the school directs at him, and he knows himself to be not one of the "best"? It's one thing to be told one's math or punctuation skills need work; it's quite another to understand that teachers regard one as a less than fully adequate person.

10. Feinberg, "The Child's Right to an Open Future," 76–97.

return; if parents come to think of their commitment to children in terms of investment, they will expect a return and they will communicate this expectation to their children. Parents may leave open the precise field in which the child is to enjoy success, but the child will be expected to return an appropriate premium on the parents' investment. Thus the child's future will not be truly open. If the parent is an investor, the child will be a worker seeking to pay off his or her debt.

II

Part of what is required to legitimate the project of producing genetically superior children is the rehabilitation of eugenics, to which the authors of *From Chance to Choice* contribute. The strategy of their approach is aptly suggested by the title of the first of their chapters devoted to eugenics, "Eugenics and Its Shadow." The question they pose is whether Nazi crimes "were inherent in the eugenic program all along" or whether "Nazi eugenics [was] a distortion, that is, a perversion, of eugenics, which stemmed not from any barbarism inherent in eugenic doctrine but from its adoption by Nazis, who bloodied and sullied everything they touched."[11] "These questions," the authors assert, "frame much of the debate over the shadow of eugenics" (38). The authors' view is that both the Nazi crimes and the involuntary sterilization programs in northern

11. According to Angela Franks, "Conflating the old eugenics with Nazism serves the ideological function of immunizing the new eugenics from critical examination"—a position with which I largely agree. See *Margaret Sanger's Eugenic Legacy*, 87. Part of the problem of evaluating eugenics may lie in the difficulty of defining just what it is. If one defines it at a very high level of abstraction—as Buchanan et al. do—as using genetic policy to produce healthier and more able human beings in the future, then it can be made to seem innocuous and the Nazi horrors will seem to be perversions of the idea. (Even under such a definition, we ought, I think, to ask how something so perverse can come from something so seemingly unexceptionable.) But if we resist framing the definition as abstractly as the defenders of eugenics tend to do, then we can see at least some elements of continuity between the Nazi experience and other eugenic practices. An alternative definition is proposed by Franks: "Eugenics is an ideology of control that views the human being more as a locus of genetic potential and peril than as a person with an innate and incalculable value and that, accordingly, seeks to shape decisions about who should reproduce or not and what kind of children are to be born or not" (67). Or, as I might propose, "Eugenics is an ideology that socializes human biology, thereby making suspect every person's genetic inheritance and inviting the development of collective identities based on supposedly shared biological traits deemed superior to those of other groups or individuals lacking these." For a rhetorical analysis of the way prominent British geneticists distance work in genetics from eugenics, see Anne Kerr et al., "Eugenics and the New Genetics in Britain," 175–98.

Europe and the United States were corruptions of eugenics, "shadows" that ought not to discredit the idea of eugenics itself. Distancing themselves from "mainline eugenicists" who "were anything but tolerant of personal and social ideals that differed from their own," they nevertheless endorse the eugenicists' goal of improving the intelligence level of the population: "Still, we would not fault the eugenicists or the authors of [*The Bell Curve*] for believing that raising the level of intellectual ability in the population would result in human betterment" (49). What merits criticism, according to the authors, is the assumption that raising intellectual ability would promote "more widespread adoption of bourgeois values" or reduce "social problems such as crime and unemployment" assumed to be in correlation to "low intelligence" (49).[12] These goals, and their concomitant assumptions, are abhorrent. Nevertheless the central aim of eugenics remains unexceptionable and appealing: "Constrained and guided by concerns of justice—the chief focus of this volume—the prospect of healthier and more able generations of human beings in the years to come is an appropriate and defensible goal of public policy on genetics" (55–56). Indeed broad eugenic policies, suitably limited by justice, may be not only defensible but "even morally required" (60) as public policy.

Detaching eugenics as idea from its worst effects in practice requires some subtle rhetorical work by the authors. The first step is to assert the need for revision in our understanding of the history. That history is much more complex than often recognized; indeed, as "historian Leila Zenderland has warned," the "history of the eugenics movement exists in two versions, an 'official' story of racist, reactionary thinkers and politicians, working with a few marginal scientists, a movement that proceeded directly from Darwin to Hitler; and a 'real' story of a bewildering array of thinkers, activists, snobs, socialists, scientific visionaries and crackpots, fascists, and architects of the Scandinavian social welfare states, divided among themselves on nearly every point of doctrine and proposed intervention" (29).[13] Later they follow Daniel Kevles in divid-

---

12. Without in any way wanting to accuse Buchanan et al. of bad faith on the matter of intelligence, I do think they and other advocates of eugenics owe us a fuller treatment of the way raising intelligence would better humanity. Eugenicists of all stripes—mainline, reform, conservative, liberal—nearly always focus on intelligence as the quality most in need of enhancement. But if humanity is to be bettered by enhancement of intelligence, then "low intelligence" must be the source of some of our current ills.

13. Zenderland's comment is from "What was Eugenics?," an unpublished paper from the American Philosophical Association, Pacific Division, 1998. It is quoted

ing eugenicists into "mainline" and "reform" groups (33). In the United States and Britain, mainline eugenicists tended to be politically conservative, troubled by social turmoil from the "unfit" lower classes, and, in the United States (and Germany) violently racist. Reform eugenicists, on the other hand, "often socialists," accepted "eugenic goals, but were unsparingly critical of the mainline eugenicists' research, biases, and proposals" (34).[14]

An important figure in the authors' redemption of eugenics is Hermann J. Muller, an American geneticist and Nobel prize winner who "insisted that natural talent could not be assessed in a society such as the

---

in Buchanan et al., *From Chance to Choice*, 29. The history of eugenics has been the subject of numerous studies. Among these are Kevles, *In the Name of Eugenics*; Paul, *The Politics of Heredity*; Ludmerer, *Genetics and American Society*; Pickens, *Eugenics and the Progressives*; and Franks, *Margaret Sanger's Eugenic Legacy*. Particularly helpful on the German experience are Proctor, *Racial Hygiene*; Lifton, *The Nazi Doctors*; Hau, *The Cult of Health and Beauty in Germany*; Weiss, "The Race Hygiene Movement in Germany," 193-236; and Wikler and Barondess, "Bioethics and Anti-Bioethics in Light of Nazi Medicine," 39-55. For studies of eugenics in places other than Germany, see Pernick, "Eugenics and Public Health in American History," 1767-72; Kamrat-Lang, "Healing Society: Medical Language in American Eugenics," 176-96; MacKenzie, "Eugenics in Britain," 499-532; Thom and Jennings, "Human Pedigree and the 'Best Stock,'" 211-34; Roll-Hansen, "Geneticists and the Eugenics Movement in Scandinavia," 335-46; Allen, "Genetics, Eugenics and Society," 105-22; and Adams, ed. *The Wellborn Science*.

14. On the "reform" eugenicists, see Kevles, *In the Name of Eugenics*, 164-92. These figures "rejected in varying degrees the social biases of their mainline predecessors yet remained convinced that human improvement would better proceed with—for some, would likely not proceed without—the deployment of genetic knowledge" (173). Among those in this group, Kevles lists C. P. Blacker, Frederick Osborn, J. B. S. Haldane, Julian Huxley, Herbert Brewer, and Hermann J. Muller. Whereas Kevles tends to identify the "mainline" eugenicists with "negative eugenics"—"ridding the world of the biologically unfit"—he associates the "reform" faction with "positive" eugenics, the use of genetic knowledge to produce improved human beings. One might ask, though, about the effect of this way of categorizing the movement on our understanding of it. "Reform" eugenicists shared with their "mainline" counterparts a concern for the degradation of the germ plasm; Brewer identified artificial insemination with "biological socialism . . . a socialization of the germ plasm," (Kevles, 190) a phrase that nearly echoes Bavarian Cabinet Minister Hans Schemm's declaration in 1934 that National Socialism was "nothing but applied biology"; Muller, Brewer, and Haldane all seemed to assume that women's contribution to the genetic upgrading of humanity was to involve primarily the bearing of the children of brilliant men (perhaps requiring only a few of the latter); and, as Kevles remarks, they "generally believed with Huxley that 'the whole progress and stability of the collective human enterprise' depended upon the gifted capable minority who might prevail against the 'dead-weight of the dull, silly, underdeveloped, weak and aimless.'" See Kevles, 192. Schemm's remark is quoted in Proctor, *Racial Hygiene*, 64.

United States, which did not offer equal opportunities for advancement to its citizens; only under socialism could the fit be identified as such and then encouraged to multiply." Cast here as an advocate of expanded and equal opportunity, Muller is later linked to an at least superficially attractive list of left social initiatives "that would provide economic security to parents, equal opportunities to women, public education in biology, and a 'socialized organization' that ensures that 'social motives predominate in society.'" Eugenics for Muller and other signees of the 1939 "Geneticists Manifesto" involved a great deal more than "the prevention of genetic deterioration"; rather it looked to a day when "everyone might look upon 'genius' as his birthright" (34–36).[15]

The authors' rhetorical strategy uses Muller to identify eugenics with progressive causes, but a further look at Muller's work suggests additional reason to be deeply skeptical of eugenics and perhaps of

---

15. "The 'Geneticists' Manifesto," signed by twenty-one geneticists, including Muller, appears in *Studies in Genetics*, 545–48. It appeared in *Journal of Heredity.* 30 (1939), 371–73. One section of the "Manifesto" suggests how the discrediting of Lamarckian doctrine may have contributed to anxiety about maintaining the better classes of people and thus to the fascination with eugenics. Noting how both heredity and environment must be understood to contribute to human development, Muller writes, "It must also be understood that the effect of the bettered environment is not a direct one on the germ cells and that the Lamarckian doctrine is fallacious, according to which the children of parents who have had better opportunities for physical and mental development inherit these improvements, biologically, and according to which in consequence, the dominant classes and peoples would have become genetically superior to the underprivileged ones. The intrinsic (genetic) characteristics of any generation can be better than those of the preceding generation only as a result of some kind of *selection*, i.e. by those persons of the preceding generation who had a better genetic equipment having produced more offspring, on the whole, than the rest"(*Selected Papers*, 546–47). If Lamarckianism had been true, those of superior advantages could count on heredity itself for a kind of continuity; inter-breeding with the lower sorts would be less threatening than under Mendelian-Darwinism, for the advantages given to those with poorer germ plasm might modify the genes themselves and be perpetuated. Lamarck's discrediting would seem to undermine commitment of the better classes to broad education for all, for if education were not combined with eugenic selection among the lower classes, those classes would slip back to their previous genetic inferiority with each new generation. For the argument that the continued popularity of Lamarckianism restrained coercive eugenic measures in Brazil and France, see Deane-Drummond, 59. This conclusion is contested by Mark B. Adams, who argues that Mendelians "sometimes found well-established and active eugenics movements dominated by their opponents" the Lamarckians. "As a rule," he adds, "the forecasts of the Lamarckians for the human future were no more hopeful, and their solutions no less draconian, than those of Mendelians." See "Toward a Comparative History of Eugenics," 218.

Progressivism itself.[16] Muller's classic, *Out of the Night*, reveals very deep distress over genetic deterioration. The argument that civilization unfortunately allows many of the less worthy to survive and reproduce has rarely been put any more bluntly than by Muller:

> For civilization affords an excellent chance to breed for many sorts of the weak, the stupid, and the vicious characters which are continually arising even among the "best" families. It might at first sight appear that this can lead to a situation little or not at all worse than that existing at present, so long as the sound and the superior also reproduce, mix with, and counterbalance the others; but this impression is erroneous and betrays insufficient understanding of the findings of modern genetics.[17]

One should note here that it is not enough simply for the "sound and superior" to "mix with" the "others"; rather there must be a more radical differentiation of these groups. Predictably Muller goes on from this point to develop the kind of logic that underlay programs of compul-

---

16. On the connection between American Progressivism and eugenics, see Ludmerer, *Genetics and American Society*, 15-19, and Pickens, *Eugenics and the Progressives*. Proctor proposes that "one might even say that National Socialism was itself progressive—if we mean by this that application of science to social problems (in a particularly 'biologistic' manner) was an important element in Nazi ideology." He goes on to suggest, however, that there may be limited value in "casting eugenicists as progressives," if the term can be made to apply to people of such widely varying ideologies—from Nazis, on the one hand, to such quintessential progressives and critics of eugenics as Franz Boas and John Dewey. See *Racial Hygiene*, 23. Proctor has assessed the possible relationship of eugenics and the new genetics in "Genomics and Eugenics: How Fair is the Comparison?" in *Gene Mapping*, 57-93. Proctor's primary worry is about justice: "The danger is that in a society where power is still unequally distributed between haves and have-nots, the application of the new genetic technologies—as of any other—is as likely to reinforce as to ameliorate patterns of indignity and injustice" (84). However one places eugenics in relationship to progressivism, Americans, in particular, should be permanently troubled by Deane-Drummond's observation that "German eugenic programmes commonly drew on American models for support." See *Genetics and Christian Ethics*, 65.

17. *Out of the Night*, 42. Further references will be given parenthetically. Troy Duster has called attention to the "sociohistorical continuity" between two periods in which "genetic reductionism" has seemed to become quite popular: the "heyday of the eugenics movement" early in the twentieth century and our own (226). Both have been periods of immense social and economic transformation with concomitant dislocation of all kinds. In the first, "the idea that social stratification and the behavior of those at the bottom of the economic order are biologically and genetically inferior was seductive enough to alter public policy, law, and the 'medical' practice of forced sterilization." Duster fears that the "seductive voice" of biological and genetic accounts of behavior is again "on the horizon" (233). See "Persistence and Continuity," 218-38.

sory sterilization, even if he does not advocate such directly. Mutations giving "rise to 'defective' or 'pathological' traits" are "relatively far more abundant than the 'beneficial mutations'" in any population. Thus, over time, the mutation process will inevitably "cause a gradual heaping up of undesirable traits ... if individuals having the defective genes are allowed to multiply merely at the *same* rate as the others" (43). The implication of this argument is that the less-sound individuals, those with undesirable traits, should be discouraged or prevented from reproducing at the same rate as the sound and superior. Moreover, there could hardly be a more serious imperative, as ultimately the health of the whole population is at stake.

If Muller believes that every child should have genius as his/her birthright, it is because he would sever the link between personal love and reproduction in order to promote much higher levels of reproduction by geniuses—specifically, *men* of genius. "Only social inertia and popular ignorance now hold us back" from putting into effect the "severance of the function of reproduction from the personal love-life of the individual" (111). To "make personal love master over reproduction," as we have, is to "degrade the germ plasm of the future generations" (112). The remedy is to "order our reproduction" so that a large part of the next generation "might average, in its hereditary physical and mental constitution, half-way between the average of the present population and that of our greatest living men of mind, body, or 'spirit' (as we choose)." In a mere century or two, "it would be possible for the majority of the population to become of the innate quality of such men as Lenin, Newton, Leonardo, Pasteur, Beethoven, Omar Khayyam, Pushkin, Sun Yat Sen, Marx (I purposely mention men of different fields and races), or even to possess their varied faculties combined" (112–13).[18]

18. With millionaire Robert K. Graham, Muller founded the Repository for Germinal Choice in southern California in 1978. Often known as the "Nobel Prize Sperm Bank," the Repository offered women the opportunity to be inseminated with the sperm of exceptional men—though not, in most cases, with Nobel quality sperm as only one Prize winner could be gotten to contribute. See Franks, *Margaret Sanger's Eugenic Legacy*, 83, and Agar, *Liberal Eugenics*, 1. According to Deane-Drummond, however, Muller quickly withdrew his support of the Repository when he realized the degree of capitalist support it had attracted. See *Genetics and Christian Ethics*, 70. Agar interestingly begins his account with the story of Graham's Repository, a narrative choice that unwittingly suggests the eugenic process—however liberal—still primarily involves human betterment through women's making wise choices about whose sperm they will allow to use their bodies. Consider, for example, the following: "In the future, a woman who wants a bril-

The means to bring about Muller's enhancement of human genetic stock include identification of worthy male donors; laboratory cultivation of "male reproductive tissues, in which the male germ cells could multiply and come to maturity" (121); and artificial insemination. Muller insists that participation in the process "will be entirely voluntary," and he is certain that as the sperm of genetically superior men becomes available, "more and more individual mothers as well as couples will become eager to participate in it [the procedure]" (117). Indeed Muller laments the past unavailability of methods for perpetuating the genes "of our departed great!" (122). No coercive methods will be necessary to promote the new process of genetic improvement by selection because properly enlightened women will be more than willing to volunteer: "How many women, in an enlightened community devoid of superstitious taboos and of sex slavery, would be eager and proud to bear and rear a child of Lenin or of Darwin! Is it not obvious that restraint, rather than compulsion, would be called for?" (122).

Two aspects of Muller's outline for a program of genetic progress are especially chilling. First is the extraordinary degree to which he is willing to objectify human beings. Even the authors of *From Chance to Choice* point out that a beginning step toward the Nazi horrors was the objectification of the Jews and others deemed unsound. But Muller himself advocates similar objectification as a necessary part of genetic evaluation: "The judgment of genetic merit, as distinguished from environmental good fortune (which can of course never be completely equalized), will become increasingly exact as time goes on, and it will be desirable, in this matter, to use methods as objective and as little susceptible to being influenced by the 'personal equation' as possible" (120). The language suggests a kind of massive and interminable Kafkaesque

---

liant child will not be restricted to the random selection of a genius's genes in the sperm that happens to fertilize her egg. She might choose to get pregnant with a genetic copy, or a clone of the genius. Alternatively, she may be empowered to search out the specific genes linked with genius, and have these engineered into her embryo" (2). The implicit anti-feminism of the valuation given male genius here, and of its claim to perpetuate itself, seems clear. What should also be noted is the degree of genetic determinism assumed, despite Agar's attempts elsewhere to distance himself from such determinism. As Agar makes much of the importance of "moral images" in giving us ethical guidance, the cover of the paperback edition of his book deserves comment. It shows three perfect replications of male torsos with only enough expressionless heads visible to suggest that there is a kind of infinite cadre of these. A strange image for a book suggesting that eugenics can somehow remain "liberal."

trial in which people would be assessed for something utterly beyond their control, "genetic merit," by a faceless panel of objective appraisers. Among the consequences of such a regime would be the destruction of all social solidarity—as everyone would come to look on others, even one's family, as in question—and the clear division of society into the genetically acceptable and unacceptable. Such a clear "objective" decision would likely encourage extravagant arrogance on the part of the acceptable and the lowering of self-esteem in the unacceptable, who would find themselves suspect in their very biology.

The second especially chilling aspect of Muller's argument is closely related to the first. Objective genetic evaluation would require an extraordinary degree of social control, itself probably dependent on the destruction of solidarity. Muller unhesitatingly endorses massive social control, advocating the kinds of "fundamental changes" being carried out by Stalin in the Soviet Union in the 1930's: "Our airy imaginings concerning the future possibilities of cooperative activity on a grand scale are brought down to earth and given substance when we turn to the great and solid actualities of collective achievement which are becoming increasingly evident in that one section of the world—the Soviet Union—in which the fundamental changes in the economic basis have already been established" (vii).[19] The degree to which Muller envisions the total rationalization and organization of society is evident in his remarks about the "individually petty operations" of the home (56). "Food preparation must be centralized," he argues, and "both clothing and housing must be rationalized" (56). Given these views—together with the conviction that personal love as the means of reproduction degrades the germ plasm—it is no surprise that Muller judges the family to be among the institutions worthy to be discarded. The progress of the race and its salvation from degeneration depend on the development of a

---

19. Muller emigrated to the Soviet Union in 1934, completing *Out of the Night* in Moscow. He presented a copy of it to Stalin, along with what Paul characterizes as a "lengthy personal appeal effusive in its praise of Bolshevism and excoriating the racist and class uses of eugenics in capitalist societies." The book failed to please Stalin, and Muller, disillusioned about the possibilities of a Bolshevik eugenics, left for Spain. *Out of the Night* was, however, well received elsewhere, both by the Left and outside leftist circles. See Paul, *Politics of Heredity*, 20–21. The degree of Stalin's rejection of Muller's theories is indicated by his "executing two of [Muller's] post-doctoral students in 1936." See Deane-Drummond, *Genetics and Christian Ethics*, 70. For a study of eugenics in Russia, see Adams, "Eugenics in Russia," 153–216.

collective order that the family and all older forms of social solidarity impede.

Muller's work reveals an odd combination of vague fear, desire for control, and religious impulse directed into salvation through the upbuilding of humanity through eugenics. The vague yet powerful fear seems characteristic of writing by eugenicists. Allowing reproduction to continue without scientific planning will, under conditions of civilization, inevitably result in the degeneration of the human race. In order to save the race, greater social control over reproduction must be implemented. For Muller what is at stake is a matter of faith, in the Tillichian sense of ultimate concern. Eugenics promises to move us *Out of the Night*, that darkness in which most of us have had the ill-fate to be conceived. As humanity takes control of its own evolution, "it will reach down into the secret places of the great universe of its own nature and, by the aid of its ever-growing intelligence and cooperation, shape itself into an increasingly sublime creation—a being beside which the mythical divinities of the past will seem more and more ridiculous, and which, setting its own marvelous inner powers against the brute Goliath of the suns and planets, challenges them to contest" (125). Such extravagant prediction seems no more rationally justifiable than the unfocused fears of contamination and degeneration that underlie Muller's positions or those of Joseph Fletcher in *The Ethics of Genetic Control*.[20] This extravagance of both fear and hope suggest that the eugenicists' purportedly reasonable positions are as much an attempt to justify extensive social control as they are proposals for rational social policy.

The authors of *From Chance to Choice* neglect Herman Muller's objectification of human beings and his willingness to endorse extensive control of society in the name of eugenics. Two further features of their telling of the history of eugenics also need brief mention. Part of the redemption of eugenics is to disassociate it from identification entirely with the political right. Thus they note how eugenics "was often

---

20. "Each of us has a genetic 'load' of three to eight defects. This could double in two hundred years if we go on spreading genetic disorders through random sexual reproduction, multiplying the illnesses and costs that result from bad genes. This increase used to be offset by death and natural selection, but now the weak are preserved and protected. Which is better, to give up sanitation and medicine and social security, or give up random reproduction? We might survive as a society with a doubled load of bad genes, but think of the enormous cost in medicine, surgery, artificial aids, and diet controls for the increased number of victims." See Fletcher, *Ethics of Genetic Control*, 29.

found in the political platforms of left-of-center political parties" such as the social welfarists of Denmark, Norway, and Canada, the Fabians in England and American Progressives. The efforts of these are described benignly as favoring "social programs that, with the help of science, applied resources available to the state to building a more humane society" (34). The authors then proceed to detail one left movement, that in Sweden, that shows "the compatibility of eugenic thinking to varied political viewpoints" (35). Noting that before the 1930s the "movement was centered in the Institute for Race Biology in Uppsala," the authors argue that later Social Democratic control led to a disavowal of racism and an emphasis on laboratory study of medical genetics. Nevertheless Swedish Social Democrats engaged in major programs of sterilization of the genetically unfit:

> The ascendancy of the socialists proved to give eugenics a second wind. The planners of the Swedish welfare state, concerned with the "quality" as well as the quantity of Sweden's then-dwindling population, were eager for the government to use natural and social science for the common good. The modernization and rational ordering of society left little room for the inferior and the deficient, and the government sought to identify and sterilize these citizens. Indeed, Social Democratic intellectuals maintained that these sterilizations were necessary if Sweden were to be able to afford the cradle-to-grave security they championed. Eugenics, in effect, was an instrument for reducing need. (35)

One would think that this sorry record of social coercion on the part of a leftist regime would cause the authors to be permanently wary of any attempt to put eugenics into practice. But this is not the direction in which the authors press the facts of the Swedish experience. While they grant that "Swedish eugenics targeted a population of itinerants (*Tattare*, or tinkers), who were imagined to be racially different," they finish their discussion by asserting that "the Swedish eugenicists strenuously denied any commonality with Nazi policies of the same era, and our current tendency to equate eugenics with Nazism distorts this historical record" (35).[21]

---

21. Gregory E. Pence notes that forced sterilization of "citizens with low intelligence or gross physical defects" continued in Sweden until 1976. From *The Elements of Bioethics*, 186.

Why Designing the Subjects of Justice Is Likely to Be Unjust   ᛤ   215

The equivocal discussion of the Swedish experience is necessitated by the two major prongs of the authors' argument. The first of these is that the failing of eugenics lay in its association with racism, as in Nazi Germany; if it can be disassociated from racism—as the authors are confident is now possible—then eugenics can be put usefully into practice for the rational betterment of human life. The second major emphasis of their historical review is to show that eugenics was espoused not only by rightist regimes but also by political parties of a progressive welfarist bent, as in Sweden. As the policies of these parties align closely with those of contemporary American progressives, the attempt is to persuade progressives to consider the value of eugenics. To put the form of the argument crudely: the authors suggest that good people like us—current American progressives—did support eugenics before the idea became suspect through its connection to Nazism. Now we should revive it and put it into practice, minus, of course, the racism that we now all recognize to be abhorrent. The Swedish experience would seem to be an embarassment for the authors, but it actually is made to support their two points: that socially democratic regimes have considered eugenics an arm of public policy and that they have recognized the need to "deny any commonality" with the kind of racist policies adopted by the Nazis.[22]

What the authors avoid is raising a much more serious set of questions suggested by the Swedish experience.[23] Perhaps that experience

22. One does not know whether the intention is to hearten or horrify in Roll-Hansen's comment on the decline of eugenics in Scandinavia: "If it is correct that eugenic thinking and practice continued without abrupt change for a considerable period after World War Two, this suggests that the experience with Nazi policies had a limited direct impact and was not decisive for the eventual abandonment of eugenics in Scandinavia." Roll-Hansen's general argument is that growing scientific knowledge of genetics, rather than the Nazi experience, diminished the appeal of eugenics in the Scandinavian countries. One wonders, though, why the Nazi experience should not have been enough, in itself, to discredit eugenics entirely. See "Geneticists and the Eugenics Movement in Scandinavia," 343.

23. Something that should be explored, too, is the degree of correlation between the most racist versions of eugenics and the heterogeneity of the populations where this occurred. Or, to ask this otherwise, did eugenics avoid the worst forms of racism primarily in those countries where there was a high degree of ethnic homogeneity? If that is the case, it calls into question the idea that eugenics can be dissociated from racism. I'm not in a position to offer a conclusion here, but it does seem that the two countries where eugenics was most clearly racist—Germany and the United States—were ones with substantial "minority" populations.

should be read as evidence that the creation of nationalized systems of health security, and the political consensus needed to support them, depends upon the minimizing of commitment to those perceived, for one reason or another, as marginally useful to the national effort. Eugenics offers a means to limit risks and to control costs. And perhaps what makes it most dangerous is its ability to accomplish these ends under the guise—unrecognized as such by its supporters—of improving society.

A final piece of the authors' argument for a eugenics of the left is to associate opposition to eugenics with that arch-enemy of everything progressive, the Catholic Church. The authors note that "the eugenicists' legislative successes in Germany and Scandinavia were not matched in such countries as Poland and Czechoslovakia," largely because of opposition by the Church, which was "virtually the only institution" to oppose eugenics "in principle." Such opposition was, however, "of a piece with its opposition to abortion and contraception: Then, as now, the Church was opposed to limitations on fertility, and its opponents were often on the left" (36). No mention is made here of how opposition to eugenics is simply a part of the Church's insistence on the right of individuals to be born free of manipulative social technique or of its defense of the family as a vital institution in the maintenance of social solidarity—the kind of solidarity that provides the best defense against ideological regimes of the right or left. Rather the Church is simply positioned as the enemy of freedom of choice in reproductive matters. Since all progressives know the Church is wrong on contraception and abortion, so, too, her opposition to eugenics must make it a good idea.[24]

---

24. Pius XI condemned eugenics in the 1930 encyclical *Casti Conubii*, "that pernicious practice must be condemned which closely touches upon the natural right of man to enter matrimony but affects also in a real way the welfare of the offspring. For there are some who over solicitous for the cause of eugenics, not only give salutary counsel for more certainly procuring the strength and health of the future child—which, indeed, is not contrary to right reason—but put eugenics before aims of a higher order, and by public authority wish to prevent from marrying all those whom, even though naturally fit for marriage, they consider, according to the norms and conjectures of their investigations, would, through hereditary transmission, bring forth defective offspring. And more, they wish to legislate to deprive these of that natural faculty by medical action despite their unwillingness; and this they do not propose as an infliction of grave punishment under the authority of the State for a crime committed, nor to prevent future crimes by guilty persons, but against every right and good they wish the civil authority to arrogate to itself a power over a faculty which it never had and can never legitimately possess." *Casti Conubii*, 34–35.

The authors of *From Chance to Choice* are convinced that eugenics can be practiced without the kind of atrocities perpetrated by the Nazis. For them the "Nazi debacle" represents a distortion of eugenics, not something inherent in eugenics itself—this despite the totalitarian arguments of Muller and the mass sterilization of the marginalized in socially democratic Sweden. For the authors, the evil distortion of eugenics is racism; if eugenics can be divorced from racism, then it can serve its original purpose of bettering humanity. Declaring the "eugenics movement . . . a creature of its time," they note that "Racism, class snobbery, and other forms of bias were openly expressed even by learned scholars; these sentiments, so obviously objectionable today, were invisible then because, of course, they were so widely shared" (45). This argument should cause us to ask what kinds of judgments might be "invisible" to us precisely because they are so widely shared as to seem unexceptionable. Whenever we discover how extraordinarily deluded previous generations or periods can be, it ought to induce in us the most serious self-reflection as to our own possible delusions. I would urge this reflection particularly as we ponder something so momentous as altering the genetic design of future generations.

Buchanan et al. argue, however, that the task now is for humanity "to accomplish what eluded the eugenicists entirely, to square the pursuit of genetic health and enhancement with the requirements of justice" (57). Despite their identification of the Nazi horrors as specifically eugenic, the authors claim "the greatest single flaw of eugenics was its failure to take justice seriously" (100). Frankly this seems an extraordinarily pallid way to describe the flaw of Nazi eugenics. One could argue, with as much justice, that the greatest single flaw of eugenics was its provision of quasi-scientific or medical justifications for policies of hatred, fanaticism, and state murder. One could argue further that its flaw lay in providing a seeming rationale for already existent German fears of degeneration in the social or national body. Or further that it lent "objectivity" to judgments about others that can never be objective (judgments that, for Christians, ought never to be entered into in the first place). Such objectivity of supposedly medical judgment prepared the way both for the destruction of social solidarity between non-Jewish Germans and German Jews and for the objectification of Jews necessary for their mass destruction. As Robert Jay Lifton's *The Nazi Doctors* establishes, the medicalization of Nazi policies was a vital step in insulating them from criticism.[25]

The goal of eugenics was "human betterment," its distinctive means "causing better people to be conceived and born, rather than ... directly bettering any people." The "already born" would benefit indirectly, through "freedom from the burdens placed on society by the unfit [and] sharing in the productivity of the gifted" (46). The language here immediately suggests the inherent problems of eugenics and its incompatibility with justice. The beginning of the evil of eugenics lies in the premise that some are "unfit." One cannot be "unfit" except for something conceived as a task or purpose. Since presumably no one would judge himself or herself as "unfit"—without the most extensive brainwashing or reeducation—then the judgment about fitness must come from without and involve standards set by others than those declared unfit. The imbalance of power between the subjects doing the judging and the objects—denied subjectivity—being judged is already total and, as such, will conduce to totalitarian forms of government or social management.

It also seems doubtful that a method claiming to produce "better people" can be consistent with justice. The goal is not simply to produce people who are more capable at certain practices. Of course some people are better baseball players than others or better mathematicians or masons or farmers or teachers. In a system of relatively just social exchange, the possessors of diverse talents complement each other in a way that benefits most, if not all. But the eugenic goal is not just to produce people who are more talented or skillful in particular ways but rather to produce *better people*. Now the authors of *From Chance to Choice* argue that eugenic production of better people could be endorsed as consistent with justice through something like Rawls's Difference Principle. As long as increased production by the "better people" redounds to the benefit of the less able, or at least does not disadvantage them, then the eugenic goal would be consistent with justice.

It's not clear, however, why "better people"—armed now with eugenic processes to produce more of their kind—would be willing

25. One of the many contributions of Lifton's book is his establishing how thoroughly the Nazi vision was a "biomedical" one. As he puts it, "Medical metaphor blended with concrete biomedical ideology in the Nazi sequence from coercive sterilization to direct medical killing to the death camps. The unifying principle of the biomedical ideology was that of a deadly racial disease, the sickness of the Aryan race; the cure, the killing of all Jews" (*Nazi Doctors*, 16).

to allow the fruits of their superiority to go to their inferiors. Rawls's Difference Principle, we should recall, derives from the original position in which all contractors are to imagine themselves without any knowledge of their social positioning. In effect, they are to act as if stripped of all external distinctions. Behind the model lies a presumption of equal worth separable from social advantage or disadvantage: worth, the right to participate as a contractor, is separate from advantage or disadvantage. But genetic superiority, that possessed by "better people," cannot be simply put off, detached from the person. Rawls can avoid having to deal with genetic advantage because he can assume it is distributed throughout the population by the natural lottery. But eugenics puts an end to the natural lottery for that part of the population who participate in it: they will never be able to conceive their "superiority" as something due in some broad way to events beyond their control and thus detachable from them. In effect, eugenics would make a Rawlsian original position impossible and it would legitimate the "better people's" refusal to assist the less able. Moreover, "better people" would consider themselves authorized to develop schemes of social cooperation in which their talents would be used to greatest advantage. Thus the genetically unimproved would find themselves ever more excluded from the world of the "better people." To the "better people" such exclusion would seem entirely legitimate, even morally required. After all, their pursuit ought to be the production of better and better people and the conditions for their flourishing. What part could the genetically unimproved play in those enterprises?[26]

III

Critical to the effort to justify extensive genetic intervention in the name of justice is breaking down the distinction between treatment and enhancement. The section on the distinction is one of the more ambiguous in *From Chance to Choice*. The authors characterize their own position as a "limited defense" of the distinction but argue that "it cannot provide a clear or unequivocal guide to the moral boundaries between what it is obligatory and nonobligatory to provide in insurance or between what is permissible and impermissible for individuals to do" (109). Much of the argument they present, however, seems to undermine the "modest"

---

26. For the Difference Principle, see Rawls, *Theory of Justice*, 75–83.

value of the distinction. This is hardly surprising, for a blurring of the distinction serves the larger agenda of the book: to argue that genetic interventions of a clearly enhancing kind be provided—and perhaps required—as a matter of justice when the technologies become available.

The authors' rhetorical strategy is to present a series of "hard cases" drawn from actual medical practice where the distinction seems "especially problematic" (109). These do not, however, make their case that the distinction is problematic. To see why this is the case requires a brief look at their examples: the cases of Shy Bipolar, Unhappy Husband, and the Short Children.

Shy Bipolar's case comes from the records of the "Harvard Community Health Plan (HCHP)," a "staff-model HMO that served more than 550,000 people in New England." After being "stabilized on lithium for some years," the patient remained shy but benefited from a therapy group not covered within the benefit plan. The plan, however, revised its benefit structure in order to pay for the treatment because the man's psychiatrist successfully argued that his shyness originated from the disorder's disruption of his adolescent development. Similarly serious shyness, the authors point out, would not be eligible for the "extended benefit" if its etiology did not include specific disorder (111). The distinction seems arbitrary to the authors: Shy Bipolar can qualify for the benefit because his treatment is a matter of therapeutic response to disease whereas Shy Normal cannot qualify because he is considered to be seeking enhancement.

Unhappy Husband was married to a woman suffering from "serious mental illness" that made her a very difficult partner. Committed to remaining married, the man benefited greatly from twenty-six sessions of psychotherapy, but these were not covered by insurance. He was undoubtedly "suffering more than many of the HMO members being treated for illnesses, and psychotherapy definitely enhanced his well-being." Given these facts, the authors ask, "What possible rationale could there be for not covering his treatment?" (111–12).

In the case of the Short Children, Johnny, whose parents are of average height, is a "short 11-year-old boy with documented growth hormone deficiency resulting from a brain tumor." Predicted adult height for Johnny is 5'3", as it is also for Billy, a similarly short 11-year-old with "normal GH secretion" and "extremely short parents" (115).[27] To treat

---

27. The case of the short children is from Allen and Fost, "Growth Hormone Therapy for Short Stature," 16-21.

Johnny, or cover his treatment through insurance, and not to treat, or cover, Billy makes "the distinction seem arbitrary." Both boys will "suffer disadvantage" from their condition; both are short "through no fault of their own" but as a result of the natural lottery; both desire to be taller not as a matter of "expensive taste" but rather because it truly is a "heightist" world in which nearly all males prefer not to be noticeably shorter than average. To regard provision of GH to Johnny as treatment and similar provision to Billy as "enhancement" seems morally arbitrary (115).

The problem with the authors' logic is that it is not necessary to regard treatment of Billy as "enhancement" at all. Here the definition of "species-typical functioning" can be quite helpful in providing clarification. Billy's shortness represents a decided departure from the "natural" or "typical" range of height for males in his society. If that range for adult males is from 5'6" to 6'4", then he might well be judged—within some specific scheme of cooperation based on justice as reciprocity—to have a claim to enough GH to bring him up to the bottom of the range. Billy is arguably "enhanced," but only by being brought somewhat closer to species typical normality. If there is anything problematic about Billy's case, it is only because the authors fail to recognize that treatment will nearly always be "enhancing" as it moves people toward more species-typical functioning. Obviously, too, it's precisely the departure from species-typical functioning (or from a group-typical norm) that causes Billy's shortness to be a matter of concern at all.

The same logic applies to the case of Shy Bipolar–Shy Normal. Therapy for extremely shy people can be understood as a matter of treatment—movement toward species-typical functioning—rather than enhancement. Of course shyness will be considerably harder to define than extreme shortness, and a decision to treat will expose a group to considerably more moral hazard than one to treat shortness. It's also far less clear that shyness is a social disadvantage than that extreme shortness in males is (and one would even like to see more evidence for the claim that shortness necessarily disadvantages one). The crucial point is that there is nothing in a cooperative group's decision to pay for therapy for shyness that problematizes the treatment-enhancement distinction: the group is simply opting—unwisely, I believe—to treat a departure from normal functioning. No enhancement is involved precisely because species-typicality operates as a norm to establish a level playing field.

The social-constructionist view of disease, as characterized here by the authors, separates the social from the natural in a too extreme way:

> Pointing to the line between treatment and enhancement is not, then, pointing to a biologically drawn line; rather, it is an indirect way of referring to valuations we make. We cannot point to such a line as the grounds or basis for drawing moral boundaries since we are only pointing to a value-laden boundary we have constructed. (119)

Judgments about height, for instance, do involve valuations we make, but surely these are rooted in the biological. If the average male height were 4'11" to 5'6", neither Johnny nor Billy would be deemed in need of treatment. The following, even more extreme version of social constructionism verges on the preposterous: "Aimed at the treatment/enhancement distinction more generally, the [social constructionist] objection is that we are being offered an apparently 'natural' baseline between disease (and impairment) and the biologically normal, when there really is none" (119). Such a view seems almost wholly divorced from bodily experience. It would have us conclude that only our "constructions"—with the assumption of full and free alterability conveyed by that word—distinguish painful, life-threatening cancers or HIV from the frustrated desires of some to be taller or brighter.

What is never acknowledged by the authors of *From Chance to Choice* is that a definition of health as species-typical functioning can have the result of leveling the playing field. The authors seem, on the one hand, to assume that only justice liberated from natural limits can assure equality of opportunity. But one could argue that the effect of adopting the social-constructionist view of health, with its abandonment of nature as a baseline, will almost surely be to exacerbate differences in the levels of care available to people of different incomes, classes, and nations. Abandoning a definition of health as species-typical functioning expands the number of conditions for which people seek assistance. Indeed desire for health care—construed as relief from as much suffering as possible—must probably be considered infinite. Competition for resources thus becomes more intense and it becomes necessary to limit claims in one way or another—either by refusal of certain kinds of claims or by limiting the number of people considered eligible to make a claim. If ideology is always rooted in economic practice, then the need to limit claims in a climate of welfare entitlement might well explain both the social constructionist understanding and the diminution of species as a relevant category in ethical discussion. Social constructionism legitimates our spending social resources on people's overcoming shyness while we ignore much clearer departures from species-typical functioning: HIV and malaria in Africa, hepatitis in Latin America, parasites and the accompanying malnutrition in Haiti, completely preventable blindness in many parts of the developing world. Surely the claim of these diseases to a greatly enlarged expenditure of social resources—by the wealthy nations—can be made much more pointedly if our operative definition of health focuses on the natural baseline of species-typical functioning. To put this bluntly, HIV in Africa is much more likely to trump shyness in Cambridge, Massachusetts, under a conception of health as species-typical functioning than it is under one that sees the production of health in a purely pragmatic way as what "we" do in hospitals and other "medical" settings.

Thus the arguments of *From Chance to Choice* do not succeed in diminishing the distinction between treatment and enhancement. What they show is simply that judgments about expensive tastes will be relative to expectations within groups based clearly on self-interested reciprocity. Whether Unhappy Husband's therapy should be covered depends on the group's expectations about marriage. If the American divorce rate goes from 50 to 80 percent, then his wanting to preserve his marriage will likely be seen as an expensive taste. Perhaps it is already seen that way, and this is the reason he has trouble being covered. It must be remembered that everybody in the group has at least two interests: one in the expansion of the number of covered conditions and a second in limiting costs (this second one is, of course, often far too indirect). Group administrators have an interest in controlling costs, of course, but they too can have an interest in expanding definitions of health if this means attracting additional clients and/or increased ability to pass on costs to employers. Under conditions of economic growth, what will surely develop is an inflationary expectation about the number of conditions eligible to be covered along with ever-closer reasoning—itself always tentative—about the distinctions between covered conditions and expensive tastes. The whole process can surely encourage the illusion that there is little difference between treatment and enhancement. The way to correct for this illusion is to direct people's attention away from their local HMO and outward toward larger groupings. If they look at the species as a group, many things covered by the Harvard Community HMO will seem expensive tastes. Maintaining a strong distinction between enhancement and treatment is a way of insisting that any meaningful consideration of justice in health care must focus on an ever-expanding circle of those considered to be within the reference group—a circle as large, finally, as the human species itself.

IV

At this point, it seems necessary to approach the theoretical issues regarding justice raised by the possibilities of genetic engineering. The authors of *From Chance to Choice* point out that the basic problem of distributive justice has traditionally been conceived as "how goods ought to be distributed among persons when their identities, at least for purposes of justice, are given independently of the distribution of goods" (85).[28] Radical genetic intervention threatens to shatter this picture, however, for now we will be confronted with determining not only how to distribute goods but also how to distribute "person-constituting characteristics in order to ensure that whichever persons do exist have equal opportunities (or equal resources)" (86). In the authors' phrase, we will embark on a large scale "colonization of the natural by the just" (82) in which we decide how to shape persons genetically in order that they can enjoy equal opportunity. Thus "equal opportunity" here is made to justify wide-scale and far-reaching shaping of human genetic identities, without, of course, consulting those to be shaped. If we should beware especially of potentially tyrannical ideas when they are presented as part of something we all endorse, then here is a place we should be alarmed.

Several disturbing questions present themselves immediately. One concerns the sheer scale of an enterprise like that apparently imagined by the authors and the degree of economic, social, and medical coordination it would require. At the moment, we trust that "personal love" found so unsatisfactory by Muller to create the persons who are part of the pool. The practices and exchanges that develop derive, more or less freely, from the needs, talents, interests, and abilities of persons whose conception does not depend on some prior judgment about how they will contribute to the established practices. This is probably to oversimplify somewhat. No doubt some American elites pair up and decide to

---

28. See Roemer, "Equality of Talent," 151–81.

reproduce with the preconception that the child will be a member of the symbol-making class, and in traditional agricultural societies, children are often produced to be additional labor. But perhaps a useful measure of the freedom of a society involves the degree to which each child can be a kind of new beginning of the world—a being who is not simply to be coerced into the already existent practices and structures but who may, in his or her own way, modify everything. Genetic design of children represents the most far-reaching attempt ever conceived to modify those coming into the world in order to fit the schemes, practices, structures, and organizations already in place. We should be particularly wary of it when it is proposed under the guise of an idea so apparently unexceptionable as that of equal opportunity.

One advantage of the system will lie in its coercion being largely hidden: those enhanced in order to be equal participants in the symbolic economy will indeed succeed in the dominant cooperative scheme and thus be unlikely to see anything coercive about it. Education will likewise be brought more into line both with the needs of the economic scheme and the talents of students now designed for the scheme. The schools are unlikely, in short, to be places where students might learn a counter-memory of how things were before genetic improvement—or of how they continue to be for those unfortunately unimproved. Part of the authors' "colonization" of the natural by the social, then, involves the possibility of unprecedented colonization of future generations by the present. As such, we might well ask whether schemes of genetic enhancement are not the logical, even necessary, outcome of the already existing colonization of future generations through our accumulation of national and personal debt. The future will have to be ever more economically and totally rationalized, in short, for the simple reason that ever-greater productivity will be necessary to service our debts. It is no answer to this at all to say that the levels of debt we have are economically sustainable. Treating debt only as an economic problem is part of the way its real effects are hidden. Those effects have to do with the kinds of choices people are able to make or are precluded from making precisely because they inherit the debt of others. Levels of debt influence the kinds of people we can be. Massive debt means ever-greater economic rationalization, with the concomitant destruction of everything that stands in its way—community or regional loyalty; local, familial, class solidarities; the particularities of "environments." If it is difficult for some to see what could possibly be wrong with widespread genetic enhancement, it is because we have been so systematically trained not to see what is lost through increasing economic rationalization. This skewed training is itself a result of debt's imperative. The debt must be paid: we cannot really allow ourselves to consider, even to see, what is lost in the process.

It's a bit difficult even to envision the kind of social arrangements necessary under the authors' more visionary projections of their society of developed genetic powers. Surely such a society would involve extraordinary coordination of information and effort among the economic, social, educational, and medical sectors: coordination required to ensure the right matches between available positions and those being designed. It should be asked whether such intentional coordination can possibly be as flexible as that arising from the spontaneous or natural exchanges of those produced without genetic design. It's also unclear how a society practicing enhancement on a wide scale would reconcile genetic equal opportunity with the maximizing interest. Are we to envision a whole society of the genetically enhanced all desirous of participating in the schemes of social coordination at the highest and most gratifying level? The potential for conflict in such a situation seems immense, and we might well see society turn for simple peace to a stratification like that of Huxley's *Brave New World* (with a somewhat more privatized version of the reproductive process itself). Such an arrangement could be justified by something like the Difference Principle. Enough advantage of the most well-off could be made to redound to the least well-off that they would be better-off than they would have been otherwise.[29]

My final point concerns the model of justice with which the authors align themselves. They call their model a "subject-centered theory of justice," contrasting it with "self-interested reciprocity" theories (294). In justice as reciprocity, the "core idea is that obligations of justice are based ultimately on rational self-interest and that consequently we have no obligations to those who have nothing to contribute to our well-being" (295). Subject-centered theories, on the other hand, constitute communities based on some quality such as practical rationality or sentience

---

29. Being "better off" in order that your life can "go as well as possible" is, of course, always understood in the terms understood by the "better off"—in short, money. To reckon what is lost in the process is beyond the calculation of this kind of economy. For a larger notion of economy, see Berry, "Two Economies," in *Art of the Commonplace*, 219–35. In this essay as elsewhere, Berry's thinking on economics is influenced by the Bible and by Henry David Thoreau.

and then insist that we have obligations of justice to all quite apart from their "capacity to make a net contribution to social cooperation" (295). The authors seek to stress the superiority of subject-centered theories in two ways. First, they identify some of the worst features of eugenics with justice as reciprocity: "the tacit acceptance of some version of justice as reciprocity may explain the strident tone of moral indignation that some eugenicists leveled at those 'inferior types' whom they regarded as 'useless eaters,' nothing but a drain on social resources" (295). Second, they identify subject-centered theories with efforts at including all within the "dominant cooperative scheme" and with human rights, held by all simply "by virtue of their humanity" (295–96).

My purpose here is not to defend justice as reciprocity but simply to point out that the argument of *From Chance to Choice* exhibits precisely the flaw that David Gauthier points to in subject-centered theories: "The demands of sympathy are quite distinct from those of rational choice, and only confusion results from treating them together."[30] In *From Chance to Choice*, this confusion is evident in the authors' claims about bettering humanity through radical genetic intervention. What they are doing, in effect, is simply guaranteeing that everyone will be able to participate in a scheme of reciprocity: everyone will be capable of benefiting everyone else, an idea that perhaps sounds unexceptionable enough when stated as a generality. But this state of affairs will be achieved by designing people to fit the cooperative scheme—all, of course, in the name of equal opportunity. Thus so-called "subject-centered justice"—when paired with genetic engineering—allows the masking of self-interest on the part of the designers. It masks inequalities of power and the fact that some people will be designing other people.

Thus, in their practices, the authors of *From Chance to Choice* operate under justice-as-reciprocity even though they fail to perceive or acknowledge it. Their logic leads ultimately to the modification of all pre-born human beings—without their consultation, of course—into ones capable and desirous of participating in the "dominant cooperative scheme." This strategy is a way of insulating the dominant scheme from change and must not be confused with an idea of equal opportunity that would seek to continually modify the scheme in response to the kinds of people who already exist. That the authors are actually operating from an unacknowledged conception of justice as reciprocity is indicated, too,

---

30. Gauthier, *Morals By Agreement*, 286.

by their confining the discussion of just health care to the United States. Despite their linking justice to rights held inherently by humanity, the authors rarely, if ever, ponder the possibility of Americans' obligations to citizens of other nations. The nation, in short, provides the boundaries of a scheme of reciprocity within which their conception of justice applies. Moreover, there is little question of our modifying the dominant cooperative scheme to bring it more into line with the realities of developing countries. The authors unequivocally state that developing countries have only one option: participation in the "industrial-symbolic economy":

> The global economy is increasingly homogenizing the dominant cooperative schemes of all societies, forging a single world society defined by a single dominant cooperative scheme—that of the industrial-symbolic economy. Most people will have no choice but to try to participate in this emerging globally dominant cooperative framework. The conflict between the interest in inclusion and the maximizing interest cannot be avoided by sorting the parties out into different, noncompeting cooperative frameworks. (293)

If this last statement means that nations—not to mention more limited localities—can no longer hope to establish viable frameworks for economic and social cooperation that are somewhat insulated, at least, from the decisions of international financial centers, then this is surely bad news for developing countries who seek to establish stable economic bases and protect their environments (which can only be understood locally). Finally, it should be noted that the authors' continual reference to the primary importance of *cooperative* schemes or frameworks indicates that reciprocity is at the heart of their practical conception of justice, whether they recognize it or not.

One can appreciate the authors' rhetorical need to gather their proposals under "subject-centered justice" rather than "justice as reciprocity." Thinking of justice primarily as a matter of reciprocity seems best suited to groups of a certain, clearly smaller, scale—family, community, locality, perhaps nation—where people can be clearly convinced that justice lies in their reciprocal self-interest and where it makes sense to speak of their agreeing on a basic framework or scheme. Sympathy supplements justice, then, by initiating relationships where no reciprocity exists—relationships that may, however, develop into reciprocal ones. The picture is of a world of diverse, bounded localities governed internally by justice according to agreed-upon rules and in the process of negotiating relations with other groups based on self-interest and/or sympathy. What the rapidly globalizing economy has done is to short-circuit this process of developing reciprocities. Suddenly people at extraordinarily different levels of "development" are brought into contact with one another, people whose ability to benefit one another is extraordinarily asymmetrical. At the same time, genetic innovations in the highly developed nations press toward the eugenic question: "What kinds of people should there be?,"[31] as Jonathan Glover expressed it, or "Why Not the Best?," as the authors of *From Chance to Choice* title one of their chapters. To raise these questions is to suggest that it is not necessary for there to be the kinds of people there currently are. It may also be to suggest that the most powerful, the most "able," the "highest functioners" need no longer develop the kinds of qualities that would bring them ultimately into relationships of reciprocity with the lower functioners. After all, if it becomes possible to produce greater numbers of higher functioners, then those lower functioners would be the kinds of people there should not be.

Under such circumstances, it may seem unwise to trust to sympathy on the part of the highest functioners to provide at least something like a "decent genetic minimum" to the lower-functioning. The development of sympathy itself may be severely limited in a society of advanced genetic powers. After all, people will no longer have to look on their talents and abilities as utterly contingent gifts; they will be seen rather as the outcome of intelligent design by their parents and society. People will be, in a way, as it has been necessary for them to be. The sense that "there but for fortune may go you or I" will cease to be relevant. Sympathy will dry up for people in difficult life circumstances as these come to be understood as the product of proper genetic allocation in a scheme designed to reconcile inclusion and the maximizing interest. Moreover, no higher functioner will ever have to worry that his or her offspring will be much "less able": pre-natal genetic screening will prevent this possibility. Distinctions among functioners at various levels of ability—judged according to the demands of the scheme—cannot help but harden. Humanity will have again managed to come under the comforting conviction that birth is fate. The rich will be able to abandon the poor with a clean conscience, provided they have received a decent genetic minimum.

31. Glover, *What Sort of People Should There Be?*

Rightly wary of the limits of sympathy, the authors of *From Chance to Choice* seek to ground their proposals in justice. Unfortunately their notion of "subject-centered" justice masks the way their real goal is a global system of justice as reciprocity in which subjects are either erased or left only as "subjects" of a new "colonization"—to use the authors' own revealing language—by those possessed of advanced genetic powers. The new eugenics will not eliminate "useless eaters" but rather guarantee that only "useful eaters" are born. All will be assimilated into the scheme, which is perhaps the best possible way to ensure the scheme against challenge and change. "Subject-centered justice" obscures the enormous existent differences in the ability of individuals to define or shape the dominant scheme—which is itself to dictate the kinds of people there shall be. Until we could provide all subjects equal ability to shape the scheme, it makes little sense to speak of it as just.

But even if this were the case, we would still need to raise the more radical question about whether eugenics can be squared with justice. If we are taught systematically to think of others as inadequate, or at least "sub-optimal," in their very biology, will we ever develop the habits of justice? Doesn't the process of becoming just involve learning to respond appropriately to others irrespective, or even in spite, of how one might want them to be or think they should be? Can one learn to give others their due—"simply by virtue of their humanity," for example—while simultaneously believing that significant features of that humanity are at least potentially alterable for the better? Does not our learning to be just depend upon accepting the limits both of others and ourselves and then coming to recognize the achievements or claims of others against that background of common limitations? If human nature comes to be seen as fully alterable, how will one know how to justly recognize another's due? Is there some point at which the "highest functioners"—accustomed to participating in the scheme with others of their ilk—cease altogether to be able to appreciate the accomplishments or claims of the "lower functioners"? Is there a point at which the obligations to one another of the highest functioning cohort become so compelling as to override all obligations to members of other cohorts? How will the competing claims of members of different cohorts be adjudicated when there is no longer an assumed background of shared human nature?

I pose these questions as a way of suggesting that the authors of *From Chance to Choice* do not successfully prove that eugenics can be squared with justice. Indeed I believe that squaring cannot be accomplished, for it would depend on overlooking the most basic flaw of eugenics: the simple assumption that the "kind of people there should be" are not those currently existing. Implicit in the eugenic question about how to improve future generations is the assumption that at least some individuals of the present are sub-optimal. We might ask, in fact, whether eugenics means the end of justice, for it allows some, at least, to imagine that they need not learn how to give others their due. Rational eugenic policy encourages us to ask how to replace existent sub-optimal individuals with better ones, and one answer will be to allow the reproductive process, with suitable genetic alteration, to take its course. But surely it will seem irrational—in light of the end of a better humanity—to allow everyone access to this process. If clear, objective distinctions can be established between the genetically superior and inferior, it will be incumbent on the latter to show why they should have access to reproduction at the price of retarding human betterment. Indeed it seems well within the scope of imagination to conceive a future regime that might, at the very least, reintroduce compulsory sterilization as a means to the greater eugenic future.

Obviously the authors of *From Chance to Choice* neither advocate nor envision any of the nightmarish scenarios I foresee. They are confident that the procedural safeguards and more enlightened views about race in today's democratic societies make any return to past horrors unthinkable. As I hope to have shown, they seem, to me, dangerously lacking in imagination about a matter on which we cannot afford to be wrong. Those who would rehabilitate eugenics owe us, at the very least, a much deeper engagement with the horrors of past eugenic regimes, one that explains why the kinds of questions implicit in eugenics are not the problem. I suspect such an explanation cannot be given. Eugenics in the name of justice should be rejected, in part to save justice itself.

8

Giving Our Children Bread

Why the Harm Conundrum Is Not Such a Conundrum

ONE EXCITING FEATURE OF reading the Bible is to hear a line or verse afresh by coming across a context where it suddenly seems dramatically appropriate. This has been my experience in reading Peter Singer's development of Derek Parfit's explorations of what has come to be called in bioethics the "Non-Identity problem" or "harm" conundrum.[1] The biblical passage I refer to occurs in slightly different versions in Matthew and Luke's gospels. It follows on Jesus's teaching that every one who asks shall receive, that all who knock shall find the door opened to them. Jesus's illustration, given in the form of a rhetorical question, turns on a request from child to parent, quoted here from Luke 11:11-12: "If a son shall ask bread of any of you that is a father, will he give him a stone? or if he ask a fish, will he for a fish give him a serpent? Or if he shall ask an egg, will he offer him a scorpion?" We know how the rest of the teaching

---

1. Singer, *Practical Ethics*, 123-25. Parfit's hypothetical appeared in "Rights, Interests, and Possible People," 369-75. Similar examples are given in Parfit, *Reasons and Persons*, 357-71. Parfit has called the problem the Non-Identity Problem because in such cases as that of Woman #2 below, there is no identity between the persons in the different outcomes. If she conceives now, A is born; if later, B. Dena S. Davis has called the problem the "harm conundrum" because it involves disabilities or conditions that could plausibly be deemed "harms" but which it seems strange to do so in light of the fact that they are inseparable from the person's existence. See *Genetic Dilemmas*, 35. A related, but somewhat different, problem is that of "wrongful life," which involves moral or legal judgments about whether a child's existence is such a burden to it that its very life could be considered a wrong. The kinds of cases treated by Parfit and Singer do not turn on questions of wrongful life but rather on how to regard harms inseparable from existence to those whose lives are well worth living.

goes: if we who are evil can be counted upon to respond to our children in these ways, how much more will the heavenly Father bestow the Holy Spirit on his children when they ask.[2]

As a father, though, I have found myself too often unable to conform even to the minimalist conception of human giving assumed by Jesus. Too often I, and other parents, give the stone rather than the bread that nourishes, the poisonous serpent rather than the fish. That we do so derives as much as anything else, I suspect, from a failure to believe in the abundant life promised by Jesus. We operate from the fear of scarcity: we withhold the life that is in us—even, at times, from our children—because we fear there is not enough for both us and them. They come asking for bread, and we give them a stone.

Rarely have I heard a clearer example of giving the stone than in the voice of a mother invented by Singer in his discussion of some hypotheticals proposed by Parfit that have been enormously influential in the bioethical discussion of the Non-Identity problem. In brief, that problem involves how we are to account for our sense that a harm or wrong has been done when a child is born with a disability that results from its being conceived as the particular child it is at a particular time or in a particular manner. Ordinarily we assess harm by comparing states prior to some harming event to those after the event. But here there is no prior state; if a particular child's disability derives from the timing of its conception or a problem in the assisted reproductive process, there just is no pre-harm condition to which it can appeal to demonstrate harm. The child's disability is bound up with its existence; there is no way for it to have existed, as the particular child it is, without the disability.

The hypothetical involves two women, each planning to have a child. The first woman is three months pregnant "when her doctor gives her both bad and good news." Her fetus "has a defect that will significantly diminish the future child's quality of life—although not so adversely as to make the child's life utterly miserable, or not worth living at all." The "good news" is that the condition in the child can be avoided by the woman's taking a simple pill that has no side effects. Following Parfit's

---

2. Verse 13, in the King James translation, reads, "If ye then, being evil, know how to give good gifts unto your children: how much more shall *your* heavenly Father give the Holy Spirit to them that ask him?" I use the King James version above for the frankly rhetorical reason that it includes all three of the metaphors: bread, fish, egg. More modern translations of Luke delete the reference to bread, which is included in the parallel passage in Matthew, which is itself without the reference to the egg. See Matt 7:9–11.

analysis, Singer concludes "we would all agree that the woman should take the pill, and that she does wrong if she refuses to take it."[3]

In the second case, a woman contemplating pregnancy but still using contraception visits the doctor and is told she has a condition that will cause a child she might conceive exactly the same untreatable defect as the child in the previous case. The good news for her, however, is that simply waiting three months will cause her condition to pass and any child she might conceive to be normal. Again we would feel strongly that this woman is wrong not to wait the three months before conceiving.

Singer asks us to "suppose that the first woman does not take the pill, and the second woman does not wait before becoming pregnant, and that as a result each has a child with a significant disability."[4] He asks which woman has done the greater wrong. Assuming the three-month wait for woman #2 causes no more hardship than taking the pill does for #1, he concludes they are "equally wrong." But Singer asks us, then, to "consider what this answer implies":

> The first woman has harmed her child. That child can say to her mother: "You should have taken the pill. If you had done so, I would not now have this disability, and my life would be significantly better." But if the child of the second woman tries to make the same claim, her mother has a devastating response. She can say, "If I had waited three months before becoming pregnant you would never have existed. I would have produced another child, from a different egg and different sperm. Your life, even with your disability, is definitely above the point at which life is so miserable that it ceases to be worth living. You never had a chance of existing without the disability. So I have not harmed you at all." This reply seems a complete defence to the charge of having harmed the child now in existence. (124)

One must grant a certain completeness to this defense. It seems as perfect, hard, and unyielding as any stone could be—and as unnourishing. Indeed it's hard to imagine how anything a parent could say to a child could do more—scorpion-like—to poison the child's life. The note of scarcity might be difficult, at first, to detect, but it is surely there. For the mother's response insists that the child should be grateful for existence on any terms and that she, the child, is owed nothing. All that the child

---

3. Singer, *Practical Ethics*, 123.

4. I've used Singer's paraphrase of the hypothetical here; see *Practical Ethics*, 123–24. Further references will be given parenthetically.

is, in short, derives from the mother, whose life is so precious that any sharing of it entitles her to dictate entirely the conditions under which it is shared. Life is scarce; it belongs to the mother; the child should be grateful to have it on any terms.

I have begun here with Singer's treatment because it helps to put the Non-Identity problem clearly before us and because I wish to respond to it by way of developing an alternative understanding of the wrongs done by both mothers. Those wrongs might best be understood, I will suggest, as failures of justice and moral seriousness involving either an inadequate or undeveloped sense of the separateness of persons and of the need for equitable sharing of burdens. Such an understanding enables us to preserve some features of a "harm-based approach," a point I will develop fully in the second part of this chapter through an engagement with Jeff McMahan's treatment of the Non-Identity problem, particularly as Parfit has developed it.[5] In the third part of the chapter, I consider several other major attempts to clarify our ways of thinking about "harm" when it is inseparable from the person's existence and about when such harm should be prevented by abortion of "defective" fetuses or by the abandoning of attempts to procreate by people at genetic risk.

First it will be helpful to explain Singer's analyses in greater detail. As he regards Woman #2 to have offered a "complete defence," he needs a way to explain his continuing sense that she has done wrong. After pondering several possibilities, Singer opts for saying that the wrong she does lies in "bringing into existence a child with a less satisfactory quality of life than another child whom one could have brought into existence. In other words, we have failed to bring about the best possible outcome."[6] The plausibility of this answer suggests, for Singer, "that at least possible people are replaceable." The relevant "question then becomes this: At what stage in the process that passes from possible people to actual people does replaceability cease to apply?" (124–25).

---

5. McMahan, "Wrongful Life," in *Bioethics*, 445–75. Quotations from McMahan will be included parenthetically.

6. An alternative way to understand the wrong done by a woman in a case like #2 is proposed by Joel Feinberg: "There is no doubt that the mother did act wrongly, but it does not follow that her wrongdoing wronged any particular person, or had any particular victim. She must be blamed for wantonly introducing a certain evil into the world, not for harming, or violating the rights of, a person." See "Wrongful Life and the Counterfactual Element in Harming," 27.

Singer never clarifies the final point absolutely, but that stage is, for him, certainly at least months after birth.

Several things need to be said about Singer's argument right at this point. First, his distinction between what Woman #1 and Woman #2 have done seems unsustainable in light of his refusal to accord either personhood or a right to be born to fetuses. Woman #1 can also argue, with only a slight modification of Woman #2's defense, that she has not harmed her child—unless, that is, there is already some being there at three months who has a right not to be harmed. Woman #1 can say to her child,

> Your sense that "you" were there at three months is merely metaphysical illusion. I was under no obligation to take any risk to assist a being whose existence I might still have chosen to terminate at any time during the next year. Your sense that "you" were harmed depends on there being some "you" prior to my so-called harming omissions of treatment, but there was no such "you" present and capable of being harmed. You, like the child of Woman #2, had only one way to be born and that is as you are, as I allowed you to be.

Singer's, and perhaps Parfit's, sense that Woman #1 has harmed her child, and can thus be distinguished from Woman #2—in what she has done, if not in degree of wrong—depends on their assuming a status for the fetus that their other assumptions deny.[7]

Second, Singer's judgment about how to understand the wrong done by Woman #2—that she has "failed to bring about the best possible outcome"—cannot help but sound like bad news to the disabled. As I

---

7. It could be argued that once the woman has decided to carry to term, she has implicitly agreed not to harm her child—through risky behaviors, for example. Yet Woman #1 does nothing to harm her child. She merely refuses a treatment that would assist it. Hers might be considered an example of what John Robertson has called "irresponsible reproduction." She might be charged with pre-natal child abuse for denying her fetus "a minimum level of care, nurture, and protection." But it's clear that the availability of abortion must undermine the ability of children to demand responsible pre-natal care, for the mother has the easy response that she has exceeded the requirements of ordinary moral behavior simply by bringing the child—in any condition—to term. As we've seen in earlier chapters, Boonin, Regan, Thomson et al. seem to imply that carrying to term is supererogatory. Robertson himself bases nearly all of his case for irresponsible reproduction on costs to society, not harms to the child. See *Children of* Choice, 75–90. When he considers Parfit's case #2, he finds the woman wrong "not because she has harmed the child," but "because she has violated a norm against offending persons who are troubled by gratuitous suffering" (76).

explore in chapter 10, Singer certainly does not intend discrimination against the disabled. He believes that the principle of equal consideration of interests should lead to an affirmative-action-style policy regarding treatment of disabled people. Nevertheless it's not difficult to see how the kind of simplistic judgments about outcomes required by utilitarianism would tend to undermine regard for the disabled. Singer apparently quite confidently predicts that the normal child will have a more satisfactory future than one disabled. Such a prediction must rest on a fairly detailed model of what the future will look like: we can only predict that A will have a happier future than B if we can say, with a high degree of confidence, that future arrangements will serve A better than B. This kind of assumption is precisely what the disabled find themselves needing to struggle against in order that future arrangements be modified so that B might do just as well as A. Furthermore, the kind of confidence required by judgments like Singer's must tend to reduce and simplify the criteria involved in the quality of life evaluation. The fewer, simpler, and more quantitative the criteria, the more certain the judgments can be made to seem. If we need certainty of judgment, we will seek few, simple, and quantitative criteria. Thus one criticism of Singer's way of evaluating lives would be that it inherently upholds and reinforces the status quo precisely because it depends upon highly predictable future outcomes. The need for high degrees of predictability will cause us to design the future in rigid ways, conformity to which can be designated success with the levels of certainty required to confirm our predictions. It is hard to see how this process can work to the advantage of any but the most normal.

Third, Singer's work helps us to see with particular clarity the link between utilitarianism and the fear of scarcity. It becomes incumbent on us to maximize the good in every action—or in every child we allow to be born—to the degree that we believe life or the good to be scarce commodities. Thus the best rhetorical strategy to make utilitarianism seem inevitable is to continually stress scarcities, and this is a standard feature of Singer's arguments and hypotheticals. Insistence on the replaceability of people serves an important "economic" function within Singer's utilitarianism. It is important to insist on replaceability in order to keep the discussion within the conditions of scarcity needed to defend and confirm utilitarian judgments. For if we recognize, or insist upon, the irreplaceability of particular people, then we will be lead to find ways—perhaps through greater cooperation to expand resources or a more serious commitment to just arrangements—to think ourselves out of the problems of scarcity. In short, commitment to the irreplaceability of persons will lead to creative economic thinking—in a very broad sense—that utilitarianism may not, particularly if it is allowed to put the very existence of individual persons into question.

My own analysis of the wrongs of Woman #1 and Woman #2 turns on questions of virtue, justice, risk assessment, moral seriousness, and the distribution of power. I wonder if, in fact, everyone would follow Singer in believing that what Woman #2 does is "as wrong" as what Woman #1 does.[8] My own sense is that #1 is somewhat more in the wrong than #2, but the difference is narrow. Woman #1 has already made the decision to care for this child; her carrying the child three months should have impressed some sense of its separateness—and her responsibility—upon her judgment. She has already assumed the risks of pregnancy but now refuses a risk-free pill needed for her fetus. The unwillingness to take such a minimal action to avoid harm to a being already living suggests a degree of selfishness inconsistent with later parental care. Woman #2 also seems selfish in her unwillingness to make a relatively easy sacrifice for the sake of the child she is to conceive. If what she does seems less wrong, it is because she does choose something good—to have a child. Woman #1 has also chosen to have a child, of course, but as her pregnancy is already a given of the case, it may seem to weigh slightly less in our evaluation of the women's actions within the cases themselves. But surely a part of the wrong done by both women lies in their demonstrating attitudes of self-concern quite inconsistent with the qualities they will need to nurture and rear their children.

Before taking up the further question of harm to the children, it seems useful to point out the serious flaws in the hypothetical cases. Without wishing to sound dismissive, I must say that these cases are clearly the work of a man, for they both treat pregnancy itself as if it were risk-free. The cases are seriously flawed by this assumption, without which they make little sense. If we factor the risk of pregnancy into the cases, then neither Woman #1's nor Woman #2's behavior makes much

---

8. Parfit's assessment is what he calls the No-Difference View. Since in both cases the result is a child with a disability, it makes no difference that Woman #1 has made the outcome worse for an already existent individual whereas Woman #2 has done so for one being brought into being. See Parfit, "Comments," 860.

sense. Woman #1 elects to take the fairly considerable risk of pregnancy—and, of course, the responsibility for the child's rearing—yet refuses a risk-free pill that will eliminate the child's disability. Obviously this behavior is so utterly inconsistent as to be unbelievable. The narrative of case #2 is perhaps somewhat more believable yet even in it the woman's behavior would seem highly unlikely if one simply wrote into the case a number of quite predictable factors. The rearing of a child with significant disability is surely, on average, a more demanding proposition than rearing a normally abled child. Yet the example expects us to believe that a woman so self-centered as to refuse the relatively minor inconvenience of waiting three months to conceive will knowingly take on a more demanding task of rearing than can be hers if she waits the three months. Again this behavior is too wildly inconsistent to be believed. The value of insights derived from comparing two such internally flawed cases seems dubious.

Indeed this problem of inconsistency in the women's behavior is even more important than I have thus far suggested. Both women clearly violate Parfit's principle of rationality: that each of us acts in such a way that his life will go for him as well as possible.[9] Both of the women in the hypotheticals act in ways that very probably will cause their lives to go less well than they would otherwise. Both act, in Parfit's terms, irrationally and in apparent disregard of their clear self-interest, assuming, of course, they intend to rear the children. Why does Parfit do this? Why does he seem, in this case, clearly unwilling to trust principle S to produce what is best both for the mother and her child? Is this because he desires to bring all beneficence within the calculation of the moral system and to argue for its impersonality? Does this intention require narratives that suggest failure in what one might almost call the archetype of beneficence: the mother's regard for her child? This is not the place for a sustained critique of Parfit's work, but I hope this analysis suggests a place to begin such a critique: with Parfit's apparent attribution of irrationality to mothers, perhaps necessitated by the uncomfortable fact that maternal care for children constitutes a dependable sort of beneficence exercised quite freely (without need of moral coercion) and in a person-affecting way.[10]

---

9. "For each person, there is one supremely rational ultimate aim: that his life go, for him, as well as possible." See *Reasons and Persons*, 4.

10. Remembering that parents do not typically need to be coerced to have children

Nevertheless we should try to make further sense of Parfit's cases, if only because they have been so influential. We have seen what Singer imagines Woman #2 saying to her child. What I would like to suggest is what child #2 can say to his/her parent:

> I am grateful to you for the gift of life and I recognize that my being disabled or differently abled is bound up with my existence. Nevertheless you failed to take seriously the risks and burdens of life to be shouldered by the one you created. I almost want to say you wronged humanity in my own person, but I don't want you to have to abstract so completely from your role as my mother to think about it that way. Rather I want to say you were unjust, for you chose to impose a significant, unnecessary, and lifelong burden on the child you were to create simply to avoid a very slight and temporary burden to yourself. I wonder if you are not existing in a condition of imaginative denial, perhaps induced by conditions of great plenty in your economic life. For if you'd had a clearer sense of the risks and burdens we all share—death, most prominently—you would have acted to minimize the additional burdens faced by the one you were to create. To put this another way, you exercised an excessive and unnatural degree of control over me (and your response to me indicates you intend continuing to do so). You certainly violated the spirit of the maxim that we ought not to use one another even if you technically were

---

may help, too, in explaining the "Asymmetry" in our attitudes toward having children, a problem commented on by Parfit, Heyd, McMahan, and others. Briefly the Asymmetry involves our sense that we have a strong duty not to have a child whose life, in Parfit's terms, "would be worth *not* living" but no correspondingly strong sense that we ought to have a child whose life will be happy and good for him. It seems, in short, that if we believe we ought not to have a "miserable child," (Parfit) we ought to have a happy one. What's overlooked in discussions of the Asymmetry is the possibility that we ought not to have any child, not because it is not good to have children, but because doing so ought not to be regarded as a duty, at least a humanly-established one. There are good reasons not to regard having children as a duty. First, it has typically not been necessary to do so: people have been quite willing to have children without coercion when they can envision a hopeful future for their children. Second, having children should be free from coercion because we want and expect parents to rear those children, and there is much greater likelihood that they will do this well if they have been conceived freely, not as a matter of duty. Third, the resentment that parents coerced into procreation may feel will likely be directed at the child, causing the child to be resentful and unable to affirm the goodness of its own existence. We need to remember that our moral intuitions about having children have been formed in the light of the need to provide for their care and rearing. This is rarely, if ever, acknowledged in philosophical treatments of the problems and paradoxes involved in "causing to exist." On the Asymmetry, see Parfit, "Future Generations," 148.

not guilty of instrumentalization because the instrument you chose to use had not yet been formed. The degree of control you exercised with regard only to your own convenience rendered me effectively a thing. Moreover, I fail to see how anyone could ever enter into relationships of trust or mutuality with one so evidently unmoved by justice in the most basic of human relations, that between parent and child.[11]

My hypothetical child has here articulated a perfectly reasonable assessment of the wrong done by Mother #2 as a failure of justice. Mother #2 has failed to give appropriate consideration to the fair sharing of burdens incumbent on us all. What makes her action unjust is the risk-free quality of what is required to have a normal child. If considerable risk had been involved in her waiting three months—or if she had required, as in a modification of Case #1, a very risky procedure—then no one would criticize her for having a disabled rather than normal child. But given that waiting the three months is risk-free, we are inclined to believe she has failed to take seriously enough the burdens all of us share. Seriousness is perhaps a difficult term to define precisely, and yet it seems a prerequisite of all moral action. We expect moral seriousness, for instance, as a necessary characteristic of authentic civil disobedience.[12] Mother #2 seems lacking in this kind of seriousness: we might legitimately be concerned about whether she could ever be expected to care sufficiently about the consequences of her action to be a moral actor. Or, to put this a bit differently, she seems inadequately aware of the deep truth of the separateness of persons. She seems not to have realized sufficiently that the being she has conceived is not a plaything but rather a separate moral subject in her own right. To the degree that we take the moral task seriously, we will see that it is unjust to ask others to bear unnecessary burdens.[13] This is

11. The child's response here seems, to me, the appropriate one as well to Heyd's "generocentrism," which he defines as "essentially the thesis that genesis choices can and should be guided exclusively by reference to the interests, welfare, ideals, rights, and duties of those making the choice, the 'generators.'" See *Genethics*, 96.

12. John Rawls argues, for example, that the nonviolence of civil disobedience is a way of signifying fidelity to law, a fidelity that "helps to establish to the majority that the act is indeed politically conscientious and sincere, and that it is intended to address the public's sense of justice. To be completely open and nonviolent is to give bond of one's sincerity, for it is not easy to convince another that one's acts are conscientious, or even to be sure of this before oneself." See *Theory of Justice*, 366–67. Feinberg discusses the "conscientiousness" of the civil disobedient in *Freedom and Fulfillment*, 154–58.

13. I want to be very clear here, though, that this is not, in my view, a reason to

particularly the case when 1) there is a very large discrepancy in power or control between those whose conduct produces the burdens and those who must bear them; and 2) when one person, here the mother, has a particular, role-given responsibility for the other. It is reasonable to say that Mother #2, like Mother #1, has been unjust and that the injustice of Mother #2 is person-affecting. It is true that Mother #2, had she been just, would have produced a different child. Nevertheless disabled child #2 is the person who is most burdened—in ways impossible to justify by reference to principles of justice—among the constellation of persons involved. Fortunately we ought not to have to worry about scenarios like that of Mother #2 very often, for in conception self-interest and justice seem ordinarily aligned. The desire to have life go as well as possible will ordinarily cause mothers to exercise justice toward their children by accepting minimal risks and inconveniences required to prevent children from bearing extraordinary burdens.

I believe the account I am developing accords better with many basic moral intuitions regarding harm and beneficence than Parfit's claim that the area of morality "concerned with beneficence and human well-being, cannot be explained in person-affecting terms."[14] To demonstrate my claim, I will look at the kinds of cases devised by Jeff McMahan to illustrate Parfit's Non-Identity problem. McMahan's own position is complex. He appears to accept part of Parfit's argument that cases such as those posed by the Non-Identity problem cannot be understood in person-affecting terms. Yet, on the other hand, he rejects some of Parfit's argument that beneficence can only be understood in impersonal terms. McMahan's position seems closest to what he calls "The Encompassing Account," according to which "person-affecting considerations and impersonal considerations are distinct and nonadditive." Neither of these kinds of considerations "is reducible to the other." Instead "both matter; both provide reasons for action. But it is not always worse if a bad effect is worse for someone; sometimes it is, sometimes it is not" (473–74). My own account will show not only why we should reject Parfit's non-per-

---

refrain from criticism of abortions justified by putative future harms to the child—biological, social, material, or otherwise. Abortion should be free from criticism on "child-centered" grounds only when we can clearly say that life itself—from the standpoint of the child—would be so unbearably painful or hopeless as to constitute a wrong. Even then we should utter this judgment with fear, trembling, and the hope to be forgiven.

14. *Reasons and Persons*, 370–71.

son affecting account of beneficence but also McMahan's "encompassing account."

All these matters will become clearer as we look at the cases. McMahan asks us to consider two, both involving a Negligent Physician. The first is called the Preconception Case. It involves a couple who seek preconception genetic screening because they suspect "that one of them may be the carrier of a genetic defect that causes moderately severe cognitive impairment." The physician who does the screening "is negligent, however, and assures the couple that there is no risk when in fact the man is a carrier of the defect. As a result, the woman conceives a child with moderately severe genetic impairments." If the screening had been done properly, a "sperm from the man would have been isolated and genetically altered to correct the defect." It would then, of course, have been "combined *in vitro* with an egg drawn from the woman." Since the "probability is vanishingly small" that this corrected sperm would have been the same as that which fertilized the egg as the couple went ahead with natural conception, the child who would have resulted from the *in vitro* process would "have been a *different* child from the retarded child who now exists" (445).

McMahan asks that we compare the Preconception Case to the Prenatal Case, in which "A physician negligently prescribes a powerful drug for a woman who is in the eighth month of pregnancy. The drug causes damage to the fetus's brain and the child to whom she gives birth is, as a consequence, moderately cognitively impaired" (446). Assuming the eighth-month fetus has begun to exist, as McMahan does, the child injured in this case is "numerically the same child as the child who would have existed had the damage not been done." Herein lies the difference in the cases. In the Prenatal Case, the "retarded child and the possible normal child are the same child in two different possible lives whereas in the Preconception Case the retarded child and the hypothetical normal child are different children." Thus the "Non-Identity Problem." The child born in the Preconception Case has a life that is limited but "not so bad as not to be worth living," and, since she would not exist apart from the physician's negligence, it is difficult to say that the negligence has harmed her or made life worse for her. This is because she is non-identical with the child who would have been born absent the negligence. This is, of course, not true for the child harmed in the Prenatal Case (446).

The problem McMahan poses, then, is how we should explain "our sense that the Negligent Physician's action" is "morally objectionable" in the Preconception Case. Clearly he harms the couple, but this does not account fully for our sense of the wrong he has done. Where my account begins to part company from McMahan's is at his next assessment:

> Most of us believe that, quite independently of the impact of the physician's action on the parents, the retarded child in the Preconception Case ought not to have been caused to exist, and that, given that he *has* been wrongfully caused to exist, the physician should be required to pay damages not only to compensate the parents for the injury done to them but also, insofar as possible, to enhance the life of the child. (446–47)

What I object to here is not the conclusion but the premise. The physician should, if judged negligent, compensate the parents and contribute to assistance for the child. But I do not agree that the child "ought not to have been caused to exist" nor, in fact, do I think that most people would accept that. To demonstrate this, I would simply ask people to consider whether they could argue thusly to the child in the second person, "You ought not to have been caused to exist." If it is inconceivable to do this, as I believe it is for most of us, then McMahan's judgment cannot be accepted. The only faint plausibility McMahan's judgment has derives from the child's being hypothetical and in comparative relation to the shadow child who would have been born otherwise. As long as the child has those statuses, it makes some sense to say it ought not to have existed. Once the child becomes actual, however, this judgment is no longer of any relevance.

McMahan notes that in discussing a pair of cases similar to the Preconception and Prenatal ones, Parfit argues for the so-called No-Difference View: that is, "given that the outcome is the same in each" it "makes no difference that in one case the outcome is worse for the individual whereas in the other case it is not" (447). Glossing Parfit's argument, which he does not fully accept, McMahan reasons thus:

> Since the objection to the physician's action in the Preconception case cannot be that it harmed or was worse for the retarded child, it follows, if Parfit is right, that this cannot be the objection to his action in the Prenatal Case either. Generalizing, Parfit claims that the fact that an effect is *worse for people*, or bad *for them*, is

never part of the fundamental explanation of why the effect is bad. (447)

Thus the "area of morality" concerned with beneficence must be "explained in *impersonal* terms" (447).

Most of us would agree, I believe, with McMahan's claim that our objection to the physicians' negligence is "equally strong" in both cases. In this sense, there is "no-difference" between the two, but this does not imply Parfit's conclusion. First an obvious point: our equally strong objections assume equal degrees of negligence in the two cases. It is not simply the comparative conditions of the children that determine our assessments but rather also the kind and degree of irresponsibility on the part of the physicians. McMahan's cases and his argument often obscure the fact that a judgment about negligence already represents a complex comparative assessment of the physician's conduct relative to standards of care or conduct. At times McMahan comes close to saying that the physician's negligence caused the child to exist in the Preconception Case or that his action actually "benefits the child . . . by causing the child's life to contain certain goods"—a point I'll return to presently (452). But what is the physician's action? Negligence is not an action but rather a description of an action based on complex distinctions from other actions the physician might or ought to have taken.[15]

---

15. The irresponsible physician here might point to something like Kavka's "Paradox of Future Individuals" to justify his actions. Basically a development of the Non-Identity problem, the paradox asserts we have only very limited obligations to future generations because any action we take will affect the patterns of procreation in the future and thus produce different sets of particular individuals, all with lives worth living. Parfit uses the example of the Risky Policy to illuminate the problem. A community debates a choice between two energy policies, both completely safe for two centuries, but one Risky farther out in time while also productive of a "slightly higher" standard of living "over the next century." We choose the Risky Policy, there is a "catastrophe two centuries later," and thousands are injured and killed. By this time, "there would be no one living who would have been born whichever policy we chose." Our choice of the Risky Policy is therefore not worse for anyone, and, if we "believe that causing to exist can benefit," our choice has actually been good for those who die, as they "would never have existed if we had chosen the Safe Policy." Our choice actually "*benefits* them." What, then, Parfit asks, is the objection to our choice?

Several responses to Parfit seem relevant. First, his way of designing the case distorts the way we must, in fact, reflect on risks involved in choosing policy options. What would be inherently uncertain to the choosers is here made a certainty. Their choice, as

Presumably the physician did not aim at harming the child. She took certain actions that were deemed to be insufficiently responsible. Perhaps she has had a long habit of taking pleasure excursions rather than reading the latest research on genetic defects. Would we then say that pleasure excursions are causally responsible for the goods of the child's life, in the Preconception Case—goods sufficiently valuable to outweigh the "deficits" of that child's life? On this view, it would seem that taking pleasure excursions at the expense of reading research is a good thing—in that it causes children to exist whose lives are of net benefit to them. Our objection to it would be simply that it is not as good a thing as reading the research, for that would lead to children whose

---

Parfit narrates it, is not about weighing risks in an inherently uncertain world but rather about instituting a policy that trades destruction of innocents distant in time for some measure of more immediate gain. It thus becomes impossible to separate our moral response from this felt injustice. Second, the causal link asserted between our choice and the existence of the particular set of victims is undermined by the very Non-Identity Problem itself. Parfit speaks of the later born as "owing" their existence to our choice, but, as the Non-Identity Problem insists, they would not owe their existence *as the particular people they are* to our choice any more than to the trillions of random acts and events involved in determining the precise timing of their conception. One could argue that the effect, then, of framing such questions from within the Non-Identity Problem is probably to make them meaningless. Since all those random events could be thought of as causing them to exist as the particular people they are, why should we focus on our choice of energy policy rather than others of these events? Still I think a wrong has been done here, and, unlike Parfit, it seems to me a wrong done to someone—primarily, of course, those who are injured or killed in the catastrophe, but also, curiously, to ourselves, particularly if we reason about it in the way Parfit does. It is worth considering whether philosophers like Kavka, McMahan, and Parfit have revealed something about the nature of wrong (and perhaps wrongful life) without being aware of doing so. Both Parfit's invented argument for the Risky Policy (which he judges, incidentally, to be wrong) and McMahan's in defense of the irresponsible physician turn on counting the existence of the victim against his claims in ways that we would never will for ourselves. We would say to the victims of the catastrophe, for instance, that the benefit of existence conferred on them by our choice outweighed any harm that came to them. This seems an outrageous logic capable of justifying our doing just about anything to others; it would be particularly outrageous if offered, as in Parfit's case, in questions of generational relationships, where one generation is so entirely dependent on another for its very existence. We would never tolerate having the good of our existence used against us by a prior generation bent on justifying harms to us. Thus, by acting in such a way as to count the good of existence against those whose good it must be (when they arrive), we act unjustly and become unjust. In biblical terms, we become like the "kings of the Gentiles" who "lord it over them" and "are called benefactors" (Luke 22:25).

lives are of greater net value. Obviously this seems an untenable account of negligence.[16]

My claim is that our objections are equally strong in the two cases because in each a person has been affected in ways that will cause him or her to bear burdens beyond those we are normally expected to bear—and because this has happened through no fault of the children themselves and through the irresponsibility of one who has failed to justly estimate the significance of two further factors: 1) that the physician here has an extraordinary degree of control over another's life; and 2) that the risks in the whole process are very disproportionately borne by the one who has no control over it, the child, while the one who has most control over it, the physician, remains risk-free absent the fear of findings of negligence. Obviously we insist on the possibility of finding for negligence in order to force physicians to assume some of the risks for their decisions. I think we might best understand the wrong done by the negligent physicians in both cases as a kind of injustice: they have failed to give sufficient due to the burdens the children must bear as a result of their inattention or lack of care.[17]

If we do not immediately understand the wrong done in the Preconception Case this way, it is only because McMahan's construction of the case causes what I will call a distortion of the risk pool. The case leads us to *think of the retarded child who is born in terms of the shadow child who is not born* and thus to see the risks and burdens to the child who is born only in relation to the unburdened child who is not born (who can continue to be unburdened only, in fact, as long as "he or she" remains purely hypothetical, unborn, and thought of strictly in "his/her" difference from the child who is born—as the "other" to that child). But once the retarded child is born, it is burdened like the rest of us. The pool that matters if we are to assess its risks and burdens no longer consists of

---

16. James Woodward has developed a similar *reductio* involving Viktor Frankl and the Nazis. Frankl seems to suggest in *Man's Search for Meaning* that his imprisonment in a concentration camp led to his developing "certain resources of character, insights into the human condition, and capacities for appreciation that he would not otherwise have had." If we "suppose, not implausibly, that Frankl's mistreatment by the Nazis was a necessary condition for the richness of his later life," it seems "wildly counterintuitive to suggest that it follows from this fact alone that the Nazis did not really wrong Frankl or violate his rights." See "Non-Identity Problem," 809.

17. I would insist again that this failure of justice is grounded in a refusal of the deep truth of human separateness. I think we might ask whether McMahan's physicians are capable of moral action.

itself and some imagined, perfect, unburdened shadow child but rather of all of us. Once we understand this, it is easy to see the child has been burdened—as the person he or she is—in a way beyond that of the rest of us. This seems to me a perfectly credible account of person-affecting harm in the Preconception Case—that is, if we understand being harmed in terms of being burdened, through no fault of one's own, in ways not true of others, and through the actions of those who have a very large degree of control over us.

Perhaps no further argument is necessary to counter McMahan's claim that "the harm based approach fails because it has no explanation of why an act that is assumed to cause a congenital harmed condition ought not to be done even when it also causes compensating benefits" (453). The account offered here has, I hope, supplied that explanation. Nevertheless it seems important to consider one further argument McMahan offers in rejecting harm-based approaches and to comment specifically on why we should reject the language of "compensating benefits." McMahan finds "untenable" the view that the Negligent Physician is not responsible "for any of the goods that the retarded child's life contains" in the Preconception Case (452). This judgment seems highly counterintuitive, and I suspect that a very great majority of us would endorse the position he rejects: that is, that the goods in this child's life "are attributable to other causes." Surely to argue as McMahan does is to blunt our ability to criticize negligence. For the physician can respond that he has created net good for the child even if not the greatest net good. Should he be required always to produce the best?[18]

Most of us would believe—contra McMahan—that indeed "there are no benefits attributable to the Negligent Physician's action that are

18. I echo the title here of Robert M. Adams, "Must God Create the Best?" 317–32. Part of Adams's wonderful argument that God need not create the best of all possible worlds is his claim that it would be an unreasonable complaint for one to say, "God has wronged me by not following the principle of refraining from creating any world in which there is a creature that would have been happier in another world He could have made" (321). The complaint is unreasonable because if God had followed the principle insisted on by the complainer He would have made a world in which the complainer would not have existed. The complainer exists, in short, only in this less than best of all possible worlds we inhabit. This is an argument appropriate for God, but not for physicians (perhaps because it is reserved for God). Physicians should do their human best—judged by established standards of the practice—to bring about good outcomes. They do not create persons and therefore cannot put in the divine claim to have benefited them even when they've clearly not done what the standards require.

capable of compensating the child for the harm that the action has caused" (452). This is not to say that the goods of the child's life cannot "compensate" it for the harms it has received. Most of us believe that the lives of disabled people are well worth living, despite their disabilities. But we would not attribute this worth, in a case like the preconception one, to the physician's irresponsibility! Nor should we regard the goods of the disabled person's life as a kind of "compensation" for that life's limitations. Physicians should "compensate" those whom their negligence burdens unjustly. But the qualities and abilities of the disabled person should not be considered "compensation" for losses. These are simply features of the person to be developed in their own right, not to somehow make up for what the person is not. What's at stake here is the process by which the disabled person becomes a subject in his or her own right, not one who is attempting to live in ways understood to be compensations for one's not being as one should have been. To think of goods in that way is to condemn one to unfreedom. Contra McMahan, the negligent physician does not cause "the child's life to contain certain goods" (452). These are, in no way, attributable to the injustice with which he has regarded the child to be created.[19]

As this last argument has commented on the matter of how to regard the "compensation" from the subject position of the injured, this is perhaps a good place to address a part of McMahan's claim for the "Encompassing Account" that turns on ascribing responses to the disabled. The position I'm developing rejects the Encompassing Account, which insists the wrong done in the Preconception Case can only be impersonal. According to it, the wrong in the Prenatal Case is both impersonal and person-affecting and thus quite probably worse than the wrong in the Preconception Case. McMahan's handling of the comparative wrongness of the two cases is a bit uncertain here, uncertainty that is itself revealing.

---

19. Part of the reason to continue insisting that harm is person-affecting is that the harms of disability must be lived out by persons. In cases involving parental or physician negligence, the disabled will have to struggle very personally not only with physical limitation but with the psychological consequences of knowing she's been harmed by others. She will have to somehow make that part of her life-story and yet in a way that it does not determine her. Moreover, while she should surely be compensated, no amount of compensation can ever guarantee her psychological freedom from the harming events.

What he offers first is an explanation of how the strictly impersonal objection in the Preconception Case "might be weaker" than the additive combination of impersonal and person-affecting wrongs in the Prenatal Case:

> In the Prenatal Case, the disabled child could reasonably (though not in practice) have this thought: "It could have been better for me." That is a bitter reflection. In the Preconception Case, the parallel thought to which the disabled child would be entitled is: "A better-off person might have existed instead of me." This is not a disturbing thought; virtually all of us could reasonably believe this of ourselves. (474)

But in order to invert the relative judgments about bitterness here, one need only attribute another equally possible thought to the child in the Preconception Case: "My parents could or should have had a child more to their liking than me. Because of my disability, I am not the child they wanted to have." This, I would submit, is easily as bitter a reflection as that attributed by McMahan to the child injured in the Prenatal Case. It concerns the child's whole being in a way that McMahan's economically accented language of "worse off" or "better off" does not. Those terms, in short, may be especially marked, in ways distorting here, by the confident assumptions of the normally abled, themselves free of serious challenge to the worth of their very existence and thus able to consider the possibility of replacement by "better off" others precisely because they have no fear that this will really happen. The bitterness of the reflection I have ascribed to the child in the Preconception Case suggests why we need strong protections against physicians' negligence. No child should have to have the thought I have attributed to the injured one of the Preconception Case. The possibility of the child's having that thought should indeed be reckoned a significant part of the person-affecting harm caused by the unjust practitioner.

One last feature of McMahan's argument requires comment. He rejects not only "harm-based" approaches to the wrongful life question but also "rights-based" approaches. My account has insisted that we can speak meaningfully of harm, in a person-affecting way, in the Preconception Case, and that the primary harm is caused by a failure of justice on the physician's part. Such an account can, I think, also capture some of the insight of a rights-based approach. It seems reasonable to say that the children in both cases had a right to just treatment on the part of the physician, a right whose violation now entitles them to compensation. As McMahan's account would deny any validity to a rights-based approach, his argument deserves scrutiny.

McMahan's objection to rights-based approaches begins by asking us to "imagine a disability—*condition X*—that is not so bad as to make life not worth living but is sufficiently serious that to cause someone to exist with condition X would be, according to the rights-based approach, to violate that person's rights." "If it is wrong to cause someone to exist with condition X," McMahan continues, then "it should also be wrong to save someone's life if the only way of doing so would also cause the person to have condition X and it is not possible to obtain the person's consent to being saved in this way." But if we imagine a late-term fetus whose life can only be saved by a treatment that causes X, it seems "intuitively clear that it would not be *wrong* to treat the fetus, thereby saving its life." Saving it, however, causes it to have X and "thus, apparently, violates its rights" (454).

Surely it would not be wrong to save the fetus in McMahan's example, and it would not be wrong precisely because it has no way of being born except with condition X. But this tells us nothing at all about its right to be born without condition X when that is possible. Another way to think about the matter is by considering the person against whom the fetus's right is to be asserted. A right seems only meaningful if there is some person against whom it can be asserted and whose duty is to fulfill it. Once the fetus is diagnosed as only savable through a treatment that will produce X, it becomes meaningless to say that it has a right to live somehow without X. There is no one who can fulfill this right. But this is not the case in the Preconception Case, in which there is clearly someone against whom the child can assert its right to be treated justly—the physician.

One problem of McMahan's presentation should probably be designated linguistic: that is, his premises and/or principles are often so detached from the contexts in which they ordinarily function as to become unhelpful. One can see this especially well in a follow-up argument to the one above designed again to suggest the insufficiency of rights-based approaches to the situation of the fetus who can only be saved by treating it in such a way that it will have X. McMahan notes that perhaps the situation of the fetus can be regarded as involving a conflict of rights. He then distinguishes positive from negative rights, arguing—soundly, of course—that "the right not to be killed is a negative right and is thus held, by theorists of rights, to be considerably stronger, other things being equal, than the right to be saved." "But if," he continues, "negative rights are in general considerably stronger than corresponding positive rights, it is at least arguable that the negative right not to be caused to be disabled is stronger, or more stringent, than the positive right to be saved" (455). But surely this relative weighing of negative and positive rights is true only because of the concerns for freedom of action and risk-taking that form the background contexts of these rights. We assume we ought to be able to act freely without the threat of others disabling us, and we recognize that there are limits on our claims to being saved by others when such saving nearly always involves substantial risks to the savers—risks we do not want to be required of us in similar situations. Moreover, the fetus can be saved *only* in such a way that it will have X. Therefore it has a clear right to be saved and a claim against us to save it, since to do so is essentially without risk to the savers. There is no conflict of rights at all, for once it can only be saved with X, it ceases to be meaningful to say it has a right not to be disabled—that is, assuming X is not so bad that life will be, for the child, so burdensome as to be not worth living.

What I hope to have offered, then, is an account of the kind of harm done by the women in Parfit's hypotheticals, from the beginning of this chapter, and the Negligent Physician in McMahan's cases. My account argues the harm is person-affecting in that the person who is created will be forced to bear burdens beyond those borne by the rest of us. He will have to do this through no fault of his own and because of actions taken by others who have been in positions where, largely free of risk or cost to themselves, they have had an enormous degree of power to determine his condition. Their failure is a failure of justice, moral seriousness and imagination, the latter because they have failed to consider sympathetically the burdens under which the harmed one must now live—and which they could have prevented through either nearly risk-free action (the mothers) or fulfillment of ordinary professional obligations (the physicians). My account is harm-based and could also be designated rights-based, as it insists the child has had a right not to be harmed when prevention of that harm was basically risk-free or a matter of ordinary professional competence.[20]

20. I believe my account also successfully answers the questions raised by Kavka's example of the slave child, which he considers a challenge to person-affecting views

In the remaining part of this chapter, I will look at four additional attempts to come to terms with the "harm conundrum," suggesting the

of harm. Briefly the example goes like this: in a society where slavery is legal, a couple who have chosen to remain childless are offered $50,000 to produce a child to hand over to a slaveholder. This seems outrageous to us and yet seems difficult to criticize on person-affecting terms because nobody seems to lose by it: the parents get the money, the slaveholder gets a slave, the child—though enslaved—gets existence and thus seems to have little reason to complain of his parents' actions, for he would not exist otherwise. Kavka claims that we must here explain the wrong done in terms of the character of the agents, and clearly their motives are responsible for a good bit of our reaction. But he, and Heyd in his comments on the example, believe "it is not the wrong done to the child which is the source of the iniquity of the deal" (Heyd, *Genethics*, 108). Here I think we should disagree, saying instead that the wrong to the child—the wrong to a person—is inseparable from our judgment about the bad character of the agents. I think we might say that what Kavka has presented is not so much a moral example in which slavery is a feature but rather a kind of description of slavery, a definition, perhaps, of what slavery is. We should test whether there isn't a kind of person-affecting assumption about wrong built into our sense of what's wrong with slavery. If slavery wrongly affected no person, would we object to it? I suppose the answer is no, but such an answer seems meaningless as we cannot imagine any slavery in which persons were not harmed or wronged. Wrong to persons is just inherent to slavery. Or we might ask the following question, that of Ursula Le Guin's "The Ones Who Walk Away from Omelas": would we consent to the slavery of even one person if it were the condition of very great good for others? Again I think we would answer no: that there is no amount of good so great as to make the slavery of even one person justifiable. Apparently our conception of what it means to be a person and freedom from slavery just are inseparable. We should go back to Kavka's example, then, to consider what is part of this paradigm of slavery. We should note how the parents in Kavka's example are not really free but rather coerced to do what they have not wanted to do by their fascination with money. Their reproductive behavior has been, in short, for sale. Perhaps we should say, then, that a fundamental condition of slavery is that those who ordinarily would be most concerned for their child's welfare can be coerced or induced to produce the child for more powerful others who are not concerned for the child in his or herself. (They could still be concerned for the welfare of the child for other reasons, as slavetraders often fed slaves well just before the auctions in order to increase their value.) To approach Kavka's example in biblical terms, we might say that it's as if all the Hebrew midwives in Exodus 1 decided to go along with Pharaoh's order to kill the Hebrew children or as if the whole rabble that became Israel allowed themselves to feed their children to Pharaoh's ambitious dreams of immortality. Surely the parent-child bond can often be disruptive of the state's good order, but perhaps it is also the best earthly source of resistance to totalitarianisms—precisely in its conserving the awareness that harm is experienced by particular persons and in ways incommensurate with that of all others. Kavka's example of the slave child is in "Paradox of Future Individuals," 93–112.

strengths and weaknesses of each. I believe the account I have developed can capture the strongest insights of these positions while avoiding some of their less persuasive features.

One important use of Parfit's hypotheticals has been made by John Robertson, defender of wide reproductive freedom for parents. Robertson echoes Parfit and Singer in judging that a child has not been harmed if its disability is inseparable from its existence—provided that disability is not so extreme as to make for a case of "wrongful life." For Robertson, the value of life to the child is so great that it outweighs nearly any consequences that could occur to the child from, for instance, the artificial reproductive process.[21] Robertson's seemingly frank upholding of the value of life will seem refreshing to those of us who share at least some of John Paul II's sense that ours is a "culture of death." Yet one wonders whether life or death has become the dominant value when it seems clear that parents would be justified, as in Robertson's scheme, in taking practically any liberties with their developing child so long as its life is ultimately not of such a burden to it as to be not worth living. Robertson's argument assumes that death is such an evil that life on nearly any terms is an advantage over it. While I would want to uphold Robertson's sense that life is a great good and death an enemy—though not one, for the Christian, to be avoided at all cost—it seems to me there is danger in his logic if it is not supplemented by a sense of justice grounded in fair sharing of risk. For one could say to the slave, as the Robertsonian parent might to a child, that existence on any terms short of continual unendurable pain is preferable to death.

Robertson's position will, in future, be tested by cases in which parents' reproductive liberty leads to harms to children whom they have sought to design or enhance using genetic technologies. These children will be able to argue that their parents' reproductive liberty extended only to the use of techniques to assist conception, not to design or enhancement. Parents will be able to offer a defense based on the Non-Identity problem: that is, that the particular child in question had no chance of being born without the kinds of genetic revision attempted by the parents. Social and legal standards of appropriate risk-taking in genetic revision

---

21. Robertson, *Children of Choice*, 76. "If offspring are not injured because there is no alternative way for them to be born absent the condition of concern, then reproduction is not irresponsible because of the effect on offspring who are born less whole than is desirable."

will have to be developed, and abortion of inadvertently harmed fetuses will no doubt become routine. Parental claims of freedom to improve life may well lead to increased destruction of life, undermining the strong valuation of life over death that funds Robertson's position. The political undoing of Robertsonians may well lie in the development of genetic technologies that allow one generation unprecedented degrees of control over the next. Surely at some point, the positive reproductive liberty of the designing generation must impinge upon the negative liberties of their children. Robertsonian libertarians may well discover that there is a natural ground of liberty in each generation's beginning the world anew—a fact deeply in conflict not only with the ethos of genetic design but also with the seeming desire of the affluent for unlimited extension of life. For it is death, after all, that has historically freed each generation from its predecessors, the new from the old.[22]

Reacting against the way Robertson defines "wrongful life," Cynthia Cohen argues that the

> comparison that parents and physicians must make when they assess whether use of [reproductive] technologies would negatively affect the good of children who might result is not between *death* and the condition of these children were they to be born with certain deficits. The appropriate comparison is between *preconception nonexistence* and their condition were they to be born with certain deficits. If preconception nonexistence, unlike death, is neither good nor bad, then any life that would be worse than it *will not have to be as bad as the life of devastating deficits set out in the wrongful life standard.*[23]

---

22. Indeed we may begin again to hear children speak in a truly "representative" fashion. The child whose parent uses the Non-Identity problem to justify harm to her caused by a botched attempt at genetic enhancement may well respond in the name of her peers. She may argue something like the following: "We could accept your claim to a very wide positive reproductive right so long as this was integral to your being able to bear children, for child-bearing seems a kind of inalienable right rooted in our nature as mortal beings fully aware of their living the mystery of time. But for the sake of children still to be born, we must limit the risks to which you are able to subject them in the search for your fantasies of perfect offspring. Perhaps you would not have allowed me to exist apart from your desire for an image of yourselves: that is no reason for me not to speak on behalf of others who might be injured by genetic revision. We recognize we must sometimes bear harms inseparable from the processes you used in order to be able to conceive; we reject the idea that we must bear harms when your object has been not procreation but reproduction of yourselves."

23. Cohen, "Give Me Children or I Shall Die!" 23–24.

I find myself partly in sympathy with Cohen's impulse here even while wanting to challenge her logic regarding nonexistence, something I'll do in a moment. Her argument has the effect of challenging, sensibly, the extreme degree of parental liberty Robertson's position would allow, at least in theory. In order to exonerate themselves from wrongful life charges, Robertsonian parents would have to demonstrate no more than that their child's existence is better than what we generally fear as the greatest of evils, death. While I applaud the "pro-life" strand of this position, it may seem inadequate to guarantee parents' taking responsibility for minimizing harm to their children. Cohen's position would do more to ensure that parents not impose the most serious of harms upon their children. It captures our intuitive sense that there is something wrong when parents harm children in preventable ways yet defend themselves by saying that life on nearly any terms is better than death. Cohen may also recognize and fear that Robertson's argument can be pressed in such a way as to justify limiting abortion, though Robertson would not want to do this. Pro-choice arguments, after all, routinely claim that all kinds of conditions more desirable than death are too harsh to be inflicted on unwanted children.[24]

24. Troubling about Cohen's argument is its seeming to invent a standard in order to justify conclusions arrived at in advance. She reacts not only against Robertson but against the strenuous standard of wrongful life put forward by Feinberg, who insists that such a life must be one of devastating deficits so thwarting to all human prospects that death would be preferable. "Many would disagree with Feinberg that children knowingly conceived with such disorders as spina bifida, blindness, deafness, severe retardation, or permanent incontinence should be considered to be suffering from devastating deficits that make their lives worse than death. However, they might well view these disorders as amounting to serious deficits that make their lives worse than preconception nonexistence. What is needed is a conceptual framework that marks off those deficits that have such a negative impact on children that reasonable people would agree that knowingly to conceive children with these disorders would be to impose substantial harm on them in the vast majority of cases." What's being proposed by Cohen, then, is a revision of the standard in order to express in principle what reasonable people know just by looking at the cases—i.e. that children with the above deficits ought not to be conceived or brought to term. See "Give Me Children or I Shall Die!" 24. Feinberg's discussions of harm and wrongful life are in *Harm to Others*, 95–104 and "Wrongful Life and the Counterfactual Element in Harming," in *Freedom and Fulfillment*, 3–36. Steinbock and McClamrock criticize Feinberg's definitions in ways similar to Cohen's in "When Is Birth Unfair to the Child?" 15–21. They argue that "even the most dismal sorts of circumstances of opportunity (including, for example, slavery, an extremely high chance of facing an agonizing death from starvation in the early years of life, severe retardation plus complete quadriplegia) fail to be covered" by Feinberg's analysis. This would seem to suggest that slaves ought not to have had children, a conclusion that seems unreason-

The weakness in Cohen's argument begins with her assertion that "preconception nonexistence, unlike death, is neither good nor bad" (24). First, it seems contradictory to place "preconception nonexistence" outside the system of evaluation signified by "good" and "bad" and yet to claim that "a life with serious, but not devastating deficits, could be bad and therefore worse than preconception nonexistence, which is neither good nor bad" (24). If "preconception nonexistence" is "neither good nor bad," then it is not worse or better than anything. It is not anything at all and thus cannot figure meaningfully in any comparative evaluation of anything.

Several more things need to be said about this comparison of death and preconception nonexistence, especially as it has been important not only in Cohen but also in other philosophical work.[25] First, I doubt if any-

---

able to me. Elsewhere Steinbock has argued that a child is wronged when she is "born with such serious handicaps that many very basic interests are doomed in advance, preventing the child from having the minimally decent existence to which all citizens are entitled." See "The Logical Case for 'Wrongful Life,'" 19.

Cohen's reasoning suggests the problems involved in the calls for a renewed medical casuistry given impetus by Toulmin's observing that ethical review boards often agreed with near unanimity on how cases should be treated even when the members disagreed seriously about matters of ethical principle or approach. Thus the call to go directly to the cases themselves. But one feature of law, exceptionless prohibition, or divine command is to cause otherwise reasonable people to arrive at conclusions they would not typically reach. Divine commands—like those of Exod 22:21–24—speak for those who are otherwise voiceless. If an ethics committee thus finds itself agreeing about cases but without agreement in principles, it might ask itself if there are voices not being heard in the room. For Toulmin, see "The Tyranny of Principles," 31–39. Toulmin and Albert Jonsen have, of course, been prominently associated with the argument for a renewed casuistry in biomedical ethics. See Jonsen and Toulmin, *The Abuse of Casuistry*. Wildes has pointed out the limitations of casuistry for a secular bioethics in *Moral Acquaintances*, 86–121. The central claim of his very convincing argument is that casuistry depends on shared moral commitments—including an account of authority—that are lacking in modern pluralistic societies. In the absence of such, for example, how does one resolve such a basic matter as the choice of cases most relevant to particular moral dilemmas? For another substantial critique of casuistry in bioethics, see Meilaender, *Body, Soul, and Bioethics*, 19–28. Meilaender argues that casuistry, like "principlism," is "a bioethical approach developed with public policy in mind" (25). He prefers principlism, as do I, because it is "open to deontological considerations" in ways that casuistry is not (27).

25. Accounts of the badness of death are inevitably involved in how we estimate the strength of Cohen's argument. One widely followed in the literature is that by Nagel, who argues that the badness of death derives from its depriving us of more of the goods of life. See *Mortal Questions*, 1–10. Kamm argues that death is a "sort of insult" and that this is one quality that distinguishes it from prenatal nonexistence. See *Creation and*

one ever gives much real thought to "preconception nonexistence" apart from philosophers seeking to justify the destruction of fetuses deemed to have "deficits" which, to the children themselves, would not make life worse than death. Second, when I have read or heard passionate pleas for nonexistence, as by Job or Jeremiah, they are really life-affirming cries that life be different—that it not mean, for instance, the destruction of all we hold precious.[26] Third, no one has ever contemplated nonexistence except from the standpoint of existence; we therefore know nothing of it except as a negation of what we know, life, and in this regard, it seems indistinguishable from death. Fourth, if, however, we understand existence as the condition on which all else depends for us, then we will perhaps come to see nonexistence as actually worse than death—though this may, in some ways, be in conflict with my previous point.

I think we know well enough why death is an evil for us. It means the end of everything we love, both for ourselves and for all of those we love. Paul aptly names it the enemy. Yet this enemy functions also to liberate our creativity: "Except a corn of wheat fall into the ground and die, it abideth alone: but if it die, it bringeth forth much fruit."[27] It would seem that the more fulfilling and joyous one's life becomes, the greater the evil of death, for one has more to lose. Yet I would suggest this is only true for people at certain stages of life. Death seems a very great evil when it comes to those who have not yet been able to fully bear fruit (not to be confused with consumerist notions of achievement). Yet it seems much less evil to one who has come to understand—and do at least part of—the work he or she has been given to do for herself and others in the upbuilding of life. For this person, nonexistence (insofar as one can imagine it) must seem a very worse evil than death precisely because it would deprive one of the opportunity to do what one must, and wants to, do to overcome death—which itself has become less an

---

Abortion, 128–30. McMahan gives extensive attention to death's badness in *The Ethics of Killing*, 95–202, 370–72.

26. Cf. Job 3:3 (and, of course, the whole of the third chapter): "Let the day perish in which I was born, / and the night that said, / 'A man-child is conceived.'"; and Jer 20:14–15: "Cursed be the day / on which I was born! / The day when my mother bore me, / let it not be blessed! / Cursed be the man / who brought the news to my / father, saying / 'A child is born to you, a son,' / making him very glad." Texts here are from the NRSV.

27. For Paul, see 1 Cor 15:26: "The last enemy to be destroyed is death" (NRSV). For Jesus's words from John 12:24, I've used the KJV.

evil and more simply part of the conditions of existence within which one works and loves. Now, of course, death seems a very great evil when it comes to children, for it outrages our sense of justice. But even in this case, our reaction is based on the sense that the child has lost something extraordinarily precious, life—itself so valuable and worthy to be lived as to outweigh the negativity of the death it ultimately must come to. Thus, even in the case of the child, it would seem that nonexistence is a greater evil than death—assuming they can be compared—for nonexistence would make impossible the life whose preciousness is what we hate the loss of in the child's death.

In short, nonexistence would seem less bad than death, I think, only if life were not considered very good. If life is considered a very great good and worthy to be lived even under the constant risk of death, then nonexistence must come to seem either evil or, as to most of us, unthinkable. I fear that Cohen's argument represents a fear of life in the face of death that may not bode well for those with "deficits." That word seems telling, for it suggests that only a life without deficits—perfection, one supposes—would be sufficiently better than nonexistence to merit the attempt of life. But none of us is without deficits, as we all are mortal. To be completely without deficits would be to be without needs, and the unneedy life is impoverished, as Kierkegaard taught us. To modify a Kierkegaardian phrase, we ought rather to learn to rest in our deficits, building up life for all and thereby running the apparent risk of making death a worse evil than it would be if our life were less joyful.[28] For one in Christ, this "apparent" risk comes, in time, to seem unreal as one comes increasingly to understand that joyful life as a gift from God, not as a possession to be lost. To adapt a beautiful metaphor from Melville, life is meant to be held lightly, in the open palm rather than the clenched fist. The remedy for death is to open the hand.[29] The real risk for the Christian

---

28. On the supreme impoverishment of regarding oneself unneedy, see Kierkegaard, *Works of Love*, 28; on the "Duty to Be in the Debt of Love to Each Another," see *Works of Love*, 171–96.

29. As the chaplain speaks to Billy Budd shortly before his execution, Billy seems—to the narrator—to listen less from a sense of "awe or reverence" as from a "certain natural politeness." Such an attitude "is not wholly unlike the way in which the primer of Christianity, full of transcendent miracles, was received long ago on tropic isles by any superior *savage*, so called—a Tahitian, say, of Captain Cook's time or shortly after that time. Out of natural courtesy he received, but did not appropriate. It was like a gift placed in the palm of an outreached hand upon which the fingers do not close." Melville, *Billy Budd*, 373.

lies not in building up our life and thereby increasing the evil of death. It lies rather in not risking our lives for ourselves and others and thereby not discovering the joyous freedom that comes from building up life that cannot be diminished by death. To not take that risk would be to live under death's dominion and to approach a life of "nonexistence" as closely as we ineluctably existent beings can do.

Dan W. Brock has addressed the "harm conundrum" with an argument grounded in the premise that "it is morally good to act in a way that results in less suffering and less limited opportunity in the world."[30] Brock claims this principle explains our sense that a wrong has been committed in a case like #2 above in which a woman conceives a child with disability when she could almost as easily have conceived one without the disability. Brock does note, however, that this explanation does not really capture our "commonsense moral judgment" that the mother has wronged the child specifically (273). My account does explain precisely this commonsense judgment by claiming that the mother wrongs the child through an act of injustice: the child is burdened in a way untrue of the rest of us, through no fault of its own, and by actions involving little or no risk or inconvenience on the part of the mother. As I argued earlier, the risk calculus is at the heart of our judgment in the matter.

It seems difficult to take exception to Brock's principle that to produce "less suffering in the world" is a good.[31] Surely no one is in favor of

---

30. "Non-Identity Problem and Genetic Harms," 273. Brock's principles give a good deal of weight to the principle of "substitution" of one child for another. In an example like Parfit's second case, the woman "acts in a morally good way by taking the medication and waiting to conceive a normal child." The normal child replaces, or substitutes for, the child with handicap who would have been conceived. Similarly "a couple acts in a morally good way by taking steps not to have a child whom they learn from genetic screening will experience suffering and limited opportunity that another child they could have instead would not experience"(273). It is difficult to see how people born with handicaps can read this without concluding that their parents have acted wrongly in failing to abort them and, at least, taking another chance to conceive a "normal" child.

31. Verhey has suggested we need to be a bit suspicious of compassion when it ceases to mean suffering "*with* another" and wants instead "to put an end to suffering—and by whatever means necessary." Under such an assumption, the commitment to suffer with others cannot help but seem masochistic; the Immanuel, a failure; and God "either unjust for allowing suffering or even less effective than a competent physician in ending it." In the manner of C. S. Lewis's *Screwtape Letters*, Verhey suggests that the promotion of modern compassion may be one of the subtlest strategies yet devised by the Devil. See *Reading the Bible in the Strange World of Medicine*, 101.

producing more suffering. But one advantage of keeping the focus on person-affecting harms—as my position does—is that it prevents our turning the principle of producing "less suffering" into a reason to avoid risk-taking. The manifest good of existence to identifiable persons—even if "suffering" and "defective"—works to prevent us from turning our admirable concern to limit suffering into a reason to allow the birth only of perfect children. We have to recognize—and I think this is particularly true of normally abled people thinking about the "dis-abled"—that our estimation of the suffering of another is always, to some extent, a judgment about the suffering we think we could bear. Obviously we must never use this fact to justify allowing others to suffer in easily eliminable ways. But this fact about suffering should put us on guard against a tendency of our self-pity, a tendency that might cause us, in the name of reducing suffering, to deny existence to those whose struggles with disability might cause us normally-ableds to feel discomfort.[32]

Perhaps the most important problem with Brock's principle involves its high level of abstraction. Surely there are kinds of suffering we should work to eradicate: that caused by serious illness, natural disasters, poverty, abuse, violence. But there are other kinds of suffering that we ought not to lessen. I want to protect my child from touching the hot burner on the stove, but when he does touch it, the suffering it will cause him teaches him a series of important lessons: touching burners hurts, other kinds of exploratory behaviors are not without risk, authoritative witnesses like parents who warn of pains to be encountered are perhaps to be taken with some seriousness. A one-hundred-sixty-pound young person may well suffer as he attempts to become a Division I football player—suffering that helps to direct his talents to other pursuits where they can be more effectively and satisfyingly used. If I grade my students' work honestly, some of them will suffer, yet that suffering may move them to give more care to their next assignments.

We should consider, too, whether too great reduction of suffering in people's lives would limit their compassion. If we take it as our overarching principle to reduce human suffering, do we risk reducing human

---

32. Particularly inadequate, in my view, is Robertson's way of explaining the wrong done by the mother in the case in question. Her wrong would lie not in harming the child but rather in her "violat[ing] a norm against offending persons who are troubled by gratuitous suffering." It seems to me dangerous to enshrine people's offense at suffering as a reason for denying existence to the sufferer. See *Children of Choice*, 76.

compassion and empathy? Do we not want rather to enable people to suffer—as they surely will—in such a way that they become more compassionate and loving by doing so? This, of course, does not mean we should inflict or create suffering in order to make people more loving—nor does it mean, as I said above, that we should not fight certain kinds of suffering with all the resources at our disposal. It does mean that Brock's premise—"it is morally good to act in a way that results in less suffering and less limited opportunity in the world"—is too general to be of much help in resolving the "harm conundrum" (273).

One last point about Brock's principle needs also to be made. Brock assumes a non-controversial correlation between acting to produce less suffering and expanding opportunity. There seems some intuitive rightness about this correlation—and I surely think we should act to expand opportunity for reasons of justice—but there are at least four problems with the connection as Brock puts it. First, expansion of opportunity for some may surely cause more suffering for others: doing justice will often hurt. Second, it may be necessary for some to suffer—at least psychologically or imaginatively—in order for them to see the need to expand the opportunity of others. Those who mourn may be comforted in part by their seeing a new gift in the chance to lovingly expand opportunities for others. Third, suffering itself, the struggle against limits, serves as an important motivation for the creativity that discovers new possibilities for human flourishing. Fourth, expanding opportunities may well mean expanding the opportunities to fail and thus to suffer. Again, this is no reason to limit opportunities: it is a reason to say that even people faced with expanded opportunities will need a stronger story about suffering than one that says it simply should be avoided or minimized.

Another approach to the "harm conundrum" is offered by Ronald M. Green, who argues that the appropriate comparison for the assessment of "wrong" done to any child is "the *reasonably expected health status of others in the child's birth cohort*."[33] On this view, preconception children are not yet particular individuals but rather interchangeable units waiting to be born into a "slot" in the cohort. When the children are born, parents compare their health to that of others in the cohort; as the children themselves grow and age, they compare their lives to other lives they "might reasonably be thought to have lived" (8) in their families and circumstances. These comparative judgments allow, in Green's

33. Green, "Parental Autonomy," 8. Further references will be given parenthetically.

view, for a way to assess "wrong" to the child: "In the absence of adequate justifying reasons, a child is morally wronged when he/she is knowingly, deliberately, or negligently brought into being with a health status likely to result in significantly greater disability or suffering, or significantly reduced life options relative to the other children with whom he/she will grow up" (10).

Green's standard has received sharp criticism from Leslie Biesecker, primarily for its failure to take into account "the realities of clinical practice" and for its much too "unitary" idea of parental autonomy. In the typical clinical situation, Biesecker explains, parents are "faced with a first- or second-trimester pregnancy where a serious condition has been diagnosed." As in "nearly all cases," the parents' "only choice is to continue or terminate the pregnancy," therefore Green's notion of parental autonomy is an "oxymoron." Moreover, such situations "involve complex maternal-fetal and parental-fetal interactions (among others) and potential conflicts"—in short, a degree of complexity that cannot be subsumed under a "unitary" concept of autonomy. To do so "has the effect of viewing fetuses and children as chattel and the parents as isolated and omnipotent decision-makers." Biesecker similarly criticizes Green's language of "fungibility" for its having little to do with the actual experience of parents. Parents think about their children-to-be in terms of "individual traits," particular roles within their families, and "other real or imagined attributes"—with, in other words, a kind of particularizing imagination very much at odds with Green's sense of conceptuses as interchangeable generic units.[34]

In Green's defense, it should be said that the standard he articulates is an attempted response to the Non-Identity problem as defined by Parfit, Singer, and Heyd.[35] Green is seeking a way to defend our commonsense intuition that a child can be wronged by parental decisions or negligence even when the child has no other way to be born except through the very acts in question. Perhaps one should say that Green's approach is overdetermined by the way Parfit and others have defined the problem and that Biesecker's criticism should be directed back at those

34. Biesecker, "Clinical Commentary," 16. Further references will be given parenthetically.

35. Green's paper may also be overdetermined by his consideration of so-called "designing for disability" questions such as those of deafness and achondroplasia. At times it's unclear whether he's thinking of these questions primarily or framing a standard for assessing harm in all births.

thinkers as well. Biesecker's assessment of Green's concepts of autonomy and fungibility resembles my own criticism of Parfit's and Singer's hypothetical narratives at the beginning of this chapter. Green's concepts, like those narratives, have little to do with the way parents typically reflect on or decide about actions potentially harmful to their children. Moreover, the operative notion of parental autonomy—in both Green's discussion and Parfit's hypotheticals—amounts to omnipotence, with the children as chattels. Biesecker's language points up what we might call the disembodied quality of Parfit's and Singer's way of thinking about the problem, one that proceeds without any reference "to maternal-fetal and parental-fetal interactions." Biesecker reminds us that parents' decisions are made *in medias res*, in the middle of an ongoing history with their children in which interests are never as polarized as they are made to seem in the narratives of Parfit or Singer. Those narratives isolate the woman in a moment of time, empowering her with a kind of illusory omnipotence, which she then exercises, as I pointed out earlier, in ways inconsistent even with her own interests.

Green's position might seem to share much with my own in that it insists that the assessment of harm involves a comparison between the health of the affected child and that of others. Our positions differ, however, in very important ways. Mine insists only that parents have the obligation, as a matter of justice, not to harm the child by burdening it in ways beyond those borne by the rest of us. The position would criticize actions of parents intended to cause such burdens or refusals to take countermeasures—as in Parfit's hypotheticals—when these involve relatively little risk to the mother. The risk pool for the assessment would be as wide as humanity itself. Green, on the other hand, uses the child's "birth cohort"—presumably those similar in national identity, class, affluence—as the pool for comparative judgments and insists a child is wronged merely by having "significantly reduced life options" (10) relative to its potential cohort members. Moreover, for him, parental wrong need not involve acts of deliberation or negligence. There is parental wrong when parents "knowingly" bring a child into being whose life options are significantly less than those of his or her fellows. "At present, for nearly all conditions," as Biesecker points out, "and for the foreseeable future for most conditions, termination of affected pregancies is the only alternative to causing the wrong [Green] asserts" (17). My position implies nothing like this.

Differences in the way Green's and my own position would play out can be illuminated by considering the case of a Down child. Green's position would seem to suggest that a Down child is wronged if "brought into being" in a cohort where amniocentesis and abortion are available. It's important to add that Green insists the parental obligation not to harm is a prima facie one and thus "not absolute." It must "always be weighed against our competing obligations and against rights possessed by other persons or ourselves, not least of all our rights as parents." Thus the right to "procreative autonomy" protects parents against government's "preventing them from having children or forcing them to have an abortion"—a right "reinforced by their right to the liberty of their religious beliefs if these beliefs oppose abortion." Religious liberty would seem to ground, too, for Green a refusal on the part of parents "to undertake prenatal diagnosis." Nevertheless "in cases where parents have no principled reason for refusing to act on knowledge of potential harms to their child ... willful refusal to undertake available testing for serious disorders becomes morally less justifiable" (10). The logic here implies that even parents who refuse testing for principled reasons wrong their children—if these are more defective than others in the cohort. The wrong can be set aside, or forgiven, for the sake of other principles, but it nevertheless remains a wrong.[36]

Thus Green's position would justify criticism of the Down child's parents—in part perhaps because the move toward cohort standards necessarily causes an implicit rigidifying of our sense of the life worth living. My position aims to keep that sense as capacious as possible. The Down child is not harmed, and the parents are not to be criticized, because they have committed no injustice. The child has not been extraordinarily burdened through some deliberate act or negligence on the parents' part. It is not required to display the potential to exercise the life options considered normative by members of its parents' nation, social class, or group health plan. Neither are parents required to ensure that potential in the child.

Green's proposal would impose a much higher standard for birth than my own. In order not to be wronged—and therefore eliminated

---

36. Green adds the important qualification that "assessing a child's expectations requires a complex global judgment that takes into account all the reasonably foreseeable circumstances of the child's life, including the willingness and ability of the parents to compensate for other less than desirable features of the child's health at birth" (10).

by parents desirous of being free of moral criticism—children, under Green's standard, would have to demonstrate themselves likely capable of living lives comparable to those of the cohort. Under my proposal, children would only be wronged if they had to bear significantly greater burdens than those species-typical burdens borne by us all—and if this were the specific result of parental or physician injustice, assessed according to typical standards of care. The great danger in Green's position, it seems to me, lies in its opening up the possibility of competitive ratcheting up of standards for "rightful birth." This possibility seems already implicit in the metaphor of the "cohort," with its suggestion of the armed military unit, particularly the Roman legion. Of course Green did not coin the term "birth cohort," which he uses in a perfectly well-accepted way. Nevertheless it's worth considering what the term may imply about our attitudes toward children. It does seem to me there is a kind of Roman imperial mentality evident in thinking of "preconception children" as "interchangeable generic units" waiting to be born into "slots" in the cohort—perhaps as those now compete for "slots" in the class of a prestigious elite university (8). The language also sets up, or perhaps simply acknowledges, the existence of groups defined as distinct from and inevitably over against other groups (hence the natural turn to the word "cohorts"). Green's approach further imposes group discipline: it becomes necessary to justify "knowingly" or "deliberately" bringing into being a child with "significantly reduced life options" relative to others in one's cohort. Surely this is right, I suppose, if one must support one's "cohorts" in the ongoing struggle against other groups.

One practical problem with Green's proposal is that it will be difficult to define cohorts with precision.[37] This seems quite fortuitously fortunate, to me, as it means that most cohorts will retain at least some diversity of various kinds, perhaps enough to keep the cohort from self destruction caused by members' envy or a kind of *rigor mortis* induced by the need to maintain exclusionary standards. Still Green's proposal seems problematic not only for the disabled but even for those people successfully entering the cohorts, maybe especially the elite ones. Perennial

---

37. Green himself recognizes the problem involved in determining "the cohort against which a child's birth condition should be measured." Perhaps he comes closest to a clarification when he states that "the health status to which the results of parents' reproductive decision making is compared is established with regard to the available life situations to which we may reasonably and rightfully aspire" (9).

unhappiness may be an inadvertent result of encouraging people to assess the possible "wrong" of their lives by constant comparison to other lives they "might reasonably be thought to have lived" (8). At some point one must live one's own life or be unhappy forever. Green's proposal looks too much like a philosophic development of the competitive envy that drives our economic life. His notion of cohorts reflects the constant striving of the ever upwardly mobile American class of achievers. Such thinking can be imaginatively impoverished if it results in a failure to see the worthiness of lives—often of great suffering—lived by those without the "life options" affluent Americans take for granted. Green has himself worked on Kierkegaard, and his treatment would be enriched by insisting on Kierkegaard's claim that a qualitatively different standard—call it the duty to love—must be in place if we are not to ceaselessly work for comparison, distinction, and, I would add, envy.[38] If we insist on the duty to love, and the absolutely equal human ability to do it since it is of God, then we will have a principle to balance Green's comparative assessment of the wrongness of lives. We could insist parents have a duty not to harm their children, either through negligence or willful action, yet maintain that this duty cannot override the child's claim to life itself, for the fulfillment of that life lies not in the exercise of any power but rather in the qualitatively different activity of fulfilling the duty to love.

---

38. Green, *Kierkegaard and Kant*. For Kierkegaard on how love of the neighbor is the only thing that allows us a certain freedom from the world's ceaseless concern for distinctions, see "You Shall Love Your Neighbor," in *Works of Love*, 73–98.

9

Why Genetic Therapy May Need Something "Very Much Like the Church"

ONE OF STANLEY HAUERWAS's contributions to medical ethics has been his insistence on the fundamental commitments and virtues necessary to sustain medicine as a "moral art" aware of its own fallibility.[1] Basic to medical practice is the willingness of the physician to be present to the other in pain and suffering. Nick Carraway in Scott Fitzgerald's *The Great Gatsby* once remarked that there is no difference "so profound as the difference between the sick and the well."[2] Yet it is "medicine's primary role," as Hauerwas puts it starkly, "to bind the suffering and the nonsuffering into the same community."[3] This is an extraordinary task, for one of the consequences of suffering is to isolate us in our own often incommunicable pain. Thus medicine—if it is to achieve its real, though limited, good of mediating between us and our bodies—must be sustained by a larger community capable of recognizing suffering and tragedy and yet also able to be present to one another. In short, "something very much like a church is needed to sustain" (65)

---

1. Hauerwas has written widely on biomedical topics and on the moral art of medicine. See particularly *Community of Character*; *Naming the Silences*; *Suffering Presence*; and, with Richard Bondi and David B. Burrell, *Truthfulness and Tragedy*.

2. After George Wilson and Tom Buchanan have learned that each of their spouses have "some sort of life apart" from them, Nick Carraway sees that in Wilson "the shock had made him physically sick." What occurs to Nick, then, is "that there was no difference between men, in intelligence or race, so profound as the difference between the sick and the well" (*Great Gatsby*, 124).

3. Hauerwas, *Suffering Presence*, 26. Further citations will be included parenthetically.

the habits of good medical practice. What God requires of us, after all, is "our unfailing presence" to one another "in the midst of the world's sin and pain." The Church can thus serve medicine in at least three ways: as an example to medical practitioners of the disciplined habits of presence; as a community that assists in binding together the well and the ill, so that the suffering and those who care for them do not become alienated in a world of their own; and as a carrier of the knowledge of tragedy together with hope, one that makes clear the distinction between salvation and health. Without the Church, we "are constantly tempted to ask too much of medicine," which can then become "a pseudo-salvific institution" whose project seems nothing less than the elimination of all suffering and limitation (53–54).[4]

Surely the practice of medicine as a "moral art" seems largely in eclipse today. To see how completely this is true, we might consider Eric J. Cassell's claim that one of the physician's duties is to teach people how to die.[5] Now I have the greatest respect for my general practitioner, but I must say she is one of the last people from whom I would expect to learn how to die. The structure of our occasional fifteen-minute interactions is simply not such that I can learn anything of this from her. My eighty-six year old father recently went through the dying process. What he had learned about how to do it seems, to me, to have come largely from his and my mother's parents and probably from his comrades during four years of service in World War II. What he had learned from all of them seemed infinitely more valuable than anything he could glean from his series of monthly visits to specialists or his brief encounters with six different doctors during as many days in the hospital. The institution of medicine is no longer organized to assist patients in the "journey with finitude," perhaps because modern therapeutic techniques actually can achieve results never imagined by practitioners during the ages

---

4. See also the chapter, "Salvation and Health," in Hauerwas, *Suffering Presence*, especially 80–82. For a terse, direct statement of the way too-great infatuation with health care can be an obstacle to salvation, see Engelhardt, "Controversies, Conflicts, and Consensus," 291–95. Waters has noted the way "emphasizing cure over care" causes medicine's embarrassment when it cannot either prevent or cure, an embarrassment that may contribute to medicine's increasing role in "identifying and destroying 'defective' embryos and fetuses, and its declining reticence to perform euthanasia and assist suicide." See "What is Christian About Christian Bioethics?" 283. Robert Song stresses the way the Church as a political society can and must unmask the idols of secular bioethics; see "Christian Bioethics and the Church's Political Worship," 333–48.

5. Cassell, *Healer's Art*, 203.

when wisdom and art were what physicians were limited to offering. Contemporary medicine is increasingly given over to what Gerald P. McKenny has called the "Baconian project" of eliminating suffering and expanding the realm of choice by submitting "nature" to the control of science and technology. Medicine no longer concerns itself primarily with assisting us to live wisely with our bodies; it seeks rather to empower us to exert control over our bodies. Its end becomes "expansion of the reign of human choice over the body" as part of the process of enabling and enhancing "whatever pattern of life" the autonomous self chooses.[6]

My only reservation about McKenny's compelling analysis of medicine's "Baconian project" is that it may abstract a little too much from the everyday process of treatment, care, healing, and endurance. Much of what people experience as illness still requires meeting the body's limitations with the wise and artful practice of health. Despite medicine's technological and pharmacological successes, people still must learn to manage arthritis, back pain, diabetes, depression, digestive disorders, migraine, tinnitus, dementia. These and many other conditions still represent significant markers in our "journey with finitude," as does, of course, the aging process itself. Thus the description of healing as learning the wisdom of the body still holds, irrespective of the direction of the medical enterprise. To ring a slight change on Hauerwas's argument, we might say that healing still requires "something very like a church," a body of people capable of being present to one another in suffering, even if our increasingly technological, specialized, and depersonalized medicine seems committed elsewhere. One of my own conclusions from this is that many more people should understand what they do daily to be a matter of healing for themselves and others. This is not to say we are all sick and in need of a physician continually (though there is a Christian sense in which this is true). But it is to say that much of what we learn about how to be well is learned from our friends, and the church is particularly well situated to promote such healing. For a healthy church is one of the few remaining places in this society where members of several generations are brought together, where the young and middle-aged can see how to be old, and the old can be refreshed by

---

6. McKenny, *To Relieve the Human Condition*, 20. For additional considerations regarding "the trajectory" from Bacon to "late modernity," see Khushf, "Thinking Theologically About Reproductive and Genetic Enhancements," 168–69.

seeing the young whose lives they have prepared. And this generational co-presence is accomplished in a place where the great enemy of all, death, is brought to light and shown to be, while terrible, finally bounded by God's love.

Obviously genetics represents one area where the Baconian project of modern medicine dominates. Genetic testing and diagnosis, with selective abortion of defective fetuses, offer parents an extraordinary degree of control over the offspring they choose to rear. This project, so central to the "culture of choice," seems logically to lead to more complex technologies of genetic enhancement or cloning. However true it is that the environment, nurture, and experiences of clones will prevent their ever being mere replications of their hosts, the argument always seems more than a little disingenuous. The goal of genetic replication is increased control. People formed to believe themselves entitled to offspring whose DNA replicates their own are very likely to exert a strong influence on their clones to repeat them (or perhaps to live out life scripts that those doing the cloning would have preferred but were themselves unable to live). In this climate of increased genetic control and choice, disability cannot help but seem highly negative, burdensome, perhaps even scandalous. How technology changes perceptions of the disabled is suggested by a comment by Dena S. Davis on her reactions to Down children:

> In my own mind I can discern a subtle shift in the way in which I view people with certain anomalies. Twenty years ago, seeing a woman in a supermarket with a child who has Down syndrome, my immediate reactions were sympathy and a sense that that woman could be me. Now when I see such a mother and child, especially if the mother is older, I am more likely to wonder why she didn't get tested.[7]

The painful thing that must be said is that the latter part of Davis's comment seems a euphemistic way of saying she wonders why this child exists, why it was allowed to be. That people sense there is something wrong in allowing a Down child to exist is suggested by a European study cited by Davis in which the investigators found that "women who decline the offer of testing are seen as having more control over this outcome, and are attributed more blame for it, than are women who have not been

---

7. D. Davis, *Genetic Dilemmas*, 18.

offered tests and also give birth to a child with Down syndrome."[8] As blame is attributed where a moral wrong is judged to have been committed, it is impossible to resist the conclusion that at least some people now see the very existence of Down syndrome individuals as a moral wrong.

Both Davis and Hans Reinders have written thoughtfully about the ethics of genetic testing and manipulation as they relate to issues of disability. Focusing most of her attention on the deaf,[9] Davis wrestles with the question of "Choosing for Disability," the deliberate use of genetic techniques to conceive children who would ordinarily be regarded as disabled (at least by those normally abled). Davis argues that a child's "right to an open future" must be the ultimate standard used to determine the justifiability of genetic manipulation. Reinders's fine study, *The Future of the Disabled in Liberal Society*, reflects throughout his deep concern that support for the rights of the disabled cannot help but be eroded in liberal society as clinical genetics progresses. As genetic advances make possible prenatal identification of an increasing number of disabling conditions, society will become less supportive of those who choose to bear disabled

---

8. Marteau and Drake, "Attributions for Disability," 1130. There is considerable decrying of "genetic determinism" in much of the literature defending genetic engineering, enhancement, and cloning. As Tom Shakespeare points out, however, the increasing "geneticising" of social experience is partly itself the result of the availability of screening techniques: "The advent of screening technology offers solutions to what is then defined as a problem: technological interventions insidiously shift the ground towards what has been variously called 'tentative pregnancy' or the 'perfect baby syndrome' or the 'supermarket syndrome', by which I mean the expectation that medical expertise will deliver a baby free from impairment or illness, and that it would be selfish for people not to avail themselves of this power. The boundaries between health and disease are altered, and social experience is increasingly 'geneticised'" (666-67). See "Choices and Rights," 665-81. The apparent prevailing valuation of a Down child is suggested by Jonathan Baron as part of an illustration of "decision analysis" regarding the "utility of fetal testing." In developing the weight of his variables, Baron notes, "The utility of a Down child for those other than the parents is probably negative (compared to no child), while the utility of a normal child might be positive, depending on the population situation." See *Against Bioethics*, 75. For an account directed at assisting pastors in their guidance of parents facing issues of genetic diagnosis and possible societal blame, see Cole-Turner and Waters, *Pastoral Genetics*, 47-70.

9. Throughout this chapter I have capitalized Deaf and Deafness when referring to those who consider Deafness a matter of culture, in accord with their usage, and used the lower case to refer to deafness simply in a descriptive way as the condition of non-hearing. Sometimes, inevitably, the choice is difficult to make and may seem arbitrary, for which I apologize.

children—and, of course, less willing to support the disabled themselves. As demands on scarce medical resources increase, the disabled are thus likely to be seen increasingly as burdens on the system. These problems so worry Reinders—rightly, I believe—that he devotes a chapter to considering whether genetic research and intervention should be limited by law precisely because they may fuel discrimination against the disabled. Reinders concludes that the "paramount value" assigned to reproductive free choice in liberal society makes unfeasible any public policy restricting genetic testing and selective abortion. He thus considers it "more than likely" that "proliferation of genetic testing among the public at large" will lead to the serious threat of genetic discrimination. One way to protect against this possibility might be to institute nationally socialized health care, but even under such a system, the danger of discrimination will not be eliminated. Indeed under such an arrangement it might take an "even more frightening" form—that is, "as an instrument of governmental policy to lower the costs of the health-care system."[10]

A key part of Reinders' argument is his examination of the so-called DPC argument, which he rejects. DPC stands for the distinction between the person and the condition—that is, for the claim that clinical genetics can treat for genetic conditions through prenatal diagnosis and therapeutic abortion without implying a negative evaluation of the lives of disabled people currently living with the conditions in question. Although she does not address the argument by name, something like the distinction between the person and condition is at stake in Davis's work, too, for this distinction is precisely what is denied by groups, like the Deaf, who insist that they should be able to use genetic technology to ensure their offspring also be deaf. Their claim is that they are at risk because they are identified with their condition, and their response is to insist that the condition is not disabling but rather simply different from the norm. One might say that the person-condition distinction has failed to hold adequately in their case.[11] If the disabled could regard their

---

10. Reinders, *Future of the Disabled in Liberal Society*, 102. Further references will be included parenthetically.

11. Part of my contention is precisely that one import of "disability" considerations is that the DPC cannot be sustained by reason alone. These issues remind us that we "reason together" face-to-face and that doing so depends on contexts of trust. My borrowing is, of course, from the King James translation of Isa 1:18: "Come now, and let us reason together, saith the Lord: though your sins be as scarlet, they shall be as white as snow; though they be red like crimson, they shall be as wool."

condition as something separable from their persons, they could see it, then, as something to be treated or prevented. But they cannot do so—rightly, I believe, under current arrangements.

My first focus here will be on the DPC and Reinders's critique of it. I am deeply sympathetic with Reinders's argument and in agreement with him on critical points. At present, the practice of genetic testing together with therapeutic abortion cannot help but presuppose "negative evaluations of disabled lives" (67). Where I differ from Reinders is on the matter of the role of abortion as the source of the problems with the DPC. Reinders claims the problem is not abortion but the negative evaluation of disabled lives. My claim is that these problems are not separable: that it is abortion that makes the problem one of negative evaluation of disabled lives. As I will try to show, abortion conditions the very way Reinders thinks about the problem, the language that he uses, in ways he does not recognize. My point is not to uphold the DPC as possible in liberal society—if that's what we are—where abortion is routinely practiced. Rather my claim is that we need a people committed to not practicing abortion in order to uphold the distinction and therefore continue to make genetic therapy a possibility. In the process, that people—something very like a church—might also be able to salvage some vestige of liberal society by preventing society from engaging too broadly in practices like abortion that destroy the very possibility of rational discussion on which liberal society rests.

My second focus here is on Davis's treatment of the difficult matter of designing for apparent disability. Unfortunately, as I will show, her concept of the child's "open future" cannot resolve the kind of issue at stake in claims by groups like the Deaf that they should be able to use available genetic technologies to ensure Deaf offspring. What Davis's argument really shows is that designing for disability can be allowable if the disability is so anomalous that it can be referred to the affected individual only—that it cannot, in other words, be claimed to represent a matter of culture, as Deaf advocates, for instance, insist deafness should be understood. For if the disability can be understood as primarily cultural, then to abort for that disability seems discriminatory (assuming it becomes possible to screen for deafness). Davis's argument is grounded in the need to contain abortion as a problem of private reproductive choice, something it can hardly seem to those currently afflicted by disabilities of all kinds which routinely qualify fetuses for termination.

What I suggest, then, is that a community again "very like the church" will be necessary if the issue of designing for what some regard as disability is to be resolved in a peaceful fashion, where no one considers him or herself simply forced to acknowledge the legality of practices he cannot accept without the deepest self-rejection.

Reinders gives three versions of the DPC argument. The first "invoke[s] the distinction between future people and actual people," maintaining that decisions made about preventing the lives of future people have no relevance whatever to those whose lives are already underway. The disabled are "persons with a name and a personal history who are included in the social networks that constitute the lives of individuals in society." "Nothing of the sort," the argument continues, "can be said of future people" (56). A closely related second version of the argument distinguishes actual or existing people from nonexistent or possible people. Here the argument insists that it is impossible for clinical genetics to convey negative evaluations of the lives of the disabled precisely because "genetics is directed at the prevention of diseases in people who do not yet exist." "Existing people cannot be the target of prevention," and "nonexisting people cannot be the object of negative evaluation" (56). The third version of the DPC grants that "preventing children with a genetic disorder from being born by aborting them in their fetal stage is, in a sense, killing potential people with disabilities." But "this is true" only "because of the use of gene technology in combination with abortion," a combination that "is not necessary." The "moral evil resides in abortion and not in clinical genetics." Once gene therapies become possible, then the "analogy with other diseases, such as cancer, will finally obtain," as it will be possible "to eliminate genetic disorders without eliminating the people whose lives are affected by these disorders." "When gene therapy becomes a real option," the charge of negative evaluation will no longer bear weight. Therapeutic treatment of fetuses to remove disabilities will then send no message of negative evaluation to those currently disabled. It is a somewhat refined version of this third form of the DPC that I will attempt to defend (58–59).

Reinders rejects the first two versions of the DPC by pointing out that the decision to terminate a fetus with, say, Down syndrome, can only be based on a "judgment about what one believes life with Down syndrome or with a child with this syndrome to be." The information required for this judgment can only come from "look[ing] at the lives of actual people with Down syndrome." Thus to prevent the life of a child with a particular disorder like Down syndrome cannot help but exemplify "a negative view of the lives of people who are actually living with it" (57). Having said this, Reinders acknowledges his analysis opens him to a counterargument by DPC defenders that we might call the "first person" defense. This counterargument again depends on a distinction "between two different modes of being," only "this time the difference is not between actual and future but between me and other." It insists we can only make a judgment about our lives "from the inside," and thus there is a mistake in "rationality" in making a decision to terminate a Down fetus based on conclusions drawn from other lives. "Evaluations of the meaning and value of life are necessarily 'first person,'" and thus "reasons for preventing the birth of a disabled child are internal to what people think about their own lives." These reasons "cannot—logically cannot—be reasons inferred from other people's lives" (57–58).

How this functions as a defense of the DPC seems a little murky. I suppose what's being said is that parents are guilty of a mistake in logic if they abort a fetus with a disabling condition based on information about the lives of those living with the condition. They may think they are operating from information about the lives of others but they are actually only reflecting a judgment about their own lives if lived under a counterfactual condition. In effect, they cannot be communicating any negative evaluation of the lives of the disabled. The disabled should recognize this fact and ignore the messages sent by abortion of fetuses bearing the disabilities with which they, the disabled, live.

The strength of this defense of the DPC lies in its insistence on the difference between first-person evaluation of lives and those by others. It sends a sharp message to parents pondering the decision whether to abort a child with a disabling condition. That message is something like the following:

> You may think you are about to make a decision about the quality of this child's life based on information you have gleaned about the lives of others with similar conditions. But you should know that the life you project for the child is really a fantasy based on your own inevitably distorting judgments about what the life of a disabled person is like.

Nevertheless this defense of the DPC fails on several counts. First, it does not seem that the couple contemplating abortion needs to make an evaluation of the whole of disabled lives in order to arrive at a decision to abort. The couple might simply assess some relatively objectifiable and predictable aspects of a disability—that is, that those with Down syndrome are unlikely to attain normal levels of academic achievement. If this is unacceptable to the couple, they may abort the child. From their standpoint, they have made no overall evaluation of Down syndrome lives. They have simply identified a feature of the syndrome that makes it unacceptable in their child.

Parents rearing Down children, however, can hardly interpret the aborting couple's action as anything but an example of negative evaluation of the lives of people with the syndrome. They will rightly point out that the diagnosis of Down syndrome in the fetus is what put its life in question. They can further insist that the aborting couple discounted every other feature of the child's possible life: that the decision to abort is tantamount to saying that nothing about this child's life could be sufficiently valuable to overcome the disability caused by the syndrome. They can also say with some justice that the aborting couple is in danger of deceiving themselves if they think the decision to terminate the fetus has been made simply on the grounds of its intellectual ability apart from its Down syndrome. Prospective parents informed that their child may have Down syndrome confront a sudden, radically changed horizon for the rest of their lives, one dramatically different from that they have likely envisioned and thus understandably strange, perhaps inconceivable. The decision to abort is likely to derive from an inability to imagine how to go on in circumstances so unlike any the couple has foreseen. To explain the decision to abort in terms of a particular feature of the disability is likely to seem a rationalization (in the strictest sense) of a choice made basically from uncertainty about entering on a way so unlike what one has envisioned. That it will appear so to those who have experienced the social estrangement often involved in rearing a disabled child seems almost inevitable.

At this point, we can see a basic problem inherent in the "first-person" defense of the DPC outlined above. The problem, occasioned by abortion's becoming the therapy of choice, lies in the difficulty of anyone offering the defense in good faith. The defense aims to reassure the disabled or those rearing disabled children that abortion of fetuses with similar conditions implies no negative evaluation of disabled lives. But who can say this in a way that it will be believed? If the normally abled person makes this argument, the disabled can with perfect justice respond that the normally abled person has never had his or her life put in question by the abortion of fetuses judged relevantly similar to him or her. (This at least has been true until relatively recently; the broadening of abortion practice may soon put us all in this category.) We must remember that the disabled have often had the experience throughout life of being identified primarily by their disability. How then can they be expected to believe that the practice of therapeutic abortion for those same disabilities sends no message to them? Can a normally abled person really attempt, in good faith, to persuade the disabled that they have nothing to be concerned about from the abortion of fetuses with similar disabilities? To put this another way: those of us who are normally abled must recognize that the abortion of a fetus with Down syndrome or fragile X appears one way to us, but quite another to those with the disabilities in question or their caregivers. No logical argument can bridge this gap. It would be irrational for the disabled to believe reassurances of support from those who have shown themselves willing to abort fetuses whom the disabled can only judge relevantly similar to themselves. No one who has felt his or her life to be put into question can be persuaded by means of logic to believe the reassurances of those whom he or she has reason to fear.

Thus the futility of the kind of argument presented by Canadian bioethicist Eike H. Kluge:

> Saying that something is a handicap or saying that it would be better if we could prevent people from suffering from a particular handicap instead of trying to find ways to deal with it after it has occurred, is not to say that those who suffer from the handicap are worthless as persons. Nor is it to brand them as second-class citizens. To say that something is a handicap is to say just that: that it is a handicap. This is not a comment about the person who suffers from the handicap but about the condition of that person.[12]

This will seem entirely convincing to those of us who are normally abled or who suffer from only minor handicaps; it will, on the other hand, be unlikely to persuade anyone whose disability has largely identified her for others throughout life and who has come to know that being disabled can come to mean continual exclusion from all kinds of socially

---

12. Kluge, *Biomedical Ethics in a Canadian Context*, 341.

valued activities—in other words, that disability too often does mean second-class citizenship. Moreover, no one is going to be persuaded by argument that he or she is not "worthless," particularly when abortion of fetuses with relevantly similar conditions is regarded as appropriate therapy.[13] If another has come to regard herself as worthless, the battle is already lost. Societies must be organized in ways that prevent any from regarding themselves as worthless.

This problem is one pro-choice advocates on abortion need to consider more seriously. Some disabled clearly feel that therapeutic abortion is directed—in discriminatory fashion—at them. This seems, to me, a reasonable fear, and pro-choice advocates need to explain why other groups—the poor, for instance—should not experience the abortion of those they judge relevantly similar to them as likewise discriminatory. Perhaps the question should be put thus: Can abortion, purely as a descriptive matter, really be privatized? How can the children of the young and impoverished—for whom abortion is often advocated—not conclude that their existence is mistaken and unjustifiable? The pro-choice advocate can argue, with entire justification, that one's choosing abortion or recommending abortion to young and disadvantaged mothers is, in no way, intended to communicate to the poor or any other group that their lives are unworthy to be lived. But—intention aside—how can the pro-choice advocate believe that he or she can control the way the message of abortion is received by those who judge themselves relevantly similar to the fetuses being killed? As I have argued above, it would be irrational for the person who judges himself relevantly similar to fetuses being killed—and who has a sense that his life is thus compromised—to believe the assurances of people who are advocating the elimination of those he deems like himself.

Pro-choice advocates like Ronald Dworkin owe us a better account, then, of how the poorest people can be expected to maintain self-esteem and even the most marginal trust in others in the face of the

13. Meg Stacey tells the story of a young woman with Down syndrome who attended "a meeting to discuss genetic screening" where a geneticist proposed "screening with the effective aim of reducing or eliminating the disease." "The young woman was appropriately angry and said so," prompting "more than one doctor" from the audience to tell Stacey after the meeting "that it had been inappropriate" for the young woman to be present. Stacey recalls one doctor in particular who "made it plain" that he "could not see her as a real person, but as a typical bundle of Down syndrome symptoms, mentioning among other things her fidgetiness." See "New Genetics," 344.

argument that abortion is "justified when the family circumstances are so economically barren, or otherwise so unpromising, that any new life would be seriously stunted for that reason."[14] If one doubts that abortion sends the social message I'm suggesting here, I'd ask her or him to consider how he or she feels about abortion for sex selection.[15] Often in the literature, otherwise pro-choice advocates balk at the idea of abortion for sex selection. I'm not suggesting such people are guilty of bad faith but rather that they are resisting the irrationality of failing to defend fetuses whom they deem relevantly similar to themselves.[16] But in every case of abortion, there can always be some group that considers itself

---

14. Dworkin, *Life's Dominion*, 98.

15. Data on the frequency of this practice in selected countries is available in *Beyond Therapy*, a report of the President's Council on Bioethics. The council notes that "generally, any variation in the sex ratio exceeding 106 boys born per 100 girls born can be assumed to be evidence of the practice of sex selection." It then goes on to give the figures for certain countries: "The sex ratio at birth of boys to 100 girls in Venezuela is 107.5; in Yugoslavia 108.6; in Egypt 108.7; in Hong Kong 109.7; in South Korea 110; in Pakistan 110.9; in Delhi, India, 117; in China 117; in Cuba 118; and in the Caucasus nations of Azerbaijan, Armenia, and Georgia, the sex ratio has reached as high as 120." The ratio "has remained stable" in the United States at 104.8. See 60–61.

16. The debate among feminists on the matter of sex selection has involved, in part, whether selection by abortion should be regulated or prohibited, or whether such regulation represents a dangerous weakening of the hard-won abortion right. Using what she calls a "modified pragmatic and feminist" approach, Cherry argues for a "restriction on the availability of fetal sex information." Her contention is that, on this question, "the importance of individual choice or preference...becomes secondary to the issue of substantive justice for women as a social group" (223). Cherry's "construction of a radical feminist analysis moves away from a view of the procedure as one of individual choice, and acknowledges sex-selection as an issue affecting women as a class" (166). I agree entirely with Cherry's position here and would extend it to all classes of fetuses targeted for abortion. Sex-selection for males sends the message to women that society devalues them; abortion of fetuses with disabilities indicates to those with disabilities that many consider their lives not worth living; advocating abortion for the poor may very well mean to many in poverty that to be poor is scandalous and indecent. See "Feminist Understanding of Sex-Selective Abortion," 161–223. Renteln comes to a very different conclusion than Cherry. She finds the practice of sex selection "morally reprehensible," but considers the "consequences of enforcing a policy of restriction" calamitous. Her major fear is that "government officials would then begin to evaluate reasons for abortions, which would be contrary to the aspirations of the women's movement." See "Sex Selection and Reproductive Freedom," 421. An observation much like my own is offered by Holmes when she points out that sex selection can be considered a paradigm case for all genetic engineering precisely because "*every* fetus is 'at risk' for sex" and therefore "every pregnancy is at risk for sex selection." See "Choosing Children's Sex," 149. All three articles contain excellent reviews of the extensive literature on the subject.

similar to the fetuses killed and thus the victims of discrimination. Let me suggest, then, that when pro-choice advocates treat abortion for sex selection as if it were an utterly different matter than other abortions—a matter of discrimination—the real force of their argument lies less in its compelling rationality than in the fact that everyone has a gender and thus a reason to sense his or her life's being compromised by killing for sex selection. In short, when the qualification for possible killing is sex, everyone sees her or himself as relevantly similar to the victims, and abortion seems a bad idea.[17]

What remains is to show how abortion is at the heart of the problem with the DPC. Following Reinders, I introduced this above as the third version of the DPC—that the problem lies in the combination of "gene technology" and "abortion"; that once fetal gene therapy for now-disabling conditions becomes successful, the analogy with other diseases will obtain; and, at that point, no negative evaluation of disabled lives will be implied by such therapy. Reinders rejects this defense of the DPC, arguing the problem is not abortion but negative evaluation of disabled lives. This position, however, divides what cannot be divided: abortion from negative evaluation. Abortion is the source of the problem in ways Reinders does not recognize. Indeed it conditions the very way he thinks about the problem, the language that he uses. Why is this important? Because maintaining some ability to distinguish person (or perhaps

---

17. Adrienne Asch illustrates the difficulty of maintaining the right to abortion on demand without signaling to classes of those relevantly like the aborted that they are without value. Asch argues her support for abortion derives primarily from the unexceptionable claim that "women's rights to full social and sexual equality with men are compromised without the option of abortion." Yet she opposes abortion for sex selection and "question[s] its use in the case of most of the impairments commonly tested for now and likely to be screened in the future." Abortion for "sex selection or disability has serious moral and social consequences that go beyond an individual woman's reproductive decisions about her own life." One of these consequences involves the social messages sent by such abortions: "To say it is acceptable to abort potential girls or boys (although probably it would most often be girls) sends a message to actual girls and boys about their worth." But this message is presumably not sent to *girls and boys* by the indiscriminate abortion of fetuses simply because they are unwanted. To believe so seems untenable to me. What matters in arguments of this type is not the motivation for the abortion but the way abortion practice is understood by those who deem themselves relevantly like those aborted—and that is beyond the control of those who choose the procedure. Without acknowledging it, of course, Asch's position turns on a central premise of the pro-life position: that abortion devalues life, not only that of aborted fetuses but of all of us. See "Can Aborting 'Imperfect' Children Be Immoral?" 386–87.

one should say "human sufferer" here) from condition seems critical to sustaining the possibility of eventual genetic therapy for now-disabling conditions. Reinders's conclusion might well undermine such therapy, and perhaps, in liberal society, it should. For he argues that the "burden of proof" is on DPC defenders to show that prevention of disabilities does not inevitably "presuppose a negative evaluation of disabled lives." In the absence of such proof, he concludes "that any attempt to distance the practices of prevention from negative judgments about the lives of disabled people is bound to fail, because it deprives such practices of the only rational grounds that people can have for pursuing them" (63). This I want to contest but not in order to uphold the DPC as possible in liberal society where abortion is routinely practiced. Rather my claim is that we need a people committed to not practicing abortion in order to uphold the distinction and therefore continue to make genetic therapy a possibility. In the process, that people, the church, might also be able to salvage some vestige of liberal society by preventing society from engaging too broadly in practices like abortion that destroy the very possibility of rational discussion on which liberal society rests.

As this is a crucial matter, it seems worthwhile to look first, in some detail, at Reinders's treatment of the third version of the DPC. He begins by asking us to consider the difference between impersonal and first-person points of view as these regard the having of a disabled child: "Suppose someone were to ask us how we would feel about having a disabled child as opposed to having a nondisabled one. From an impersonal point of view, it is clear that people would prefer the latter. Thus we would say, 'Of course, I would rather have a healthy child!'" (59). One problem with Reinders's argument is immediately evident here from the language itself. It seems impossible to take an "impersonal" point of view on this question, as is clear from Reinders's own framing of the question: he addresses a first person "us," thinks of the answer in terms of the highly personal language of feeling and preference, imagines a response from a first person "we," and ultimately formulates the response as the statement of an "I." What he shows is that the question is an inherently first-person one, incapable of being addressed from an impersonal point-of-view. I would argue he only needs to invoke the language of impersonal points of view because he is pondering how the argument will play in a liberal society, where one needs to assume the fiction of impersonality in order to formulate arguments capable of compelling all rational minds.

My point is that Reinders's very language is more fully captured by liberal assumptions than even he, as one quite critical of liberal society, recognizes. The strangeness of argument on the question as it is driven by such assumptions emerges in a further question he poses just after the piece cited above: "If the question is asked in general—'Would you rather have a child with or without a genetic disorder x?'—then the answer appears to be fairly obvious. Personal relations being absent, it is rational to prefer a child without a genetic disorder" (59). But as soon as one imagines the question, it becomes a first person one, as it is impossible to imagine rearing a child under a condition where "personal relations" are absent. Moreover, I simply do not know what it means to say it "is rational to prefer a child without a genetic disorder" (59). Does this mean we should regard as irrational someone who gives birth to and rears a child with Down syndrome? Does it mean, under the regime of abortion, as I fear it might, that it would be irrational for parents not to abort a child deemed defective if there were reason to believe they could conceive a normally-abled "replacement"? I want to be clear in what I'm contending here. I am in substantial sympathy with Reinders's overall argument, and I do not think he means the implications I have just pointed out. Nevertheless it seems to me they are implicit in his way of framing the questions, one dictated in ways he may not perceive by liberal assumptions themselves. It seems, to me, that on the kinds of questions he has posed, it might be better to say there are only first-person points of view, taken from a variety of levels of information and experience.

On further reflection, Reinders suggests there is no paradox in the responses of the parents of the disabled. It is the "fact of sharing the life they live together" that "makes all the difference." When asked, hypothetically, and with no reference to a particular child, if they would choose to have a child with, say, fragile X syndrome, they will likely say no, but their actual life with a child with fragile X is something they would not want to have missed. One way to put this is that the DPC "reduces the parental perspective on a disabled child to an impersonal point of view" in a way that simply makes no sense of such parents' experience with their child. If the parents of James, "a young man with fragile X," are asked, "If your son could be cured, would you not prefer to have him without fragile X," they could say little, as James without fragile X would not be James. James's "identity cannot be distinguished from the bodily existence that is characterized by his genetic condition." The parents of James cannot make the person-condition distinction because, to do so, involves "rejecting their life with their present child because of what that child is" (60–61). The direction of the argument has, in effect, been suggested by a powerful quotation from Dick Sobsey that Reinders uses as an epigraph for his chapter:

> Any artificial attempt to split my child from his disability is dishonest, dissociatively psychotic, or without any knowledge of my child. It is like saying, "I like your child; it's just his body, mind, and spirit that I don't like." David's disability is global. It is part of him just as much as his species or gender. It affects every aspect of his existence. It is not like a pair of shoes that he can take off. Without it, he would be a total stranger to me.[18]

Reinders's conclusion, then, is "that any attempt to distance the practices of prevention from negative judgments about the lives of disabled people is bound to fail, because it deprives such practices of the only rational grounds that people can have for pursuing them" (63).

This is a serious charge. If we accept it, we might well discontinue attempts to develop gene therapies for disabling conditions, as doing so seems inseparable from expressing negative judgments about disabled lives. If we argue for the continuation of therapeutic genetic development, we must do so while fully honoring Sobsey's insistence that the lives of people with certain disabilities cannot be separated from those disabilities, and it is wholly dishonest to do so. We must, one might say, discover a way to continue developing therapies for syndromes like fragile X without, in any way, diminishing the lives of those who live with the syndrome. If we can do this, we can perhaps discover different "rational grounds" for genetic therapies than those rightly castigated by Reinders above.

A way to begin an alternative analysis to Reinders's is by showing how his treatment is framed by abortion's becoming the therapy of choice for prevention of disability. Two points seem critical. First, at present disabling conditions for which there is no genetic therapy must be, as Sobsey's remarks make clear, lived out, made sense of, in a way, through the whole of one's life. This understanding seems implicit in

---

18. Sobsey, "Family Transformation," 13–16.

the very concept of disability, which names a kind of condition that must be made a part of life in a way that other, eliminable conditions do not require. But when it becomes possible to treat a particular, now disabling condition with genetic therapy, it will no longer be something that requires living out as a continuing feature of one's existence with which one must reckon. To treat such a condition therapeutically, then, will imply nothing whatever about the lives of those who have lived, or continue to live, with a condition which for them was not eliminable but rather something to be lived and given meaning within a whole life's story. In short, to ponder treating fragile X as a condition eliminable through genetic therapy seems threatening now to those with fragile X or their caretakers because, at present, the syndrome can only be made a part of one's whole story—in a way that will not be necessary once the therapy becomes possible.

Secondly, the effect of abortion in framing the whole discussion is evident in such recurrent phrases of Reinders's as "negative evaluation of disabled persons" or "negative judgments about the lives of disabled people." This is not a criticism of Reinders; I am in utter sympathy with his position. My point is that this language of totalizing judgment about the whole of a person's life or the person herself reflects the fact that abortion has become the therapy of choice. Therapeutic abortion puts into question the lives of the disabled. The defense, then, must be at the level of the whole life. Abortion denies that such a life can be good. The disabled and their parents necessarily respond that "disabled lives" are good. Again, *contra* Reinders but in service of his larger point, abortion forces the framing of the discussion as one about the worthiness of whole lives in a way that makes the DPC fail.

Thus it may paradoxically fall to those who are committed to resisting abortion to uphold the distinction between condition and person necessary to genetic therapeutic development. A body of people committed to opposing abortion could help to keep the debate from being framed as one in which whole lives are brought into question and the disabled must respond to vindicate themselves in ways no one should ever be asked to do. The scope of Jesus's admonition to "Judge not, lest ye be judged" is sometimes a matter of debate, but in the context being discussed here, its application seems clear. No one should engage in judgments about the whole of anyone else's life. We might be called to judge particular acts for purposes of punishment or particular practices or even traits of character. But this is quite different from engaging in the "negative evaluation of disabled lives" that is the logic of therapeutic abortion and that rightly worries Reinders. Paradoxically it is those who care for, rear, and support the disabled who uphold the ability for a meaningful distinction between person and condition to be made. For that distinction can be made only when there is no reason for the disabled to feel they must defend themselves against the consequences of the distinction.

As Hauerwas has argued that medicine needs the Church, I am suggesting the challenge of the disabled points to genetic therapy's need for the Church. The problem is clear: how can we simultaneously address potentially disabling conditions through genetic therapies without, in any way, diminishing the lives of those currently living with these conditions? First by providing honor, support of every kind, and solidarity for the disabled and those who choose to rear disabled children. Second, by insisting that our primary identity as Christians is one given from above and is perhaps infinitely different from any the world gives: that of fulfilling the vocation to love. This vocation embraces, indeed *crosses*, the normally abled and the disabled. Third, the church must be a community capable of acknowledging and bearing suffering so as to be an alternative to the impossible secular project of banishing all suffering—a project too easily given, in its worship of efficiency, to banishing those who suffer. We must acknowledge our fear of suffering, our tendency to banish it from our midst, and make of the church a place where the disabled feel fully accepted—on the same and only grounds as the normally abled—as the irreplaceable persons in Christ they are called to be. If the disabled can come to feel that their lives *cannot* be diminished, then perhaps the discussion of therapies can focus on other "rational grounds" than those considered and dismissed by Reinders.

We might specifically address the matter of therapy for disabling conditions as a question of relieving suffering. Because we know we inevitably suffer in all kinds of ways, it seems reasonable to remedy suffering where we can: this has meant the development of medicines and therapeutic techniques to address conditions once thought irremediable. Genetic therapy for now-disabling conditions can be seen as a continuation of this practice. Such therapy should in no way demean those disabled, or their caregivers, who have made living with now irremediable conditions fully a part of their life stories. It is not aimed at eliminating disabled lives but rather only at remedying conditions now disabling in order to allow those who might be disabled to live lives in which the condition does not need to be incorporated in the whole of one's story—in which another life can be lived. We would do this not from any belief that we are eliminating suffering, for we know that to be impossible short of the last day, but rather from the fallible knowledge that we are attempting to remedy a kind of suffering that seems unnecessary. Part of such fallible knowledge would be to recognize that our remedy of one condition may open the person to suffering of a different kind or on another level. One practical value, it seems to me, of thinking of genetic therapy for the disabled as a matter of reducing suffering is that it helps avoid the polarization between genetics, on the one hand, and social means of addressing the problems of the disabled, on the other. If our goal is to reduce suffering, then we can, and must, be simultaneously committed to genetic therapy for disabling conditions and to elimination of the social factors that currently afflict disabled people.

The gap opened by therapeutic abortion between the normally abled and those regarded "disabled" is perhaps nowhere more evident than in the vexing debate over whether the "disabled" should be allowed to use genetic techniques to design or guarantee children with similar "disabilities." Much of the literature on this question has focused on the Deaf, among whom a growing Deaf culture movement insists that deafness constitutes a "cultural identity rather than a disability," one that must be "nourished and maintained."[19] From this viewpoint, abortion of deaf fetuses would be regarded as discrimination or even genocide rather than therapeutic medicine. Deaf pride advocates insist they have "a cohesive community, a rich cultural heritage built around the

---

19. Davis's treatment of deafness under the chapter title, "Choosing for Disability," revealingly begs the question at hand, for the issue for Deaf is precisely whether deafness should be regarded as disability or culture. Even treating the issue as a "genetic dilemma" rather than a cultural one brings it within the thoroughgoing medicalization of modern life that Deaf see as oppressive. On the "construction" of deafness as "Disability vs. Linguistic Minority," see Lane, "Constructions of Deafness," 171–89. Lane's article is also helpful for its Foucauldian depiction of the way the "troubled-persons-industries" influence the construction of deafness and thus the treatments and policies regarding deaf/Deaf. For an extensive study of "representations" of deaf people, see Lane's *Mask of Benevolence*. One of the emphases of Lane's book is on the way representations of the deaf, measurement practices, special education, and surgical approaches all act in interrelated and interlegitimating ways—in Lane's view, ways determined by the audist establishment.

various residential schools, a growing body of drama, poetry, and other artistic traditions, and of course, what makes this all possible: ASL."[20] Developing this cultural heritage and pressing their claims for equal access and opportunity in the redistributionist state obviously depend upon maintaining a certain critical mass of the Deaf. Deaf parents are themselves sometimes inclined either not to have children if they will be born hearing or to abort hearing fetuses. Another option in cases where the connexin 26 mutation is responsible for deafness in parents would be to use in vitro fertilization and preimplantation genetic diagnosis to transfer only deaf embryos to the uterus. This may make pregnancy more difficult to achieve and add to the costs of IVF, but for some deaf parents, the guarantee of having a deaf child makes this an attractive approach.

Several points need to be made before I examine one extended attempt—that by Dena Davis—to grapple with the issues raised by this apparent selection for "disability." First, as Davis points out, "not all deaf people adhere to the notion of deaf culture, and some find the analogy to racial and ethnic groups 'nonsensical'" (57). Second, complicating the issue is the often intensely debated matter of cochlear implantation. Should cochlear implants become sufficiently perfected, Deaf culture will be seriously impacted, as "90 percent of deaf children are born to hearing parents," (55) who could be expected to overwhelmingly elect implantation for their children. Third, to the normally abled person who first comes upon these dilemmas in reading medical ethics, it must seem bizarre, at the least, that some parents would choose to have their children "disabled" in some way. What that reader should ask, I suggest, is whether he might not feel similarly if he had been identified by others through much of life by a condition that either does now or will in future likely qualify fetuses for abortion.[21]

20. See D. Davis, *Genetic Dilemmas*, 56–57. A good introduction to Deafness as culture is Padden and Humphries, *Deaf in America*. See also Dolnick, "Deafness as Culture," 37–53. A place to begin study of the history of the Deaf is Lane, *When the Mind Hears*. A strong critique of the Deafness as culture position is offered by Balkany et al., "Ethics of Cochlear Implantation in Young Children," 748–55. The layman will find extremely helpful Boothroyd, "Profound Deafness," 1–33. Boothroyd explains such matters as the categories of profound deafness, distinctions among educational environments, and the groupings of profoundly deaf by ages at which deafness began and the length of time one has been deaf.

21. I am aware that I may here put the Deaf in too defensive a position—by suggesting that Deaf identity is somehow a reaction against the disability construction. Deaf

Davis offers one of the fullest attempts to struggle with the issues of selecting for disability, but it is, in my view, unsuccessful. Following Joel Feinberg, Davis bears heavily on what she calls the child's "right to an open future." Defining just what this phrase means is difficult, but it seems to imply primarily that "parents ought not to make decisions about their children that severely and irreversibly restrict" their future choices (27).[22] An example, for Davis, of such severe and excessive restriction is presented by the Amish. She cites the 1972 Supreme Court case of *Wisconsin v. Yoder*, in which a group of Old Order Amish successfully argued that they should be exempt from sending their children to school past the eighth grade—in contradiction to Wisconsin's requirement that all children attend school until age sixteen. On the one hand was the Amish interest in maintaining their own culture and community; on the other, the state's interest in making sure "its citizens could vote wisely and make a living" (26). Davis notes that Feinberg, like the majority of the justices, "felt that the difference between leaving school after eighth grade and at age sixteen (only two more grades for many children) was not enough to justify the state in putting such a heavy burden on the Amish parents' religious beliefs" (27).[23] Her own "instincts," however, "go in the other direction": if Wisconsin believed its students entitled to schooling until age sixteen, then the Amish children "were entitled to that minimum as well, despite their parents' objections" (27).

I have no strong conviction about the court decision. It seems to me the two-year difference is narrow enough that one could come down on either side of the question. What is disturbing about Davis's argument, however, is the way she refuses to consider the Amish as presenting a valuable alternative to mainstream American culture. It begins to look like the child has a right to an open future but not if that child is reared

---

might prefer to say simply that their desire is to be members of the culture in which they, like everyone else, find themselves: in their case, that of the Deaf-World.

22. See Feinberg, "Child's Right to an Open Future," 76–97.

23. Interestingly, Feinberg seems to have approved of the Kansas courts' decision in a 1966 case to refuse "to permit an exemption for Amish communities from the requirement that all children be sent to state-accredited schools." "Child's Right," 81. The case in question was *State vs. Garber*, 197 Kan. 567 (1966). For Feinberg's treatment of *Yoder*, see 83–87. In discussing the Kansas case, he invokes John Stuart Mill in a way quite unlike Davis, noting that the public interest in that case might be with the Amish, for we all "profit from the example of others' 'experiments in living.'" (82). On this point, see Mill, *On Liberty*, 124.

in a culture sufficiently cohesive and different from the mainstream so as to constitute a real alternative. The Amish might well argue that there is no openness of future for anyone who must come to accept the killing of other human beings as a necessity of life in the state. Or that openness of future is an illusion if it is predicated on an economic life that systematically destroys the land on which we ultimately depend. However one regards these matters, they are serious questions put to the mainstream by Amish culture.

Davis, however, consistently portrays the Amish only as repressive and limiting. She depicts the justices as ducking the question of "whether the liberal democratic state owes all its citizens, especially children, a right to a basic education that can serve as a building block if the child decides later in life that she wishes to become an astronaut or a playwright, or perhaps to join the army." The final phrase suggests just how fully an education in the state is at odds with Amish convictions. Davis's rhetoric often suggests that for her an "open future" means primarily one of economic success. In criticizing the court's decision, she notes, "As we constantly hear from politicians and educators, without a high school diploma one's future is virtually closed. By denying them a high school education or its equivalent, parents are virtually ensuring that their children will remain housewives and farmers" (26).[24] Elsewhere she remarks that John Stuart Mill "would abhor" the situation of "the Amish communities in *Yoder*, which unabashedly want to give their children as few choices as possible" (30). The notion that the Amish represent choices barely conceivable by mainstream American culture—choices for non-violent Christianity and sustainable environmental practice—is not explored or even acknowledged by Davis. Later she calls the Amish a "narrow-choice community" and reverts to the tired argument that some people need the "fit" of "an authoritarian community based on tradition, where one is freed from the necessity of making choices" (30). Nowhere does Davis display the willingness to consider the strengths or virtues of the Amish way of life *as they might appear to the Amish*. She

---

24. It has been a consistent theme of Wendell Berry's that industrialism's promise to relieve human beings of work has lead to the unfortunate denigration of physical labor of all kinds. Presenting a serious alternative to our current arrangements would necessarily involve coming to afford greater dignity to physical work. See, for example, "Racism and the Economy," in *Art of the Commonplace*, 47–64. The superiority of Amish to industrial agricultural practices is an emphasis of Berry's novel, *Remembering*, in *Three Short Novels*.

does assert finally that a regard for diversity means liberals "should tolerate even those communities most unsympathetic to the liberal value of individual choice" (31). But her rhetoric everywhere seems at odds with her tolerance, at least insofar as the Amish are concerned, and there is no possibility she might hear the deepest Amish criticism: that a society reliant ultimately on violence has already preempted its citizens' most important choice.[25]

Davis draws a very close parallel between the Amish and deaf parents who desire deaf children: "The Amish are an example of a group guarding its ability to shape the lives of its children; deaf parents wishing to ensure deaf children are an example of families pursuing the same goals" (31–32). Davis provides a fuller account of Deaf culture's own claims than she does for the Amish, but ultimately she discounts these claims as insignificant relative to the child's right to an open future. "If deafness is a culture," she concludes, "it is an exceedingly narrow one," and "although deaf activists correctly show that many occupations are open to the deaf with only minor technological adjustments, the range of occupations will always be inherently limited" (63–64). Such a "narrow choice of vocation is not only a harm in its own sake, but also is likely to continue to lead to lower standards of living" (64). Thus Davis concludes that "deliberately creating a deaf child counts as a moral harm." In fact, she contends that "less rides on where you come out on the disability-versus-culture debate than first appears." If deafness is a disability, the

---

25. Davis's argument seems an illustration of what Engelhardt has called "liberal cosmopolitanism," to be distinguished, very importantly, from "libertarian cosmopolitanism." See Engelhardt, *Foundations of Christian Bioethics*, 134–55. Engelhardt endorses the libertarian position as a default option for societies that rightly recognize themselves to be without a content-full moral view that can be subscribed to by all. This position would allow "individuals with diverse moral commitments in their own moral communities to act with common moral authority and live peaceably within a larger secular society" (135). It is a "procedural" position only, whereas liberal cosmopolitanism is actually a content-full or substantive way of life masquerading, we might say, as a procedural one. It conceives the "thisworldly life project[s]" (140) of individuals to be the source of ultimate value; its central affirmation is of "equality in liberty of choice and in the pursuit of satisfaction or fulfillment, which affirmation gives flesh and substance to moral rationality" (140). Liberal cosmopolitans are committed to living "in conformity with a particular concrete, canonical moral understanding that gives centrality to liberty, equality, and personal fulfillment" (140–41). Thus, as Davis does with the Amish, they will consider suspect, perhaps even "morally deficient, moral communities that do not recognize autonomous self-determination as the keystone of moral flourishing" (141).

harm to the child lies in limiting its choice of careers or marriage options; if it is a culture, the harm lies in confining the child excessively "to a narrow group of people." The concern for autonomy "that grounds the ethics of genetic counseling" should prevent any genetic counselor from acquiescing to parental choices that so confine a child's economic and cultural choices. On the related issue of cochlear implantation, Davis argues that parents "have an obligation to have their children implanted" if the technology improves sufficiently (65).[26]

Unfortunately Davis's arguments discount rather than answer the claims of the Deaf. The Deaf will respond, with entire justification, that Davis's judgment about Deaf culture's narrowness represents little more than a kind of cultural imperialism expressed by one who does not know the culture from the inside. Similarly, if deafness has meant a narrower range of vocational choices and lower standards of living, this is, at least in part, because of the very kinds of exclusion and discrimination against which the Deaf contend. If marriage options for the deaf are limited,

---

26. Much of the debate over constructions of deafness turns on the issue of cochlear implantation. Lane and Grodin point out, for instance, the problem caused by the surgery and habilitation's delaying the "child's acquisition of ASL and therefore . . . the time that child has any full language at his or her command" (236). See "Ethical Issues in Cochlear Implant Surgery," 231–51. For a study that suggests the age of acquisition is critical for later proficiency in ASL, see Mayberry and Eichen, "Long-Lasting Advantage," 486–512. Elsewhere Lane has pointed out some of the problems regarding parental surrogate decision-making regarding implantation. There may have been "prolonged lack of communication between parent and child," and unless the child has acquired ASL and been with Deaf children and adults, he or she will have little ability to know what a future without implantation might look like. Thus it may be very difficult to get anything like an informed opinion from the child. There may also be a conflict of interest between parent and child, one unrecognized by even the most responsible parent: "The morally valid surrogate must not have a conflict of interest with the patient's best interest. Painful as it is to acknowledge, parents may have such a conflict of interest; for example, they put more weight on their child acquiring extremely limited communication in their primary language than on the child acquiring fluent communication in ASL." Lane, *Mask of Benevolence*, 233–34. On the other hand, Tucker claims that "most children, and people who become deaf later in life and have memory of normal hearing, do very well with cochlear implants, thus reducing (if not eliminating) the need for special schools, interpreters, and other costly accommodations. Such individuals who refuse today to have cochlear implants, yet demand costly accommodations, should, in this author's opinion, be viewed as acting unethically" (13). See "Deaf Culture, Cochlear Implants, and Elective Disability," 6–14. The article contains a useful summary of studies indicating the positive results of cochlear implants. For representative examples, see Horn et al., "Audiological and Medical Considerations," 82–86; and Cohen, "Ethics of Cochlear Implants in Young Children," 1–2.

this, too, is because the hearing are too often unwilling to accept the Deaf as equally interesting and valuable human beings. In short, every harm Davis mentions will likely appear to the Deaf as evidence rather of discrimination than of anything inherent in deafness itself.

What Davis means by an "open future" is interestingly clarified by another example of genetic selection she ponders and which she contrasts somewhat with deafness. She begins her chapter on "Choosing for Disability" with an account of Celia, an achondroplasic woman who served as clinic coordinator in the genetics department at Johns Hopkins. When Celia and her achondroplasic husband wanted to have children, it was not possible to test for the achondroplasia gene, "a double dose" of which "is always fatal" (50). Thus she and her husband adopted an achondroplasic child, who, like her, is very involved in Little People of America (LPA). If Celia and her husband were now beginning a family, they might well, Davis opines, "approach a genetics counselor for assistance in ensuring that they had a child with achondroplasia, possibly by using in vitro fertilization and preimplantation genetic diagnosis to retain only embryos carrying one copy of the relevant gene." (51) Thus Davis frames this case of selection for achondroplasia as a matter for ethical reflection, one she treats in a revealingly different way from deafness.

What's puzzling about Davis's treatment of the case are the things she does not say. Elsewhere she articulates a firmly Kantian sense of the maxims that ought to guide conception: "Deliberately creating a child who will be forced irreversibly into the parents' notion of the good life violates the Kantian principle of treating each person as an end in herself and never as a means only" (34). But this Kantian test is not applied to the maxims under which an achondroplasic couple would choose for a child with the condition. Surely achondroplasia is irreversible and will likely cause the child to be more influenced by its parents—for good or ill—than the normally abled child is influenced by its parents (with obvious exceptions). What should actually be more relevant to the strict Kantian, of course, is the *maxim* under which the action is being taken. In this case, it seems at least arguable that they are treating the child as a means, even if the parents can respond that they are acting *also* with a sense of the child as end in herself. If Davis does not apply this test strictly to her achondroplasic couple, it may be because her account of conception is incoherent from a Kantian point-of-view. She argues that "the decision to have a child is never made for the sake of the child—for no child then exists. We choose to have children for myriad reasons, but before the child is conceived, those reasons can only be self-regarding. The child is a means to our ends" (34).

Davis's Kantianism does not apply the test for the categorical imperative where Kant insisted it must be applied: to the maxim under which action is taken. If she were to do so, then she would have to conclude that no one should conceive children, for in doing so, they regard the child as means only—at least on her account. For Davis the decision to conceive is wholly self-regarding on the part of parents, who must then come, later in life, to regard the child as utterly an end in herself. This seems neither a description of any possible psychological change nor of the way most parents regard their children, either before or after they are conceived. It should be understood rather as the schizophrenic justification of a form of life combining abortion on demand—with its assumption that the child is at its parents' disposal until birth—with the conviction that autonomous economic success is the prime determinant of identity.[27]

Arguably, then, achondroplasia might be considered just as irreversible, determinative, limiting, and stigmatizing as deafness. Yet Davis is not willing to draw the conclusion that parents' ensuring achondroplasia in their children counts as moral harm. Rather she finds it a "much more difficult judgment call (perhaps only because less has been studied and written about the world of 'little people' and the extent to which their cultural, social, and career choices are constrained by their condition)." Thus she does not urge genetic counselors to refuse to assist parents like

---

27. Perhaps Davis's way of thinking about parental motivations for having children should be understood as an indication of the way instrumental rationality has simply colonized all discourse in bioethics: in other words, in order to be taken seriously in talking about parents' reasons for having children, she must present it in a way understandable to those accustomed to thinking of action as always directed toward instrumentality of some sort. What's happened is that other descriptions have simply been excluded from consideration. I find much more credible, for instance, Gabriel Marcel's description of parents "who, in a sort of prodigality of their whole being, sow the seed of life without ulterior motive by radiating the life flame which has permeated them and set them aglow." See *Homo Viator*, 88. Or, to adapt a phrase from Thoreau, it seems to me that having children springs from a "simple and irrepressible satisfaction with the gift of life." Thoreau said that he found such satisfaction recorded "nowhere," but perhaps—though he understood much—he failed to understand what moves ordinary people everywhere to have children. See *Walden*, 122.

Celia and her husband, for it is unclear that the adult achondroplasic will find "momentous pieces of his adult life" foreclosed by his condition (66).

My point here is not to argue that either the deaf or achondroplasics do "moral harm" in ensuring their children are deaf or achondroplasic. In both cases, a great deal of what is "disabling" about the conditions must be attributed to discrimination and other fully alterable social factors. What I want to point out and account for is the seemingly counterintuitive way Davis distinguishes the two groups. The reason for that distinction is suggested paradoxically by Davis's comment that less rides on the understanding of deafness as culture or disability than is often thought. This is because *culture is a disability* for Davis if it is, in her view, too constraining. In other words, deafness poses a different problem for Davis than achondroplasia precisely because the Deaf claim to have a culture fully as rich and valid as others. Achondroplasia is rare enough that it can be treated as an anomaly and the designedly conceived achondroplasic child regarded primarily as an individual. Quite unintentionally, Davis's language of "little people" tends to press achondroplasics toward the category of curiosities. What is important to note is that achondroplasia is sufficiently rare that allowing achondroplasic parents to elect for achondroplasia in their children will have no effect on mainstream reproductive practices. This is not true of deafness.

As Davis points out, 90 percent of deaf children are born to hearing parents. Every one of us is also subject to the possibility of deafness through accident or age. These are important facts to see. They mean that all of us who are hearing have a strong stake in technologies or therapies that would eliminate what we regard as a threatening and disabling condition. Yet this condition is precisely what those who are deaf must learn to live out, and in a way that could perhaps be less determinative of their identities if mainstream culture were less fearful and more accommodating. The Deaf respond by coming to understand Deafness as a culture rather than a disability. It is difficult to see how they could respond otherwise when deafness constitutes such a determining feature of their lives. After all, what else is a culture but a way of speaking about a distinctive group's pattern of responses to determining conditions? But this point—that Deafness be understood as culture—is precisely what Davis cannot accept, and she cannot accept it because it does seem the strongest argument in favor of the Deaf's being able to ensure deaf children. Thus, in regard to deafness, she blurs the culture-disability distinction. The rather underdeveloped counterexample of achondroplasia allows her to indicate she is not simply opposed to designing for difference from the mainstream. What it actually does is highlight the fact that she opposes designing for difference where the difference can be described as cultural. She must do this in order to protect abortion on demand from the charge that it amounts to discrimination when the fetus is eliminated for suspected deafness. Abortion must be contained as a problem of private, individual reproductive choice: to grant that a child is aborted because of a particular *cultural* identity would be tantamount to approving discrimination. Thus, on the complementary issue of designing for "disability," such genetic design can be allowed as long as the condition is anomalous enough to be referred to the affected individual only—as in achondroplasia. If the condition is broadly enough distributed that those affected by it could constitute a culture, then designing for it cannot be allowed—for to do the opposite, to abort for what is effectively a "cultural" identity, would be discriminatory.

Thus we arrive at a seemingly unbreakable impasse. Surely anyone is rightly entitled to desire hearing for herself or her children. The Deaf, on the other hand, can, with equal rightness, claim that the pattern of their responses to the condition constitutes a culture. Once again perhaps we can see how genetic therapy will require the Church—that is, if the church is capable of being a people committed to resisting abortion. For it will require a people committed to opposing abortion to prevent the issues regarding deafness from becoming ones in which whole lives are put into question and the Deaf respond in the only way that they can: by asserting that their lives are fully as worthy and valid as anyone else's. Without, in any way, meaning to indicate that the impasse I mentioned above can be easily broken, I will close with some modest suggestions about how the church might provide a context in which the hearing and the Deaf can approach their differences.

Perhaps the most important thing the church can say to the hearing and the Deaf is that one's most determinate identity is to be the person-in-Christ one is called to be. One's vocation is to love God and the neighbor, to work, serve, and know in ways always ordered to love. This is a vocation equally open to the normally abled and the disabled.

We are to care for the fetus and for the child irrespective of its worldly abilities precisely because it carries at all times the potential to fulfill this vocation that is qualitatively different from any the world gives. Loving God and the neighbor cannot be a matter of somehow doing more than someone else, of being more than someone else. It is to relinquish the act of distinction. To put this in a more rigorously theological way, one can find release from the project of ceaselessly resisting a colonizing normality by resting in the "difference established by God" in the Christian body.[28] Thus if hearing and Deaf are able to understand themselves as being, in their most determinate identities, reconciled in a common vocation, perhaps they can begin to speak about deafness as a condition, as one feature among many, and not as the overriding determinant of their lives.[29]

If the development of charity can come to be the most determinate vocation of our lives, then a condition like deafness can perhaps be seen not as dis-abling but rather only as differently-abling. If the deaf can see their condition as something that does not determine their identities, perhaps they can begin to enter into conversation with the hearing over whether the condition should be seen as limiting in a way that ought, when possible, to be remediated. The hearing, however, will have to be absolutely willing to entertain the possibility that deafness is not limiting to the Deaf. It goes without saying that the hearing should cultivate appreciation for the achievements of Deaf culture and recognize the real risks on the part of deaf parents who have hearing children. For deaf parents to have hearing children is to risk a degree of difference from those children, a potential alienation, that is quite unlike anything

---

28. Shuman, "Desperately Seeking Perfection," 148. Shuman points out that difference is not simply to be tolerated or appreciated in the Christian body; the Christian body is "*comprised* by difference," a fact "rooted first of all" in the triune godhead. Shuman delineates three qualities of life in the Christian body that might guide decision making about uses of medical genetics, which must be ordered, in his view, to a Christian perfection of the body "shaped finally by the cross and resurrection of Christ" (149). These three qualities of life in the Christian body are affirmation of the "fundamental interdependence of the body's members and an irreducible respect for the differences among them"; a "commitment to be present as servants to weakness and suffering within and beyond the body"; and a recognition of the particular authority that belongs to "its weakest and most dependent members" (148–49).

29. Suggesting the possibility of a "hearing and deaf partnership in deaf education," Lane comments, "For that partnership to be forged, both parties must bring their cultural frames into consciousness, construct a mutual understanding of those frames, and make an empathic leap, trying to position themselves at each other's 'center.'" See *Mask of Benevolence*, 200. Something like this process is what I'm suggesting the Church might enable.

normally abled parents confront. The hearing must do everything they can to reduce the possibility that deafness be seen as disability—to be responded to, then, through the development of a separate culture. If social arrangements can be such that the Deaf/deaf are not forced to see themselves as disabled—in the eyes of the hearing—then possibly they can come to understand deafness as a potentially limiting condition, perhaps more radical but not different in kind from other limiting conditions on us all.

10

On Peter Singer's Silencing in Germany

Or, What's Wrong with Asking "What's Wrong with Killing?"

ATTACHED TO THE SECOND edition of Peter Singer's *Practical Ethics* is an appendix entitled "On Being Silenced in Germany." Here Singer gives an account of the disruption or forced cancellation of several academic gatherings scheduled in Germany during the 1980s and 90s where the issue of euthanasia was to be discussed. At some of these he was to be a participant; at others, other prominent critics of the sanctity of life doctrine, like Helga Kuhse, were to be featured. Opposition came from what Singer styles as "radical disability groups," most prominently the "Cripples Movement." One case is particularly instructive. Singer himself had been scheduled to speak at a European Symposium on "Bioengineering, Ethics, and Mental Disability" at Marburg in June, 1989, and on "the subject 'Do severely disabled newborn infants have a right to life?'" at the University of Dortmund during the same summer. The prospect of Singer's appearances raised a storm of actual and threatened protest that caused *Lebenshilfe*—"the major German organization for parents of intellectually disabled infants" and the organizer of the Marburg conference—to withdraw his invitation to speak. *Der Spiegel* soon published an attack on Singer's views, "illustrated with photographs of the transportation of 'euthanasia victims' in the Third Reich, and of Hitler's 'Euthanasia Order.'"[1]

---

1. Singer, *Practical Ethics*, 345. Further references will be given parenthetically.

Singer's written defense was rejected by *Der Spiegel* on the grounds of insufficient space, yet the magazine did find space for a later critical account of his views on euthanasia, a lengthy interview with one of his opponents, and "again, the same photograph of the Nazi transport vehicles" (345). Singer tells the whole story as illustration of the sorry state of academic freedom and public discussion regarding such matters in some areas of Western Europe. He rightly points up the irony of his being told that he "lacked the experience with Nazism that Germans had had": Singer is "the child of Austrian-Jewish refugees," and "three of [his] grandparents had died in Nazi concentration camps" (346). On one occasion in Zurich, a protesting audience's cries of "Singer *raus!* Singer *raus!*" caused him to feel "what it must have been like to attempt to reason against the rising tide of Nazism in the declining days of the Weimar Republic." Indeed, at that event, he was assaulted: "Protesters came up behind me and tore my glasses from my face, throwing them on the floor and breaking them" (357).

What Singer tells is truly an amazing story. A Jew is again silenced in Germany, only this time for advocating liberalizing views on matters such as euthanasia and infanticide stringently prohibited precisely because of the Nazi experience. Singer's censoring may perhaps have had as much to do with his simply breaking silence on proscribed topics as it did with the specific positions he articulates. He gave voice and face to the arguments, making a distinction, where a kind of forced unanimity prevailed.[2] In the process he discovered a felt link with his own particular

---

2. Eric B. Brown ("Dilemmas of German Bioethics," 37–53) has commented on some of the further consequences of the "Singer Affair" for bioethics in Germany: "Singer's ideas were depicted as the vanguard of Anglo-American bioethics—a dangerous form of instrumental rationality and a deceptive ruse by which Darwinist fascism would reintroduce itself in Germany. The study of Anglo-American bioethics was suspended in many German universities, and many bioethics scholars were forced from their teaching posts. In the state of Baden-Wurttemberg, Social Democrats pushed for a formal government declaration that the thought of the 'Anglo-Saxon institutes such as the Kennedy Institute of Ethics, the Hastings Center, or the Center for Human Bioethics (in Australia),' be considered 'incompatible with the norms of the Constitution'" (46). Brown sees the "Nazi taboo" beginning "to fade in Germany," but remains unsure "what will ground German bioethics in the years ahead" (52). Arnd T. May ("Physician-Assisted Suicide, Euthanasia, and Christian Bioethics," 273–83) also sees a shift in Germany "from traditional to post-traditional moral commitments" (280). He cites a 2001 poll indicating that "64–80% of the people in Germany" support active euthanasia, evidence of an "emerging majority interest in autonomy" influenced, in part, by "recent developments in the Netherlands, Belgium, and elsewhere" (274). For a strong critique

identity, despite his being a strong and consistent advocate of an ethical universalism. This, however, is an irony that Singer perhaps does not see. It's noteworthy that Singer's blocked or disrupted appearances involve lectures, speeches, presentations involving an "I" speaking directly to an audience of "yous." One irony of his experience—and this I believe he is not aware of—is that it can be read as confirmation that doing ethics is a matter of an "I" and a "you." This is something Singer specifically denies in his opening chapter of *Practical Ethics*: "Ethics requires us to go beyond 'I' and 'you' to the universal law, the universalisable judgment, the standpoint of the impartial spectator or ideal observer, or whatever we choose to call it" (12). Now, of course, ethics requires our correcting our own subjectivities by some measure or other, but Singer's easy movement toward universalizability seems precisely what his disabled opponents denied. For the disabled, there can be no easy move of abstraction from their particularities, precisely because the particularities of their conditions play such a strong role in both their own self-understanding and their identity for others. While I, in no way, would want to endorse the denials of Singer's right to speak or the manner in which he was treated in Germany and Switzerland, I do think a general defense of the disabled's reaction to Singer can be offered.[3] That reaction can be seen as the response of a people vividly aware of their particularity rejecting what they cannot help but hear as the potential tyranny of a universalizing voice—even if it is utterly unmeant in that way, as I believe it was and is in the case of Peter Singer.

Singer's work is marked by a deep and sincere desire to limit suffering. He has argued persistently, in an admirably honest and compelling way, that suffering qualifies one for moral regard and that the suffering worthy of such regard is not only that of human beings but also that of other animals. His strategy has been to put all human beings and the

---

of Singer's work by a German advocate for the disabled, see Tolmein, "Case of Peter Singer."

3. My own view on the need for open discussion is in substantial accord with the following comment by Singer: "If a sound ethic cannot be discussed in public because it will lead to genocide or the murder of people with disabilities, we are in dire straits indeed. I am not so pessimistic. As compared with placing a taboo on discussions of the basis of human equality, an open discussion seems to me much more likely to lead people to a compassionate ethic that is at the opposite end of the spectrum to Nazi attitudes to racial minorities or to those with disabilities." See "A Response," 294. Singer has commented on these matters, too, in "German Attack on Applied Ethics" and "'Singer-Affair' and Practical Ethics."

members of at least the most neurologically complex other species on a single scale of suffering, and then to argue for utilitarian balancing and weighing when we are forced to make choices about who lives and who dies. Thus his well-known disdain for speciesism, that drawing of a line, or circle around all human beings and attributing to them special moral worth simply by virtue of membership in the species. Speciesism, like racism or sexism, simply allows us to disregard the suffering of a whole category of beings, in this case, the other animals.[4] Honest assessment of the ability to suffer—or of such personhood characteristics as sentience, awareness of continuity in time, understanding the possibility of ceasing existence in death—suggests that non-human higher mammals are more worthy of moral regard than human infants. Thus absolute prohibition of human infanticide seems irrational to Singer as long as we continue to regard the higher mammals in instrumental fashion. Even though I would treat these issues quite differently, it must be said for Singer that he has primarily used the comparison of human infant to higher mammal to raise the status of non-human animals and not to diminish the status of human infants.[5]

It has also seemed irrational to Singer to allow abortion of "disabled" fetuses—and, more generally, abortion on request—while preventing parents from deciding to euthanize disabled infants. Since Singer be-

---

4. For a representative statement of Singer's on speciesism and its analogy to racism, see chapter 3 of *Practical Ethics*, "Equality for Animals?" 55–82. As an anecdotal matter, I will add that African-American students have sometimes provided the strongest resistance to Singer's analogy when I have taught his "Animal Liberation." The objection generally comes in the form of a question much like this: "Does he mean that the relationship between the white slaveowner and my ancestor was like my relationship to the steer whose meat I consume in a hamburger? If so, I reject that as ludicrous and demeaning." One problem for the students involves the way Singer conceptualizes the extension of the circle of moral concern; his model, as well as the racism-speciesism analogy itself, leaves little room for the vigorous assertion of rights by the victim of racism herself. He/she is reduced to passivity by the very conferring of previously denied status. See "Animal Liberation," 138–51. A further difficulty with the analogy lies in the fact that recognition of human beings as a species provides a—perhaps *the*—primary argument *against* racism or sexism.

5. Singer insists, of course, that Darwinian thinking demands understanding the relationship between humans and other animals as a "continuum" not only "with respect to anatomy and physiology, but also with regard to their mental lives." Darwin has knocked "out the intellectual foundations of the idea that we are a separate creation from the animals, and utterly different in kind." "Sadly," the "revolution in our attitudes to nonhuman animals" made possible by Darwin has not yet occurred. See *Darwinian Left*, 17.

lieves no morally significant distinction can be made between fetus and infant, it seems irrational to surround the Down syndrome infant, for example, with a kind of protection denied the fetus diagnosed with Down syndrome. Singer makes this argument from within what seems to him a reasonable estimation of parental practices. In many cases, he believes, preventing parents from euthanizing a disabled infant—by definition, a non-person—precludes their having another child. The disabled child substitutes for one whom the parents would otherwise have and whose overall life prospects could reasonably make for less suffering and greater overall happiness. The animating concern of Singer's argument is the humane reduction of suffering and promotion of happiness.

Despite their humanity, Singer's positions cannot help but seem troubling to the disabled. To see why this is the case, we can begin by considering the response he made to *Der Spiegel* in the midst of events in 1989. Here is Singer's account of that response:

> I sent a brief reply in which I pointed out that I was advocating euthanasia not for anyone like themselves, but for severely disabled newborn infants, and that it was crucial to my defense of euthanasia that these infants would never have been capable of grasping that they are living beings with a past and a future. Hence my views cannot be a threat to anyone who is capable of wanting to go on living, or even of understanding that his or her life might be threatened. (345)

Singer's formulation here echoes his handling of the relationship between the indirect, classical utilitarian reason against killing and infanticide. The indirect, classical utilitarian argument against killing holds that we ought not to kill because doing so causes all to be threatened and thus diminishes their happiness. In Singer's view the argument does not hold as a reason against infanticide "because no one capable of understanding what is happening when a newborn baby is killed could feel threatened by a policy that gave less protection to the newborn than to adults." On this matter, he follows Jeremy Bentham, for whom infanticide was "of a nature not to give the slightest inquietude to the most timid imagination," for, in Singer's language, "Once we are old enough to comprehend the policy, we are too old to be threatened by it" (171).[6] Singer's reassurance to the disabled follows the same logic: the very fact the disabled can

---

6. Bentham, *Theory of Legislation*, 163.

understand it and want to go on living is tantamount to proof they have nothing to fear from the arguments for euthanasia and infanticide.

Several features of Singer's response seem curious. First is the irony of the impartial or universalist ethicist's making such a straightforward appeal to what he assumes to be the solely self-interested motives of those who oppose him: their fears and objections are to be allayed by the simple reassurance that he does not mean to advocate killing people like them. Or perhaps we should put this slightly differently: Singer may believe that what he is making is an ethical argument in his intended communication to *Der Spiegel*, but it cannot help but appear as an appeal to the self-interest of the disabled he is addressing. Singer is fond of asking, "What's Wrong with Killing?," and this interchange with the disabled may offer one way of beginning to respond to that question. One thing that's wrong with killing is that it makes rational discussion impossible. Participants in rational conversation must believe that they are not subject to being killed: if they are in need of being reassured on this matter, then the possibility of such conversation has been lost. Singer's continual putting into play the question of who shall be killed cannot help but undermine rational discussion, which can only take place when all the participants believe—perhaps on the basis of a word stronger, more enduring, more trustworthy than the inevitably self-interested assurance of one player—that their very existence is not at stake. Now Singer may believe himself disinterested, but any participant in conversation with him can reasonably say that he has never disinterestedly contemplated questions about who shall be killed—for he has always, knowingly or not, exempted himself from those whose lives are put in question.

It seems important to ask, too, what the rhetorical effects of Singer's position might be. Does it not implicitly encourage the disabled person to renounce his/her identity as disabled? Note the logic is that s/he need not fear being killed because s/he is not like those disabled newborns for whom euthanasia is "advocated." Would insisting on solidarity or identification with disabled newborns negate this logic, thus exposing the disabled to being killed? In Singer's defense, his proposed response to *Der Spiegel* goes on to offer what must seem to him a clear empirical definition of the kind of infants for whom he advocates euthanasia—those who "would never have been capable of grasping that they are living beings with a past and a future" (345). Still it seems extraordinarily naïve of Singer to believe that he can control the way an audience of disabled people will hear definitions of disability that mark one either as a candidate for euthanasia or not. His response to *Der Spiegel* seems to ask of the disabled a nearly impossible abstraction from their own bodily, as well as social, experience. For those disabled bodily, the experience of the body is not something easily dismissed. Moreover, those disabled in any way must continually reckon with the way their disability identifies them for others. It must seem hollow indeed, to the disabled, to be reassured by a normally abled person that she will not be judged to be like other disabled people (in this case, newborns)—when, in fact, her disability has identified her for the normally abled throughout her experience.

I think we should revisit here one of Singer's ways of paraphrasing Bentham on infanticide. Infanticide, according to Bentham, ought not to disquiet even the "most timid imagination" because, as Singer explains, "no one capable of understanding what is happening when a newborn baby is killed could feel threatened by a policy that gave less protection to the newborn than to adults" (171). Perhaps I am guilty of having a timid imagination, but I suppose I want to say that I'm not sure anyone is really "capable of understanding what is happening when a newborn baby is killed." Surely it's somehow relevant here to say that any understanding of what's happening in infanticide must be a matter largely of imagination, and that imaginations are more or less timid relative to life experiences in a world of very unequal powers. Some of us of timid imagination—but also aware of our own fears of dependence and capacity to kill—might say that part of what is happening when newborns are killed is a rejection of weakness, of a dependence that frightens us. We must be careful about diminishing the force of established prohibitions against killing precisely because human beings have shown such a predilection to kill. Thus I would want to offer the following modifications of Singer's principle articulated above. First I'd be inclined to say that "anyone capable of understanding what is happening when a newborn baby is killed should feel threatened by policies giving less protection to newborns than to adults." Or second, "we should feel threatened by policies giving less protection to newborns than to adults if they are formulated by those who believe themselves capable of understanding what is happening when newborns are killed."

Singer, of course, does not believe there is any reason for the disabled to be threatened by his positions. The principle of equal consideration of interests protects them, and Singer advocates an affirmative action approach to policy for the disabled based on the recognition that they have been victims of discrimination akin to racism and sexism. In *Practical Ethics*, he confronts directly the contradiction, sensed by some, between "recognition of disabled people as a group that has been subjected to unjustifiable discrimination" and his positions on abortion and infanticide for disabled fetuses and newborns. He grants his argument for infanticide is based on the assumption that "life is better without a disability than with one," but rejects the claim that this is simply a prejudice held by normally abled people and "parallel" to racist or sexist prejudice:

> It is one thing to argue that people with disabilities who want to live their lives to the full should be given every possible assistance in doing so. It is another, and quite different thing, to argue that if we are in a position to choose, for our next child, whether that child shall begin life with or without a disability, it is mere prejudice or bias that leads us to choose to have a child without a disability. (53–54)

Singer claims, in effect, that we can simultaneously will to regard disabled people as full equals and yet act to eliminate children with disabilities through infanticide. I doubt it is possible to maintain both these positions simultaneously, either as a matter of personal belief or political conviction.

What Singer fails to recognize is the change in plausibility to his arguments caused by easily available abortion and his case for infanticide. It does seem plausible to hold that we can simultaneously value the disabled as full equals and yet prefer to have children without disabilities as long as strong prohibitions against abortion and infanticide are in effect. When those prohibitions are in place, the risk of having disabled children, and thus of needing special social assistance, applies to every potential parent in the population. The distinction between the disabled and the normally abled cannot be fixed in the way that becomes possible with abortion and infanticide. Singer is fond of reminding his readers that prohibitions against infanticide are simply irrational holdovers from Judaic and Christian practices.[7] But the arguments he makes

---

7. Michael Tooley makes a similar argument about infanticide, claiming that one cannot regard its prohibition as evidence of "moral progress" without holding "that the underlying theological assumptions"—Judaic and Christian—"are reasonable ones" (322). Tooley, of course, does not believe such theological assumptions reasonable,

above seem decidedly dependent on those practices he rejects: it is one thing to say our choosing to have children without disabilities implies nothing regarding our attitudes toward the disabled when that "choosing" means no more than that we hope to have normal children but will accept disabled children without even the thought that we might kill them. It seems quite another to tell the disabled we regard them as equals when we make it clear, through abortion and infanticide, that we will kill new human beings with similar disabilities.[8]

Singer offers the following example as further evidence of his claim that it's not simply a prejudice to believe life is better without disability: "If disabled people who must use wheelchairs to get around were suddenly offered a miracle drug that would, with no side effects, give them full use of their legs, how many of them would refuse to take it on the grounds that life with a disability is in no way inferior to life without a disability?" (54). There are several important things to be said about the way Singer puts this question. First, while I do not believe Singer wants to suggest the lives of the disabled are inferior, it is difficult to see how the disabled could possibly understand him otherwise. Second, if this is offered as evidence—as testimony on the part of the disabled themselves—that the inferiority of disabled life is not a matter of prejudice, then how are we to regard that belief? Is the intention to establish it as warranted conclusion, even as fact, that life with a disability is "inferior" to life without disability? What is the goal or consequence of establishing such a comparative judgment as fact? This should cause us to ponder further Singer's use of the term "inferior." What are the kinds of assumptions under which it becomes necessary or desirable to assess lives as

---

a position he assumes is shared by most philosophers. See *Abortion and Infanticide*, 309–22.

8. Francis Fukuyama makes a rather different argument about infanticide that should be read as a corrective to Singer's: "The more closely one looks at the actual practice of infanticide, the more it becomes clear that it is motivated by exceptional circumstances that explain how the normally powerful emotions of parental care can be overridden. These circumstances include the desire of a stepfather or new mate to eliminate a rival's offspring; desperation, sickness, or extreme poverty on the part of the mother; a cultural preference for males; and an infant that is sickly or deformed. It is hard to find societies in which infanticide is not practiced primarily by those at the bottom of the social hierarchy; where resources permit families to raise their children, nurturing instincts dominate.... Infanticide is thus like murder more broadly considered: something that occurs universally but is universally condemned and controlled" (*Our Posthuman Future*, 142).

superior or inferior—and to establish these with a kind of certainty? Ought we not perhaps to reject categorically any such uses?

I can well imagine that all the wheelchair-bound people of Singer's example would take the new wonder drug. But I doubt any of them past adolescence would think of what they're doing as leaving an "inferior" life. Even if they thought of life as no more than preference satisfaction, I'm sure they would have realized that satisfaction of preferences is largely an individual matter and that people develop preferences in relation to their situations in life. Moreover, they would not simply cease being the people they were previous to taking the drug: they'd still be the same people, with largely the same interests, commitments, and sources of enjoyment, only now more mobile. They might well describe themselves as more fulfilled, perhaps even happier, but I doubt many could be brought to describe their own previous lives as "inferior" in any way. I suspect many would say their new lives are better in many ways, less good in some, presumably fewer, ways. But I believe they would nearly all say that their new life would be less good if it threatened to cause them to be less compassionate for others who are disabled as they were.[9]

Something else is important to note about Singer's treatment of infanticide. He *advocates* euthanasia for infants who, as he wrote to *Der Spiegel*, "would never have been capable of grasping that they are living beings with a past and a future" (345). This is a very limited class: only those severely disabled infants who will never develop the characteristic features of personhood—sentience, consciousness of continuity in time, awareness of the possibility of ceasing to exist. His larger arguments, however, press for the removal of prohibitions surrounding infanticide for a much wider class of infants and the granting of increased discretion to parents in making judgments about whether to accept or kill their children. Such arguments cannot help but be disquieting to disabled people, particularly when Singer combines them with a blend of arguments emphasizing three points: 1) infanticide raises basically the same issues as abortion; 2) judgments about whether to abort or sustain fetal and infant life should consider the matter of replaceability, that is, that parents will forego having a future child or children in order to care for those they elect to accept; and 3) judgments about the matter

---

9. For a Christian critique focusing on Singer's very limited conception of value, particularly that of suffering, see Jeffreys, "Euthanasia and John Paul II's 'Silent Language of Profound Sharing of Affection,'" 368–71.

of potentially replacing one child with another should be guided by the utilitarian directive to bring about the greater good.[10]

Singer's position on abortion turns on denial of personhood to the fetus, as it lacks rationality, self-consciousness, or awareness of itself as a distinct being. He acknowledges the difficulty "liberals" on abortion have "in pointing to a morally significant line of demarcation between an embryo and a newborn baby," (169) and solves the question by denying personhood to children until they are at least one year old (and possibly longer). If we put aside the "emotionally moving but strictly irrelevant aspects of the killing of a baby," Singer claims, "we can see that the grounds for not killing persons do not apply to newborn infants" (171). Singer maintains "we should certainly put very strict conditions on permissible infanticide," but it is not clear why this should be the case. Singer suggests it may "owe more to the effects of infanticide on others than to the intrinsic wrongness of killing an infant" (173). Surely disabled people are right to be troubled by these positions. The defense of infants is made to depend on the effects killing them will have on others. The force of such a defense lies in others' identification with the infants whose lives are in question. If others do not identify with disabled infants, they are more likely to be justifiably killed—and, of course, it is disabled people who understand the degree to which the normally abled do not identify with them.

Singer forthrightly defends infanticide on grounds that it enables the replacing of one child with another likely to experience greater happiness. The argument begins with the assertion that killing infants, as we have seen, "cannot be equated with killing normal human beings, or any other self-conscious beings" (182). In language considerably more problematic for disabled people than the formulation offered in his intended reply to *Der Spiegel*, Singer adds, "This conclusion is not limited to infants who, because of irreversible intellectual disabilities, will never

---

10. For an argument for "replaceability" quite similar to Singer's, see Hare, *Essays in Bioethics*, 185–91. One particularly distressing feature of Hare's treatment is his invention of a conversation between an extant "abnormal" fetus and a purely theoretical child waiting in the queue but likely to be born only if the fetus is terminated. Hare's fetus is made to say to the theoretical Andrew, "All right, we'll make a bargain. We will say that I am to be born and operated on, in the hope of restoring me to normality. If the operation is successful, well and good. If it isn't, then I agree that I should be scrapped and make way for Andrew" (190). Here the fetus consents to its own replacement, implicitly declaring itself to be worthless in the disabled state.

be rational, self-conscious beings" (182). We must remember, too, that Singer has ruled out as morally irrelevant any defense of infants on the grounds that they are human beings. To make that argument would be to indulge in a speciesism akin to racism or sexism.

Singer recognizes a difference between infants whose lives will be "so miserable as to be not worth living" from their own "internal perspective" and what he calls the "more difficult problem" of those whose "disabilities ... make the child's life prospects significantly less promising than those of a normal child, but not so bleak as to make the child's life not worth living" (184). Actually I find it unclear why he characterizes this as a potentially "difficult problem," for he resolves it quite simply. Singer suggests that hemophilia probably presents the kind of dilemma he's deemed difficult. While a very serious condition, hemophilia does not ordinarily impose such burdens on its sufferer that he finds life not worth living. Nevertheless fetuses are routinely aborted if they are discovered to have hemophilia. If this is done by a mother who has "previously decided to have a certain number of children, say two, then what she is doing, in effect, is rejecting one potential child in favor of another." She could offer as a defense the argument that "the loss of life of the aborted fetus is outweighed by the gain of a better life for the normal child who will be conceived only if the disabled one dies" (188). We accept such "replaceability" when death occurs before birth, and since "birth does not mark a morally significant dividing line," Singer "cannot see how one could defend the view that fetuses may be 'replaced' before birth, but newborns may not be" (188). On the total utilitarian view, which Singer defends, the hemophiliac or Down infant can be killed justifiably when it will be replaced by another child who is more likely to experience greater total happiness than the one replaced. On these matters Singer is unequivocal: "When the death of a disabled infant will lead to the birth of another infant with better prospects of a happy life, the total amount of happiness will be greater if the disabled infant is killed. The loss of happy life for the first infant is outweighed by the gain of a happier life for the second. Therefore, if killing the hemophiliac infant has no adverse effect on others, it would, according to the total view, be right to kill him" (186).

Finally, there are three additional points of Singer's argument that cannot help but bring uncertainty to disabled people. As part of his challenge to "the virtually unchallenged assumption that the life of a newborn baby is as sacrosanct as that of an adult," he argues, "Indeed, some people seem to think that the life of a baby is more precious than that of an adult. Lurid tales of German soldiers bayoneting Belgian babies figured prominently in the wave of anti-German propaganda that accompanied Britain's entry into the First World War, and it seemed to be tacitly assumed that this was a greater atrocity than the murder of adults would be" (170). Here we might ask whether we should discount our emotions as a source of moral insight in the way Singer asks us to do.[11] It is perfectly possible to hold that the killing of a noncombatant adult is every bit as bad as killing a baby, while at the same time insisting there is an important moral insight in our horror at the bayoneting of the baby. Surely the particular horror of that crime is caused by the baby's defenselessness, by the overwhelming disequilibrium of power between killer and victim. We would probably call such a crime "heartless" and in doing so, we are saying something important, namely that one must particularly—and probably willfully—deny one's emotional center in order to ignore such a total imbalance in power between killer and victim.

11. Richard J. Arneson ("What, if Anything, Renders All Humans Morally Equal?," 103–28) has raised an interesting problem concerning the role of emotion in Singer's work. Arneson is particularly concerned with the matter of human moral equality and how it can be maintained in light of what he dubs the "Singer problem"—which "arises if one accepts that the morally significant cognitive capacities that are relevant to the determination of the fundamental moral status of a being vary from individual to individual by degree" (105). In short, if "cognitive capacities" largely define personhood, how do we argue for moral equality when these capacities are not held equally by all humans? Having reached no satisfactory answer to this problem, Arneson suggests that perhaps we have, like Singer, focused too exclusively on cognitive abilities in thinking about "the normative basis of human equality." Thus he proposes we widen the consideration of what makes humans moral actors to include "affective capacities," the emotional qualities that make us "attend to the interests of other beings." Finally, however, Arneson discounts this move as helping much with the Singer problem, for, as he concludes, "After all, if I am very cognitively deficient by comparison with the Einsteins of the world, I am also very affectively deficient by comparison with the planet's Mother Theresas" (127). One thing Arneson overlooks is that Einstein could claim his cognitive capacities to be his in a way that Mother Theresa would never assert of her compassion—hers only by the grace of Christ and thus never elevating her over anyone. In his "Response" to the essays in this volume, Singer singles out Arneson's as the one that speaks most directly to the real issues that may have motivated some of his German attackers: "To the extent that the attacks focus on anything at all that is really to be found in my writings, however, it is to be found in the line of argument that Arneson discusses. As he remarks in his opening paragraph, that argument forces us to rethink the basis and nature of the moral equality of all humans. In most of the world, this seems a reasonable philosophical enterprise" (293).

We would be rightly appalled that people could be brought to the point of making total frontal assault on an infant, looking fully into his or her face without pity or the recognition of solidarity that would restrain murder. What is distressed in us about such an attack is the same thing that distresses Singer—and that he appeals to in his readers—when he is attacked in the face and has his glasses broken by the Zurich crowd. Murderous assault against the defenseless must rightly distress us. Perhaps our horror at killing the defenseless stems from fuller memory of ourselves as defenseless. Thus to argue that the defenseless need no special protection is a way to deny the uncomfortable fact that one was once defenseless and utterly dependent on the good will of other human beings.

I offer my next point as an extremely painful but I hope healing speculation. Perhaps Peter Singer's utilitarianism should be seen as a kind of response to the Holocaust—that is, as a commitment to an ethical scheme so abstracted from particularities that it offers the greatest possible protection against any marking of distinctions that would position one group as ever dependent upon the good will or pity of another. To make the marking of distinctions impossible we must even become such abstract actors as to express only the perfectly just amount of horror at the bayoneting of the infant—the amount due to every sentient creature, not even just human beings. Unfortunately, in addressing the problems of ethics, Singer cannot avoid making distinctions, and he makes a strong one between the normal and the disabled. Now I do not want to position disabled people as defenseless or dependent or as necessarily in need of the emotional solidarity of the normally abled. Surely disabled people have had to work against precisely these kinds of judgments in order to achieve self-realization and dignity. Nevertheless it seems unlikely to me that the political purposes of disabled people can be advanced without some solidarity from the normally abled—and it also seems inevitable that the normally abled's response to the disabled will be, in some sense, emotional. It will be grounded in a response perhaps not wholly unlike that we have to the German soldier bayoneting the infant: it is outrageous, wrong, unjust, heart-rending that some should be so disadvantaged, in power, relative to others. This might, of course, lead to pity, and I'm perhaps as inclined as Nietzsche to detest pity. But the way to overcome pity is not by becoming pitiless but rather by working to overcome conditions that make one group subject to another's pity. We overcome pity by working to create conditions of greater equality where our feelings for one another are those of compassion, suffering with, rather than the kind of condescension implied by pity. Singer's minimizing emotion as a guide to moral action bodes no particular good for the disabled. I fully appreciate the desire of the disabled not to be regarded as objects of pity or even as the recipients of compassion. Moreover, I would insist that the normally abled should come to regard the expansion of opportunities for the disabled as something to which they are entitled and not as a kind of compassionate gift. But that recognition of the rightness of full opportunity for the disabled will, in many cases, only come for the normally abled after an extended period of experience and reflection grounded in a strong emotional response to a perceived radical disequilibrium in powers (however erroneous this perception may actually be).

A second emphasis of Singer's that should concern the disabled is his tendency to treat abortion as a routine matter. As we have seen, infanticide raises for Singer no moral questions not already raised by abortion. One might find this point relatively untroubling, I suppose, if strong prohibitions or, at least, limitations on abortion were in place. Singer, however, tends to treat abortion as a relatively routine, even casual, matter—particularly in his examples. He sees the broad abortion right to be essential to women's self-determination, which may well be the case under the current economic and social order shaping gender relations. Nevertheless this can hardly be good news for infants: if infanticide is morally equivalent to abortion, and abortion is simply a routine matter, then why should infanticide seem much different? Of course most parents who bring their children to term do want those children and would have no motive or desire to kill them. But this might not be true of parents of disabled children, or, in a more genetically progressive age, even of parents whose infants somehow seem not to have acquired the full intended benefits of their engineering.

Singer's examples routinize abortion, and perhaps, in this case, philosophy simply follows practice. As in the example discussed in chapter 2, Singer presents the decision to abort as little more than a consumer choice: if the presence of a two-month fetus conflicts with a scheduled mountain-climb, a woman need think no further about aborting. If she intends to conceive a replacement child later, she cannot be accused of depriving the world of a rational person. One child is as good as another.

The particularity of the child to be aborted no longer carries any weight; the child has truly become a commodity, a product of parental fantasy, a supplier of pleasant experiences. Sadly the child ultimately born to this woman will have to continually justify itself to her: he or she will have to prove constantly more compelling than alternative consumerist pursuits. No doubt even the most skillfully performing child will find this impossible to accomplish. The disabled probably need not even apply, particularly to this parent.

Sometimes "ethics" in Singer seems to have run amok, governing every choice. All that seems involved in the abortion decision is a highly abstract calculus of suffering. Since the fetus has been invalidated as a sufferer, it can be disposed of for any reason whatever. There is even a curious flatness of affect—intended, I think—in Singer's telling of his illustrative narratives. The real point of the argument is contained in the narrative, and it is to persuade us to regard the abortion choice as one involving nothing more important than the timing of vacations. This choice, like others, is simply a kind of consumer decision, involving preferences about how to spend one's time. This time, abortion and mountain climbing, next time, parenthood and TV.

There seems an odd tension between such absence of narrative affect and Singer's concern for suffering. Singer puts suffering at the center of our moral deliberation yet depicts people whose ability to suffer is difficult to conceive. Now surely Singer's mountain climber can experience pain as a neurological phenomenon, but I find it somewhat difficult to believe in her ability to suffer. I wonder if there has not been a deadening in the capacity for suffering—whether consciously chosen or economically induced—in one who can frame the choice to destroy a particular fetus as a matter to be weighed against giving up a pleasure trip. I'd argue, in fact, that there's a general failure in Singer's work to adequately distinguish suffering from pain. Mostly when he writes of suffering he seems, to me, to mean pain.[12] This too simple conflation

12. Consider the assumptions, for instance, in the following argument of Singer's regarding pain and suffering. He begins by asserting that "human speciesists do not accept that pain is as bad when it is felt by pigs or mice as when it is felt by humans." Then he invents a possible objection to this position. Some people will be prompted to reply, "Surely pain felt by a mouse just is not as bad as pain felt by a human. Humans have much greater awareness of what is happening to them, and this makes their suffering worse. You can't equate the suffering of, say, a person dying slowly from cancer, and a laboratory mouse undergoing the same fate." Finally, Singer indicates he "fully accepts"

derives, in part, from the rhetorical and ethical task of raising the moral status of the non-human animals. The non-human animals more clearly experience pain than more complex kinds of suffering (this is *not* to say they do not suffer.) The non-human animals can therefore be made to seem more like human beings to the degree that a focus on pain can be made to substitute for questions about suffering. Singer's conflation of pain and suffering, however, does not simply reflect the task of raising non-human animals' status; it *also derives from* his perceiving human beings and the non-human animals to be more similar than they have traditionally been conceived to be in the Western tradition of Judaism and Christianity. Seeing human beings as more like non-human animals may well cause one to miss those aspects of suffering unique (perhaps) to human beings: life-long unhealed grief, for instance, for the absolutely unique child lost by parents who fully understand the irrecoverability and, might I say, irreplaceability of the dead.

Singer's pressing abortion in the direction of consumer choice and his emphasis on the replaceability of children illustrate something Simone Weil warned about regarding the so-called sanctity of human personality. Weil considered it a "grave error of vocabulary" and thus almost surely a "grave error of thought" to speak, as Personalism did, of the sanctity of the human personality. The error lay in separating the sacredness of the human being from his or her particularity. "There is something sacred in every man," she writes:

> but it is not his person. Nor yet is it the human personality. It is this man; no more and no less.
>
> I see a passer-by in the street. He has long arms, blue eyes, and a mind whose thoughts I do not know, but perhaps they are commonplace.
>
> It is neither his person, nor the human personality in him, which is sacred to me. It is he. The whole of him. The arms, the eyes, the thoughts, everything.
>
> Not without infinite scruple would I touch anything of this.

---

that in this case "the human cancer victim normally suffers more than the nonhuman cancer victim." We must notice how this assumes, however, that the human being and the mouse suffer essentially the same thing, distinguishable primarily in quantity. But such quantitative comparison seems clearly inadequate. The human being does "undergo fate" here, aware that things could have been otherwise, in a way that the mouse is unlikely to sense. Surely this is a source of suffering for the person, particularly when she knows that the fate toward which she is tending is the negation of all that she has known thus far. See *Practical Ethics*, 58.

Almost directly anticipating Singer's many arguments undermining the "sanctity of life," Weil notes "it is impossible to define what is meant by respect for human personality." It could not be defined nor properly conceived, and thus to set up the sanctity of the personality as a "standard of public morality" was "to open the door to every kind of tyranny."[13] What we can learn from Weil is that thinking about the sanctity of life cannot be separated from practices honoring the inviolable sacredness of particular persons. "Sanctity" rhetoric divorced from the sacredness of particular human beings can easily be undermined, as Singer's work shows, and paradoxically no set of terms may have more effectively produced that divorce, that fatal abstraction, than those of personality, person, personhood.[14]

A third, and final, feature of Singer's treatment of infanticide concerns the kind of protection against it that he builds into his utilitarianism. As we have seen, Singer regards the "*intrinsic* wrongness of killing the late fetus and the *intrinsic* wrongness of killing the newborn infant" to be "not markedly different." He claims, however, that this is only true "when those closest to the child do not want it to live." "Killing an infant whose parents do not want it dead," he maintains, "is, of course, an utterly different matter" (173–74). But what makes it "utterly different"—altogether other or wholly other? What brings the parent-child relationship under the rubric of the "utterly different" where it is given immunity from the consequentialist calculation of the rest of the moral system? Let us suppose society could be brought to so fear overpopulation that nearly everyone regarded children beyond the replacement level as an ominous threat. Under such a circumstance, it might well be possible for so much happiness to be effected by killing a child that it would outweigh the suffering of the parents who did not want it to be killed. Moreover, such killing would reinforce the beneficial rule that families ought not to have more than one or two children. Can Singer assure us that there is no condition of scarcity under which we would void the prohibition against state killing, let us say, of children even against parental wishes? Can any "matter" really be "utterly different" under Singer's utilitarianism, which constantly asks us to engage in comparative judgments of value under hypothesized conditions of scarcity? In the abortion ex-

---

13. Weil, "Human Personality," 314.

14. For a particularly sharp criticism of Singer's attacks on the sanctity-of-life doctrine, see Thomasma, "Sanctity-of-Human-Life Doctrine," 68–69.

ample treated above, for instance, killing a fetus and mountain climbing were not "utterly different matters" but rather experiences whose values could be estimated according to a common metric. Singer has himself supplied the metric—suffering—and there must surely be some measure of general suffering that would override the suffering caused parents by having their children killed.

Finally, the particularistic emphasis of Singer's defense of parental rights not to have their sub-optimal infants killed seems at odds with what might be called the educational side of much of his work. Singer has typically argued that moral progress in the West has involved continually widening the circles of moral concern as those on the "inside" of some group have come to recognize those on the "outside" as being more like them. In other words, he has been suspicious of various forms of particularistic concern.[15] He has attacked speciesism as akin to racism, sexism, and homophobia, each of which represents a form of exclusionary particularism that once seemed "natural and inevitable"[16] but now seems unjustifiable. So, too, the argument goes, we must and will eventually come to understand speciesism, the unjustifiable preference for our own species. But why, we must ask, does Singer invoke another standard of concern when he considers the parental-child relationship? He cannot accord this most preferential of relationships any particular moral status on the grounds that it is "natural and inevitable," for he has consistently argued that every other form of unjustifiable exclusionary discrimination was once so understood.

It would seem consistent with Singer's overall emphases, then, to argue that moral or state educational policy should be directed at breaking down parents' preferential and exclusivist regard for their own children, at least when these are sub-optimal. Such regard might be the appropriate object of rational therapy, designed to help parents understand their attachment to the sub-optimal infant as a purely emotional response that ought not to be allowed to exclude the child's replacement—one capable of a manifestly "superior" life (given the disabled's own testimony to their lives' "inferiority" in some regards)[17] and a greater contribution to the balance of happiness for sentient beings. Infanticide by such par-

---

15. Singer, *Expanding Circle*.

16. Overcoming what has come to seem "natural and inevitable" seems the necessary task, for Singer, of all liberation movements. See "Animal Liberation," 139.

17. Cf. *Practical Ethics*, 54.

ents, too, would have the additional beneficial effect of demonstrating that even the most powerful forms of particularism can be transcended. Rational state policy might honor such parents as precursors to a utilitarian paradise, for they will have demonstrated, where it matters most, that each, to them, has been one and no one more than one.

11

Repugnance, *Frankenstein*, and Generational Injustice

A Consideration of Reproductive Cloning

WHATEVER ONE THINKS OF cloning intellectually or ethically, one must admit that the reaction against the possibility of human reproductive cloning has been intense. After Ian Wilmut announced the successful cloning of Dolly in 1997, the Clinton administration moved immediately to organize a council to consider the issue, and the council predictably recommended against cloning for reproductive purposes.[1] Under the Bush administration, the President's Council on Bioethics, chaired by Leon Kass, unanimously voted for a ban on reproductive cloning, going significantly beyond the earlier council's reasoning in its presentation of arguments against the practice. Kass himself accurately characterized the spirit of public reaction against cloning as repugnance.[2]

---

1. The 1997 commission's primary argument against reproductive SCNT emphasized its dangers to the one cloned. Many commentators on both sides of the issue thus rightly saw the matter as still unresolved. If SCNT could be made as safe—for the cloned person herself—as other forms of artificial reproduction, then the issue would have to be discussed, on more complex grounds, than those the 1997 group had used to justify its conclusion.

2. Kass and Wilson, *Ethics of Human Cloning*, 18–20. The book consists of two pieces by each author, the first of which is Kass's "Wisdom of Repugnance," 3–59; this is followed by another article originally written independently of the volume, Wilson's "Paradox of Cloning," 61–74. Written expressly for the book, the final two pieces, one by each writer, expand their original positions and comment on one another's views. Interestingly, Wilson's chapters seem open to limited reproductive SCNT, but in 2002 he joined all the voting members of The President's Council on Bioethics—chaired by Kass—in voting against reproductive cloning. He was, however, among those on the council who supported regulated research on cloned embryos. The report, *Human*

He has been criticized, in fact, for claiming that repugnance has about it a kind of wisdom in itself. Surely some practices once found repugnant by great numbers of people—interracial marriage, for instance—now seem perfectly reasonable, justifiable, and normal. Unexplained and unjustifiable repugnance can look a great deal like simple prejudice. On the other hand, we may not want to discount the moral wisdom of repugnance altogether. Certainly we are right to regard soldiers' bayoneting children with repugnance, as I argued in the last chapter. We now find repugnant the very kind of racism that would, in an earlier day, have found interracial marriage repugnant. Thus repugnance in some cases may carry wisdom with it. What we need, I suppose, is a repugnance we are able to examine in order to see if it contains an otherwise justifiable moral leading. To be clear about my own feelings on the matter of reproductive cloning, I would say I share Kass's repugnance at the idea, or at the assumptions that lie behind it, but I would certainly feel no repugnance at the presence or existence of persons created by SCNT (Somatic Cell Nuclear Transfer). It is not open to me as a Christian to feel repugnance at anyone's existence.

Richard Dawkins, of "selfish gene" fame, has asked forthrightly, "But is it so obviously repugnant that we shouldn't even think about it? Mightn't even you, in your heart of hearts, quite like to be cloned?"[3] While I think I can honestly say I would not want to do this, I suspect there is something in Dawkins's simple question that may explain the "repugnance" which greeted the possibility of human reproductive cloning. However one regards the theories of evolutionary biology, it does seem true that part of our profoundest dilemma as creatures fully cognizant of mortality is that involving our continuity beyond death. The simplest, most straightforward approach to that problem would be to shape our children fully in our own images. As its defenders have pointed out, SCNT would not create replicas of the persons whose genes are reproduced. Children created through SCNT would be exposed to different influences than their parents, grow up in a different time, de-

---

Cloning and Human Dignity: An Ethical Inquiry is available online at www.bioethics.gov.

3. The line immediately following the quote is well worth citing: "As Darwin said in another context, it is like confessing a murder, but I think I would." "What's Wrong with Cloning?" 55.

velop other preferences, and so forth.⁴ Still, this defense seems a little disingenuous. The motive behind SCNT would be to reproduce the host in some fashion. Donors would be chosen with some expectation that the offspring will bear strong resemblance to them. One's genetic twin would be much more likely to resemble one closely than the child created through heterosexual intercourse. Of course SCNT would not solve the problem of mortality, immediately at least—so long as something like the Abrahamic notion of life as a journey to the distance remained. But if parenthood became less a going along with the children one loves and more a matter of watching oneself unfold again, under one's own scrupulous care, then perhaps death would have lost its sting.⁵ If I can see that I will be repeated, I do not lose myself to death in the same way as I do if I regard my life as a unique, unrepeatable history—a step-by-step journey from a specific beginning point to an unknown place in the distance.

Perhaps we know, then, that there is something profoundly attractive about reproducing through SCNT, and thus we must maintain a very strong prohibition against it. Perhaps we feel the lure of SCNT's promise of our continuance in a way of our own devising while simultaneously knowing that we'd regard such parental preemption of our own identities to be the most odious tyranny. Writers like Kass, Hans Jonas, and Dena Davis have stressed the way SCNT may contribute to closing a child's future.⁶ Jonas warned that the child created by cloning would live

---

4. For a representative argument of this type, see Green, "Much Ado About Mutton," 124–25.

5. The scrupulous watching of the clone unfold—not as oneself but as a possible repetition of a lost lover—is the motif of Martha Nussbaum's Jamesian "Little C," in *Clones and Clones*, 338–46. One can only imagine what the Master would have done with such a theme.

6. Kass's arguments have been made in *Toward a More Natural Science: Biology and Human Affairs*, especially in chapter 2, "Making Babies," 43–79; in *Ethics of Human Cloning*; in the introductory matter of the President's Council on Bioethics report of 2002; and in *Life, Liberty and the Defense of Dignity*, particularly in chapter 5, "Cloning and the Posthuman Future," 141–73. Jonas's extraordinary treatment of "biological engineering" is in "Biological Engineering: A Preview," in *Philosophical Essays*, 141–67. Dena S. Davis takes ultimately a more moderate stance on reproductive cloning than those of Kass or Jonas, though she shares many of the fears expressed by Jonas. She recognizes that some parental motivations for cloning are likely to harm children, but sees "some uses of human cloning as ethically acceptable in the right situation." See *Genetic Dilemmas*, 128. The kind of SCNT Davis could endorse she calls "logistical"; the kind that troubles her more seriously is "duplicative." In the first, the parents simply

always under the shadow of parental expectations. Defenders of SCNT like Greg Pence argue that these harms to the child are far too speculative to count as reasons against the procedure. Besides, they add, parents shape their children's futures and identities in all sorts of ways. Why should SCNT be regarded any differently?[7] The concept of an "open future" has also proven very difficult to define with any precision, so much so that pragmatist Glenn McGee excludes the possibility: "No child has an open future, and even a cursory examination of the changing history of parenthood makes clear that it is not individuality but rather correct forms of responsible relation that is the goal."[8]

If our response to McGee's claim is repugnance—as mine is— we might begin by trying to understand why we react in that fashion. Certainly it is part of good parental care to teach children to relate responsibly to others, but to make that the whole of what parents do seems to me a formula for universal heteronomy. McGee's comments overlook the imbalance of power between generations, extending to parents, as cloning would, an unprecedented ability to determine the future of children. That parents see their children as individuals and rear them to be so is surely one of the guarantees of personal and social freedom—of necessary resistance, for instance, to the "correct forms of responsible relation" when these become authoritarian and life-denying. To deny one an open future and subsume all of one's life under "forms of responsible relation" would seem to deny that the self has a unique relationship to itself. It is to deny, in effect, that there is a dimension in which each of us is uniquely him or herself. It is to deny that each of us possesses a unique inwardness, known at least as difference from all others, if in no other way. For those are the things we are asserting when we claim an "open future." To claim an "open future" is to insist that there is a dimension of my life to which I relate in a way that no one else can. To ring a change

---

seek SCNT to conceive a child, and the "duplicative element" is a "side effect." In the second, "the genetic replication itself" is "the attraction" (115). It still seems problematic, however, to be concerned about "duplicative" SCNT when one claims that to believe clones will be mere replications of their hosts is to subscribe to a mistaken genetic determinism. Why should one be concerned about parents' conceiving children under mistaken notions?

7. For Pence's arguments in favor of SCNT, see especially "Will Cloning Harm People?" 115–27; "Arguments against Human Asexual Reproduction," 119–50; and *Brave New Bioethics*, 57–86.

8. McGee, *Perfect Baby*, 152.

on a phrase by Derrida, it is to insist on "the gift of death"—the gift of "my death," which is also the context for my working out my salvation in "fear and trembling."[9] We may find cloning repugnant for the paradoxical reason that we believe it will rob clones of their deaths. Whether this will be the case for clones is something it is difficult to know. Clones will die, of course, but it is not clear that they will experience death as the loss of a unique and unrepeatable history—especially since they will be understood as products of a baby-making process whose goal is the production of those capable of responsible relations. What we fear for clones is always, in short, what we fear as we imagine it affecting us. Cloning threatens our unique relationship to the lived context of all that we are—our bodies. If I understand that my body can somehow be "replaced" or duplicated, then I do not lose to death the whole of everything that I am in quite the same way as I expect to now. I am deprived of the reality that makes my actions meaningful: the knowledge that my being is toward death, that I am here once for all only, that my history will never be fully knowable to another (and is largely hidden even from me).

What we find repugnant in cloning can be illuminated further by a look at Dawkins's comment on his motivation for desiring to be cloned:

> The motivation need have nothing to do with vanity, with thinking that the world would be a better place if there was another one of you living on after you are dead. I have no such illusions. My feeling is founded on pure curiosity. I know how I turned out, having been born in the 1940s, schooled in the 1950s, come of age in the 1960s, and so on. I find it a personally riveting thought that I could watch a small copy of myself, fifty years younger and wearing a baseball hat instead of a British Empire pith helmet, nurtured through the early decades of the twenty-first century. Mightn't it feel almost like turning back your personal clock fifty years? And mightn't it be wonderful to advise your junior copy on where you went wrong, and how to do it better? Isn't this, in (sometimes sadly) watered-down form, one of the motives that

---

9. For Derrida, there is an inescapable aporia in responsibility, which "demands on the one hand an accounting, a general answering-for-oneself with respect to the general and before the generality, hence the idea of substitution, and, on the other hand, uniqueness, absolute singularity, hence nonsubstitution, nonrepetition, silence, and secrecy." See *Gift of Death*, 61. Derrida is critical of the proponents of correct forms of responsible relation, "the moralizing moralists and good consciences" who too often forget that alterity and singularity "constitute the concept of duty as much as that of responsibility" (67–68).

drives people to breed children in the ordinary way, by sexual reproduction?

Dawkins's "pure curiosity" points to the rightness of Augustine's criticism of that vice (as he understood and Dawkins exemplifies it). For Augustine, curiosity involves a dialectic of possession: things can take possession of the soul, the desire to see and to know can itself become an act of taking possession.[10] Dawkins seeks to possess what he is himself possessed by: himself. What, we might ask, would Dawkins's "small copy" be watching while being so watched? Would he not be watching himself being watched? Would he not be watching his body develop, inevitably, into a copy of his father, the very one he would need to differentiate himself from in order to have his own life? Knowing, with considerable exactness, the trajectory of his bodily development, would he be deprived of a sense of serendipity, possibility? Would he have the sense that his future was already exhausted, having been lived in advance by the one who had produced him in order to turn his own clock back fifty years?

What, too, would be the possibility of love and trust between Dawkins and clone? Would there be adequate distance between them for love to be required and possible? My sense is that the relationship as Dawkins describes it would preclude love. How could the clone ever trust that anything Dawkins did was for its own sake? How could Dawkins ever do anything for the child that was not moved by his own self-reflexive curiosity? Love exists where there is separation; it exists to bridge separation. It depends, if you will, on two beings whose futures are open, whose deaths are their own deaths. It is crushingly hard for parents not only to face their own deaths but to acknowledge the ultimate deaths of those who mean more to them than their own lives—their children. Parents must learn to give their deaths in order that children can live free of guilt for replacing them and without the need to reenact what their parents have been.[11] The children learn, in turn, how to give their own

---

10. Dawkins, "What's Wrong with Cloning?" 55. On curiosity in Augustine, see *Confessions* 10.34–35 (Pine-Coffin, 239–42).

11. What I mean by learning to give one's death here is coming to understand it—for the Christian, through the Cross—as the condition for one's loving others as neighbors. Death remains the enemy, but if, in the work of love, one can come to see it as the condition of a neighbor-love empowered by God through faith, then one can live free of the need for consolation. One's children will then be free to live without needing to compensate one for anything lost.

deaths in order that their children might also be free to live their lives and to love. Perhaps what we find most repugnant in cloning is its seeming to circumvent this whole generational work of love. The parent who makes reproduction contingent on the child's offering the best possible "package of experiences," to quote John Robertson, has already refused the beginning of the way of love—at least as it has been understood in its fullness by those of us with open futures.[12]

༄

I will make an argument against SCNT for reproductive purposes later in this chapter. The argument is closely related to the concerns expressed by Jonas and yet cannot be attacked for depending on speculative judgments about the possible harms to children of excessive parental expectations. But first I'd like to use a piece of literature to illumine some of the problems inherent in reproductive SCNT. The text is one frequently cited in medical ethics, Mary Shelley's *Frankenstein*, but I know of no reader who has used it in quite the way I will. Usually the novel is cited briefly as a warning against "playing God," either by those who take that notion seriously or those who want to debunk it. Citation of the novel, or other works of fiction, is often accompanied, too, by warnings that we must remember to distinguish clearly between rational arguments and "mere science fiction" examples. By this point in this book, I hope to have cited enough of the counterfactuals or imagined examples of philosophers to suggest that their narratives also frequently need to be scrutinized as works of fiction. Indeed since those narrative examples are designed with the specific purpose of illustrating arguments arrived at in advance and by other means, it might well be suggested that they offer less insight into the actual effects of moral and medical practices than the best works of imaginative literature—assuming, as I do, that an identifying mark of such works is that they are *not* designed to illustrate ideas arrived at otherwise. *Frankenstein*, in fact, has come to have a life of its own in the philosophic literature as a source of philosophers' examples. What this signifies is itself a matter worth considering.

What does it mean, for example, that on at least two occasions in *Life's Dominion*, Ronald Dworkin cites Frankenstein's creation of the monster as if it offers a normative account of pregnancy? Dworkin uses comparisons between the fetus and the monster to establish that the fe-

12. Robertson, "Liberty, Identity, and Human Cloning," 1390.

tus has no "interests of *its own*" and thus no right to protection against being aborted. "Imagine that," Dworkin begins:

> just as Dr. Frankenstein reached for the lever that would bring life to the assemblage of body parts on his laboratory table, someone appalled at the experiment smashed the apparatus. That act, whatever we think of it, would not have been harmful or unfair to the assemblage, or against its interests ... stopping the experiment before it *came to life* wouldn't be harmful to it—even if Dr. Frankenstein had designed the procedure to work automatically unless interrupted, and that automatic procedure had already begun.[13]

Of first importance here is that Frankenstein's creation of his monster is no longer a bizarre aberration but rather a kind of norm by which to understand the development of all fetuses. Second, comparing the fetus to a collection of body parts obscures its existence as an already unitary being, however we decide to regard its moral standing. The comparison leads to Dworkin's clearly non-biological or anti-biological assertion that the fetus has not yet "come to life." Third, the concept of the fetus as a collection of already existing body parts denies the way in which each child represents an absolute new beginning of the world. Here the analogy stresses the child's continuity with the past at the expense of its newness—the new is, in fact, an ill-fitted, even monstrous, combination of what has already been. Fourth, the analogy's likening conception to a technological procedure destroys any awe we might feel in the presence of mystery; we certainly do not have the same reluctance to alter, stop, or reverse "procedures" as we do in destroying the natural. People on all sides of the abortion question often revere nature in ways they cannot feel about technology: many of us are reluctant to cut down trees, change the course of a river, or contribute to a species's extinction. Fifth, Dworkin's presentation of the Frankenstein story has the effect of raising the importance of active beneficence at the expense of non-maleficence, often regarded the more important duty. For Dworkin, there is nothing here without "help," the active beneficence he regards "essential." But one could certainly argue, with greater biological accuracy, that there is

---

13. *Life's Dominion*, 16. Dworkin again uses the comparison of fetus to Frankenstein's monster on page 19. One wonders if the primary rhetorical effect is not to move the fetus to another category of being, one to which we feel the tie but in which we only partially recognize ourselves, a recognition we would prefer to deny.

something there in the fetus that will—without active interference or some happening construed as beyond human control—develop into a full fledged human being. As to the fetus's having "interests," everything about its behavior suggests it is entirely interested in continuing to live.

Clearly Dworkin's citation of *Frankenstein* is not simply a neutral philosophic example that illuminates fetal interests but rather a specific rhetorical move reflecting a particular understanding of fetus and pregnancy and designed to press us toward a specific conclusion.[14] That the example resonates with readers does suggest, however, how much we have come to think of pregnancy as more like a directed technological process than a natural one. My own use of the novel is frankly rhetorical and is based on an assumption similar to Dworkin's about the work's pertinence, though I obviously draw very different conclusions from it.[15] *Frankenstein* has become familiar enough to help us see where we are going and yet I hope it still remains strange enough to challenge us. As reproduction through SCNT becomes possible, new significations can be seen in the novel. On my reading, Mary Shelley's work bears specifically on several matters directly related to reproductive cloning: the possible

14. Susan Winnett's reading of Frankenstein's creation experience is one that seems ironically relevant to Dworkin's use of the story. She argues that Frankenstein exhibits a characteristically male way of retrospective sense-making in his reaction to his creation: "His indulgence in the retrospective mode of 'male' sense making keeps him from acknowledging his ongoing responsibility to the birth he clones as well as from seeing that henceforth his plot inevitably involves the consequences of an act that he regards as a triumph in and of itself. That creation would demand anything of him *beyond* the moment when scientific genius culminates the trajectory of its intellectual self-stimulation seems never to have occurred to him." Following Winnett here would lead to recognizing inaccurate and deeply gendered assumptions in Dworkin's use of the Frankenstein analogy. See "Coming Unstrung," 510.

15. Dworkin has himself written about cloning in chapter 13 of *Sovereign Virtue*, "Playing God: Genes, Clones, and Luck." For him the practice of extensive genetic engineering threatens the possibility of a "kind of moral free-fall" because it would undermine the distinction between chance and choice on which our ideas of responsibility are premised. Dworkin does not, however, oppose the extension of research in SCNT from fear that it will radically reshape our moral notions. "Ethical individualism," in fact, commands the continuation of research and freedom for the scientists who choose to do it." See *Sovereign Virtue*, 442–52 especially. Justine Burley has subjected Dworkin's prediction of a "moral free-fall" to extensive criticism in "Morality and the 'New Genetics,'" 170–92. The thesis of her critique is that the coming of "genetic control" poses the possibility of moral free-fall only if one conceives of morality along the lines of Dworkin's liberal egalitarianism (172). Dworkin replies in detail to Burley in the same volume, 362–66. Burley defends both therapeutic and "human cloning" in "Ethics of Therapeutic and Reproductive Human Cloning," 287–94.

confusion of relationships toward parents for the person produced by SCNT; the motives behind and consequences of using SCNT to produce "replacements" of lost loved ones; the possible reactions of parents at the failure of the delayed twin to meet expectations; and the possible closing of a child's future through excessive parental determination, even that motivated by "love."[16]

Feminist critics of *Frankenstein* frequently focus on the doctor's failure to nurture his monster. All readers of the novel will surely remember the scene in which Dr. Frankenstein abandons his new creation, leaping from bed amidst a dream of bestowing death on Elizabeth with a kiss and holding his mother's corpse in his arms. If Dr. Frankenstein had accepted, nurtured, and loved his creation, so this reading goes, the monster might well have become at all times the gentle being he often seems by nature. The failure to care on Frankenstein's part, together with the other rejections suffered by the monster, lead to the story's dreadful events.[17] But perhaps we should ask whether Dr. Frankenstein can really be expected to care for one with whom he has no bodily connection. If child-making becomes the production of a preconceived idea, is one likely to be horrified when the bodily presence inevitably fails to conform to the idea? Advocates of SCNT often reassure opponents by pointing out that its products will not really be replications of existing individuals but more like delayed twins who will develop uniqueness through their own experiences. But replication seems certain to be at least part of the

---

16. Dena S. Davis contrasts the Frankenstein story with Jewish legends of the Golem, especially those concerning Rabbi Loeb of Prague, who creates the Golem Joseph as a protector of the Jewish people. In calling the Golem into being, Loeb is "participating in an act of co-creation that is not only permitted, but required by Judaism." From this Jewish sense of humanity's role as "co-creator," Davis deduces the possibility of a much more positive attitude toward cloning than that reflected in accounts grounded in the Frankenstein myth, with its much stronger implicit prohibition against humanity's usurpation of divine prerogative. See "Religious Attitudes Toward Cloning," 519. For a different reading of the Golem legends in relationship to genetic matters, see Zoloth-Dorfman, "Mapping the Normal Human Self," 180–202.

17. Anne K. Mellor, for instance, argues that "*Frankenstein* portrays the consequences of the failure of family, the damage wrought when the mother—or a nurturant parental love—is absent." See *Mary Shelley: Her Life, Her Fiction, Her Monsters*, 39. Ellen Moers finds the novel "most interesting, most powerful, and most feminine" in the "motif of revulsion against newborn life, and the drama of guilt, dread and flight surrounding birth and its consequences. Most of the novel, roughly two of its three volumes, can be said to deal with the retribution visited upon the monster and creator for deficient infant care." See *Literary Women*, 93.

producer's intent, for without the expectation of replication, how would one choose the host to clone? Thus products of SCNT may experience *more* rejection because they are more like delayed twins than immediate replications. One could object that parents now routinely accept children who do not conform to preconceptions. But one must remember that this acceptance is rooted in the conviction that it is good for children to develop toward identities not determined in advance—toward open futures, as Feinberg puts it.[18] Reproductive SCNT, as well as genetic enhancement, would profoundly alter that assumption, thus increasing Dr. Frankenstein-like rejections of what may well seem "monstrous"—one's idea embodied and standing before one in a form unlike one intended.

The association in Frankenstein's dream of Elizabeth and his mother contributes to the novel's repeated pattern of substitution as a means of consolation. Frankenstein's father, a public spirited man of strict justice, married Caroline Beaufort two years after he comes "like a protecting spirit to the poor girl" on the death of her father, Frankenstein's good friend.[19] She in effect replaces his friend Beaufort, while he cares for her in a role at least as much fatherly as spousal. Elizabeth, then, is adopted quite abruptly from the peasant family, with whom she, a Milanese nobleman's daughter, is living. She can apparently be simply lifted from one family and placed in another.[20] The language Shelley uses to describe Frankenstein's mother's "presentation" of Elizabeth to Victor further stresses the girl's objectification: "'I have a pretty present

18. Feinberg, "Child's Right to an Open Future," 76–97.

19. *Frankenstein*, 18. Further page references will be to this widely available text of the novel, which reprints the 1831 edition. They will be included parenthetically.

20. This is not the place for a detailed discussion of the arguments regarding the relative merits of the 1818 and 1831 versions of *Frankenstein*. One of the most interesting of Shelley's revisions, however, concerns the adoption of Elizabeth. In the 1818 version, she is a cousin of Victor's, in the 1831, a foundling. Mary Poovey suggests the change was "no doubt partly to avoid insinuations of incest," but that it also emphasizes "the active benevolence of Frankenstein's mother, who, in adopting the poor orphan, is now elevated to the stature of a 'guardian angel'" (134). It might be added that the change stresses not only the active quality of Caroline's benevolence but also its Godwinian impartiality. In the 1818 version, Elizabeth is the daughter of Alphonse's sister and an Italian gentleman whom she has married. When the mother dies, the Italian Lavenza plans to marry again and wishes to send Elizabeth to Switzerland to be educated. In effect, he refuses to parent her, turning her over to Alphonse to regard as his own. For discussion of the revisions between the two texts, see Poovey, *Proper Lady and the Woman Writer*, 133–42. Also helpful is Jacqueline Foertsch, "Right, the Wrong, and the Ugly," 697–711.

for my Victor—tomorrow he shall have it.' And when, on the morrow, she presented Elizabeth to me as her promised gift, I, with childish seriousness, interpreted her words literally and looked upon Elizabeth as mine—mine to protect, love, and cherish. All praises bestowed on her I received as made to a possession of my own" (21).

Caroline's death involves a complex pattern of substitutions and consolations. First Elizabeth catches scarlet fever and Caroline is warned not to attend her. But as Elizabeth's illness becomes life threatening, Caroline does attend her. Elizabeth recovers, but Caroline, her "preserver," dies—in effect, in the place of the one whom she has "saved." Caroline, on her deathbed, then binds Elizabeth and Frankenstein's future: "My children ... my firmest hopes of future happiness were placed on the prospect of your union. This expectation will now be the consolation of your father." Next she charges Elizabeth specifically with replacing her, "Elizabeth, my love, you must supply my place to my younger children" (28). This charge creates an impossible double bind for Victor: to console his father—to compensate him for his loss—he must marry the woman who now substitutes for his own mother.

Victor creates the monster in order to do, free of possible reproach, what he desires to do—to free himself from the tyranny of a family that has preempted his future. That tyranny is evident not only in his mother's arranging for Victor's marriage to be his father's consolation but in other subtle ways as well. Of his parents' rearing him, Victor says:

> With this deep consciousness of what they owed towards the being to which they had given life, added to the active spirit of tenderness that animated both, it may be imagined that while during every hour of my infant life I received a lesson of patience, of charity, and of self-control, I was so guided by a silken cord that all seemed but one train of enjoyment for me. For a long time I was their only care ... (19)

There is no mention of affection or love for Victor here: the seemingly total attention and care of his parents derives from their active sense of duty and their own tenderness rather than from love *for him*. Moreover, as "every hour" of his life becomes a lesson, he recognizes that while all seemed enjoyment, he was really being continually "guided" by a silken cord. Victor again, perhaps unknowingly, reveals his parents' subtle domination of his development in a later comment on his childhood happiness: "We felt that they were not the tyrants to rule our lot according to their caprice, but the agents and creators of all the many delights which we enjoyed" (23). Here again is guidance with a silken cord: not parental rule by caprice or will—will that could be challenged by the child as part of the process of differentiating and defining him or herself—but rather the subtler, all encompassing rule that works by creating *all* the child's enjoyments.[21]

The novel's pattern of substitutions and dis/replacements continues with the stories of Justine Moritz and the murders of William, Clerval, and Elizabeth. In her own household, Justine is the favorite of her father, but "her mother could not endure her" (50). Victor's mother observes Justine's plight after the death of M. Moritz and brings Justine to live with the Frankensteins. When Justine's siblings die one by one, her mother begins "to think that the deaths of her favourites was a judgment from heaven to chastise her partiality" (51). She calls Justine home, where she transfers her sense of guilt to Justine, accusing the girl "of having caused the deaths of her brothers and sister" (51). When her mother dies, Justine returns to the Frankensteins, only to live out in reality the substitutionary role earlier envisioned for her by her own mother. When the monster kills William, Elizabeth first blames herself but ultimately the entirely innocent Justine is executed for the crime.

Justine's execution occurs despite Victor's sure knowledge of her innocence. Victor affirms her innocence but never offers the story that could potentially free her and direct the guilt toward himself: that of the monster's creation and slaying of William. His "first thought" is to do precisely this: "to discover what I knew of the murderer and cause instant pursuit to be made" (61). But on reflection he changes his mind, and for several good reasons: no one will believe his tale; he will be regarded insane; "the strange nature of the animal would elude all pursuit"; and

---

21. For a reading of Victor's childhood similar to my own, see Zimmerman, "*Frankenstein*, Invisibility, and Nameless Dread," 135–58. Zimmerman asks whether Victor's should be regarded an "ideal 'infant life'": "'Lessons,' passively received every hour, preempt any sense of authentic being. The lesson of 'patience' entails the imposition of an alienating structure of time, a premature violation of the sense of early omnipotence; the lesson of 'charity' precludes the infant from spontaneously having something to give, so that the claims of otherness disallow those of selfhood; the lesson of 'self-control' thwarts playfulness and passion. What kind of self can develop in the face of such an onslaught? Even—or especially—the murderous rage (and guilt) that such self-obliteration is likely to fuel has no standing, cannot be spoken, must be split off and disowned (as the monster)" (139). For a contrasting psychoanalytical reading of Victor's childhood and especially his father, see Veeder, "Negative Oedipus," 365–90.

pursuit would itself be useless, as "Who could arrest a creature capable of scaling the overhanging sides of Mont Saleve?" (61). In short, Victor has created the perfect way to enact crime without having to pay for it. Creation of the monster enables Victor to commit the crimes he desires, to lacerate himself with guilt, and yet to avoid being called to account by others for either his desires or their results. That the monster enacts what Victor desires is clearly indicated by the way Shelley reveals the identity of William's killer through Victor. After seeing a large vague figure "in the gloom," Victor asks himself whether his monster could be the "murderer of my brother." The presence of the idea itself becomes "irresistible proof" of the fact: "No sooner did that idea cross my imagination than I became convinced of its truth" (60). Surely Victor is so easily convinced precisely because the monster enacts what he has at some level of personality imagined doing. Victor himself "consider[s] the being whom [he] had cast among mankind ... nearly in the light of my own vampire, my own spirit let loose from the grave and forced to destroy all that was dear to me" (61). Victor has given life to the monster not only through the galvanic process but also by imparting his desires.[22]

But why should Victor consciously or unconsciously desire the death of William? The answer may lie in the preferential language the Frankensteins use for William. Victor learns of his brother's death through a strangely formal, even somewhat reproachful letter from his father that repeatedly refers to William as his "sweet child," his "lovely boy," and "his beloved." The same letter reports Elizabeth's crying out, in self-reproach, "Oh, God, I have murdered my darling child!" (56–57). This cry must surely add to Victor's inner conflict, for here Alphonse himself casts Elizabeth in the role of replacement for Caroline. Thus now, for his father's consolation, Victor is to marry the woman who has replaced Caroline not only as mother to his brothers but also as "wife" to his father. The family's especial fondness for William is evident, too, in Ernest's referring to him as "our darling and our pride" (62).

---

22. Joyce Carol Oates presses questions about the relationship between Victor and his creature that are similar to my own: "But if Frankenstein is not to blame for the various deaths that occur, who is? Had he endowed his creation, as God endowed Adam in Milton's epic, with free will? Or is the demon psychologically his creature, committing the forbidden acts Frankenstein wants committed?—so long as Frankenstein himself remains 'guiltless.'" She argues, too, that "in one sense the demon *is* Frankenstein's deepest self." See "Frankenstein's Fallen Angel," 547, 551.

Deep psychic anger at William may thus derive from Victor's sense of displacement within the family; he may long again to be the "sole care" of his parents, particularly his mother. A desire for sole possession of the lost mother is suggested by the circumstances of the murder itself: the monster has taken from William a valuable miniature portrait of Caroline that William had teased Elizabeth into letting him wear on the night of his death. Desire for the mother's portrait suggests an attempt to retrieve her psychically from death, a move that would also help untie the knot she has created for Victor by her death-bed commands. Moreover, to retrieve his mother would be to reestablish relationship with the one who knows him—as an embodied being—as distinct from all others, as unsubstitutable.

Resurrecting the dead has been part of the motive for Victor's scientific researches from the first. As he seeks the animating principle of matter, he reasons that he "might in process of time (although I now found it impossible) renew life where death had apparently devoted the body to corruption" (39). Images of bodily corruption occur frequently in the novel, contributing to the emphasis on death as a power that hangs over all. Pondering grief after his mother's death, Victor notes that a "time at length arrives when grief is rather an indulgence than a necessity; and the smile that plays upon the lips, although it may be deemed a sacrilege, is not banished" (29). Here mourning seems forever incomplete; the smile is not banished but it nevertheless remains a sacrilege after the loss of the other. Going on seems understandable only as a duty: "my mother was dead, but we had still duties which we ought to perform; we must continue our course with the rest and learn to think ourselves fortunate whilst one remains whom the specter has not seized" (29). We are not fortunate to be alive here but rather must learn to think ourselves fortunate while there is still one whom death has not conquered. Surely to live in such a way is to live under death's dominion.

The all-dooming power of death is emphasized, too, in the most dramatic confrontation between Victor and his monster. Overcome with such "rage and hatred" that he is, "at first deprived ... of utterance," Victor threatens the monster with violence he simultaneously realizes to be pointless: "And, oh! That I could, with the extinction of your miserable existence, restore those victims whom you have so diabolically murdered" (83). The monster's perspicuous response bears especial attention: "'I expected this reception,' said the demon. 'All men hate the wretched; how, then, must I be hated, who am miserable beyond all living things!'" (83). Is it true that human beings hate the wretched, and if so, is it because they remind us of our own wretchedness? Moreover, if we do hate the wretched, are we moved to render some people or group of people wretched in order to hate them? Responding further to Victor's threat, the monster challenges his creation to do his duty toward him; if Victor will do so, the monster will "leave [the rest of mankind] and you at peace, but if you refuse, I will glut the maw of death, until it be satisfied with the blood of your remaining friends" (83). If the monster represents Victor's double or alter ego, then this tremendous threat would seem to indicate a rage in Victor capable of destroying all of humankind. Repeatedly during the scene he speaks of his own rage; it makes him troubled, deprives him "of utterance," and is finally "without bounds" when he springs onto the creature, "impelled by all the feelings which can arm one being against the existence of another" (83).

The boundlessness of Victor's rage recalls his earlier insistence that "nothing in human shape could have destroyed" William and that "indeed every human being, was guiltless of this murder" (60, 64). Despite the obvious humaneness often displayed by the monster, Victor's statement rightly points to his creature's acting out psychic demands and feelings that can usefully be called extra-human. His mother's appropriation of his life for his father's consolation, his incomplete mourning and concomitant sense of death's dominion, and his parents' well-disguised but tyrannical shaping of all his motives and desires leads to a more-than-human striving for perfection whose other side is the boundless rage acted out by the monster. One could argue that Victor's purpose is nothing less than the salvation of all humanity, which he, at the level of psychological fantasy, indeed manages to do while simultaneously ridding himself of the one whose existence causes his worst double-bind—Elizabeth, his wife-mother but also from the first, his possession, "since till death she was to be mine only." When the monster first asks Victor to create a mate for him, Victor consents, though requiring from his creation a "solemn oath to quit Europe forever, and every other place in the neighborhood of man" (133). But later Victor begins to fear the prospect of the monster's producing children, a "race of devils... who might make the very existence of the species of man a condition precarious and full of terror" (150). He now "shudder[s] to think that future ages might curse me as their pest, whose selfishness had not hesitated to buy its own peace at the price, perhaps, of the existence of the whole race" (151). He has now, in effect, elevated himself, at least in fantasy, to the position of destroyer or savior of humankind. To refuse to create a bride for the monster becomes a matter of solemn duty to save the human race.

Victor's response to the monster's curse at this point suggests his complete self-centeredness. The monster responds to Victor's denial of his request with a threat that resonates with Christ's eschatological language: "It is well. I go; but remember, 'I shall be with you on your wedding-night'" (153). Victor hears these words as an announcement of "the period fixed for the fulfillment of my destiny. In that hour I should die and at once satisfy and extinguish his malice" (153). Having created a potential destroyer of humanity, he will now, in Christ-like fashion, die at his appointed hour in order to make satisfaction. Especially curious is his complete failure to consider the possibility that his creature's threat is directed at Elizabeth. His concern for Elizabeth reveals the way his apparently self-denying other-regard actually masks intense egocentrism. He is brought to tears pondering how Elizabeth will suffer from being deprived of him!

> When I thought of my beloved Elizabeth, of her tears and endless sorrow, when she should find her lover so barbarously snatched from her, tears, the first I had shed for many months, streamed from my eyes, and I resolved not to fall before my enemy without a bitter struggle. (153)

Curiously Victor never considers the possibility that the monster's threat is directed at Elizabeth. So apparently bent on his own destruction is he that he refuses Elizabeth's epistolary offer to release him from any marital commitment to her. The letter brings the creature's threat vividly to mind yet Victor responds by resolving to bring about the marriage immediately. On the wedding night, Victor entreats Elizabeth to go to bed, then paces the passages of the house looking for his adversary while simultaneously leaving Elizabeth exposed and vulnerable to the monster's attack. Thus Victor contributes to bringing about what he wants and needs, the death of Elizabeth, the forbidden desire that cannot be thought and thus can only be enacted by his alter ego. Victor resolves whatever guilt he may feel about marrying the mother-substitute; destroys a sibling rival whom his mother termed her favorite; and reclaims his life from its appropriation for his father's loss of his mother. He can continue to proclaim himself guilty of the worst of crimes yet remain outside the reach of law or accountability to others. And he can claim to have lost a victim "far dearer" to him than himself and yet remain conveniently alive.

Just before Victor's marriage, his father asks him if he has "some other attachment," to which Victor responds, "None on earth" (174). "Attachment" refers primarily here to romantic affection, but the interchange nevertheless points also to Victor's near complete freedom from "attachment" of any kind after Clerval's death. Victor seems without connection to his brother Ernest, and his father prides himself so completely on his impartiality that one can ask whether he's capable of particular attachment to anyone. Indeed in the same conversation, Victor passionately vows to "consecrate" himself, "in life or death," to Elizabeth, only to be warned by his father not to "speak thus." We ought rather, Alphonse explains, to "transfer our love for those whom we have lost to those who yet live" until a later time at which "new and dear objects of care will be born to replace those of whom we have been so cruelly deprived" (174). Alphonse Frankenstein's advice seems nearly wise except for the almost mathematical neatness of the process by which one "transfers" affection and later "replaces" one set of objects of care with another. Surely we do not simply transfer love for the dead to others "not yet" dead—death here seeming to be the normative condition, with life a temporary exception. Rather we extend or enlarge our love to include both those dead and those living and we recognize as well that no one loved can really be replaced by another. "Objects of care" can perhaps be replaced but not loved and loving human beings.

"Such were the lessons of my father," Victor tersely and non-committally glosses the advice we've just examined. The phrase in this context suggests how *Frankenstein* can be read as Mary Shelley's own response to the lessons of her father, William Godwin, author of *Political Justice*. Godwin is perhaps best known for a hypothetical question he developed in defense of utilitarianism and against all forms of preferential love. If one could rescue only one's mother or Archbishop Francis Fenelon from a burning building, Godwin asked, which should one save? Godwin argued that there were no reasonable grounds on which to defend the rescue of one's mother here and that the defensible choice was to save Fenelon, who would produce a much greater quantity of good for humanity.[23] One feasible way to respond to Godwin is by asking a series

---

23. "Supposing the chambermaid had been my wife, my mother or my benefactor. This would not alter the truth of the proposition. The life of Fenelon would still be more

of questions. Why should I have to justify a preference for my mother? Who has the authority to ask me to justify a preference for my mother? What sort of being would I be if I could not simply accept preference for my mother as a given requiring no justification? My mother's carrying me and her extended period of care for me are the very bases of my existence as an embodied being with a particular history. Would not saving Fenelon in the hypothetical be to discount an irreplaceable part of my own history? Would I not become something unhuman, a stranger to myself, perhaps a monster?

A related way to approach Godwin's analogy might be to ask about the ability to care of agents who would easily choose Fenelon over those closest to them. Rodger Beehler has argued that "caring about others is integral to the moral point of view."[24] It is not something we can choose but rather is simply given as a background and practice that makes moral discussion intelligible. "You cannot decide to care about others," Beehler argues; caring is itself beyond discussion. Now surely Godwin's argument for saving Fenelon reflects care for others. Godwin's judgment rests precisely on the ground that Fenelon will do more good to others than one's mother. Yet surely each of us learns to care through close loving relations with our parents, siblings, spouses, and children. To consistently subordinate our particular loyalties to these people might be simply to produce people with little ability to care at all—and thus without the background commitments necessary for moral discussion. To form people committed to continually choosing against benefiting their mothers for the sake of universal humanity may lead only to the creation of what C. S. Lewis called "men without chests."[25]

---

valuable than that of the chambermaid; and justice, pure unadulterated justice, would still have preferred that which was most valuable. Justice would have taught me to save the life of Fenelon at the expence of the other. What magic is there in the pronoun 'my,' to overturn the decisions of everlasting truth? My wife or my mother may be a fool or a prostitute, malicious, lying or dishonest. If they be, of what consequence is it that they are mine?" *An Enquiry Concerning Political Justice 1793*, 1:83.

24. Beehler, *Moral Life*, 155.

25. That is, men and women who have no idea that certain features of the universe "merit" our respect and reverence, or that responses to situations can be "just," "appropriate," or "ordinate." Lewis quotes Traherne's asking, "Can you be righteous unless you be just in rendering to things their due esteem?" I believe one should simply declare Godwin's question regarding Fenelon or one's mother to be unworthy of an answer, but if I were pressed, I should like to answer it along Lewis's lines: "I am saving my mother because to do so is to render her the esteem she deserves." See Lewis, *Abolition of Man*, 25–26.

One might also ask whether it is really possible to weigh the good my mother does me against the general good done humanity by a great benefactor like Fenelon. The good I receive from my mother could not have been accomplished by any other. She has sustained me in the womb at some risk to herself and cared for me through the extended period of development required by a human being—again at some risk to herself and with inevitably some sacrifice of other goods. The time she has given me, in love, can never be restored to her. I cannot repay or compensate her, for I can never give her back what she may have missed while caring for me. I would say I remain forever in her debt except that she makes clear that an understanding of the relationship in terms of debt and payment is wholly inappropriate. She has freely given me her life, and I can do no more than stand forever grateful and astounded at my wholly undeserved good fortune. The good my mother has done me cannot be quantified in such a way as to weigh it against the good a great benefactor does humankind.

Frankenstein, on the other hand, depicts the domination of one generation by another through the "strict justice" of Victor's Godwin-like father. Much as Hans Jonas has warned about regarding children born of SCNT, Victor's life is largely preempted by the choices of his parents (and in ways difficult for him even to identify, much less resist). In fact, we might even see Victor's act of creation as flowing directly from the logic of Godwin's famous hypothetical regarding Fenelon and one's mother. If the particularity of Victor's connection to his mother must be discounted as completely as Godwin insists upon in the hypothetical, then the creation of new humanity might just as well take the form of Victor's creating the monster. If the unique connection to one's mother means so little, then surely we can no longer think of each human being as a radically new beginning to the world, to cite Hannah Arendt.[26] Godwin's doctrine means that none of us counts very much as the particular, embodied being she is. Each of us is a replaceable "object of care,"

---

26. *Totalitarianism*, 177: "Beginning is the supreme capacity of man; politically, it is identical with man's freedom. *Initium ut esset homo creatus est*—'that a beginning be made man was created' said Augustine. This beginning is guaranteed by each new birth." Arendt identifies the quote as being from *De Civitate Dei*, book 12, chapter 20, but it seems closest to a line from the end of chapter 21: "Hoc ergo ut esset, creatus est homo, ante quem nullus fuit"—"In order that there might be this beginning, therefore, a man was created before whom no man existed." Augustine *City of God* 12.21 (Dyson, 532; Latin is from *De civitate Dei libri XXII*, 1:548).

a death waiting to happen in a nihilistic world where the best we can do is to continually transfer care from one lost object to another not yet taken. Given these realities, why not fashion the bodies now wandering the earth from those who have done so previously? Nothing new is really possible anyway. If to care is the best we can do, why not form today's "objects of care" directly from yesterday's?

The argument I will offer against SCNT is based on its inherent generational unfairness. I share the concerns of people like Jonas and Kass who have claimed a right of ignorance for each child. Their warnings against excessive parental expectations of children produced through SCNT seem to me entirely reasonable. I am not convinced by its defenders that SCNT poses no threats to children's individuality that are not posed already by institutions established precisely to shape children in ways designed by parents and others.[27] Genetic shaping is unlike education, socialization, or training in that these latter can all be undone, resisted, or played off against one another. Clearly this may be very hard to do in some cases, and I do not want to suggest that all training is something the liberated adult learns to put aside as a mark of freedom. As Stanley Hauerwas has so nicely said, that version of liberal freedom as escape from any defining story simply leaves people to be their own tyrants.[28] Nevertheless, genetic shaping is different from other kinds of shaping in its irreversibility. Before turning to SCNT, we should think very hard about the effects on a person of knowing that his or her identity has been chosen in advance by others to a degree not true of non-clonants. It seems to me very likely that the product of SCNT will be continually at war with herself: attempting to form an identity "of her own" while knowing that her sense of "ownness" will never be quite the same as others. Intense resentment seems the likely result.

27. Gilbert Meilaender's critique of John Robertson's "reproductive liberty" seems relevant here. Meilaender has stressed the difference between "begetting" and "making" children, which would be widely allowable under Robertson's version of libertarianism. For Meilaender, only the child who is "begotten, not made" can finally be regarded as our equal in dignity rather than "a product at our disposal." See *Body, Soul, and Bioethics*, 84. Chapter 3 of this book offers an extended critique of Robertson; see 61–88.

28. "The modern conception has made freedom the content of the moral life itself. It matters not *what* we desire, but *that* we desire. Our task is to become free, not through the acquisition of virtue, but by preventing ourselves from being determined, so that we can always keep our 'options open.' We have thus become the bureaucrats of our own history, seeking never to be held responsible for any decisions, except for those we ourselves have made" (Hauerwas, *Peaceable Kingdom*, 8).

Nevertheless, as SCNT's defenders maintain, these harms are too speculative to make reproductive SCNT illegal, particularly when it has quite possible benefits—presuming that it can be made as safe to the product of SCNT herself as other forms of reproduction. Thus I would prefer that those considering SCNT consult "speculative" works of fiction like *Frankenstein* to see consequences undreamt of in the philosophies of medical ethicists. But I think an argument based on generational justice can be made against reproductive SCNT without any speculation about the procedure's psychological consequences at all. Whether reproductive SCNT should be banned in all cases is a difficult call. Its most justifiable use seems to me the cloning of a child in order to use it as a donor for purposes of histocompatibility—of bone marrow, for instance. This presumes, absolutely, that the child will be accepted, reared, and loved by her family—difficult things for the law to guarantee.

Because I believe my argument has a kind of libertarian or liberationist dimension, I will try to make it against one of the fullest and best defenses of reproductive cloning—that by libertarian John Robertson. Robertson's argument is premised on SCNT's having become efficacious and at least as safe for the product herself as other forms of reproduction. This I freely grant. He proceeds then to argue that "reproductive liberty," a core human interest, should include the right to utilize SCNT unless a compelling case can be made that it involves "special risks or problems." He begins by defending SCNT as a "technique to assist infertile or genetically at-risk couples to have healthy children or to procure tissue or organs for transplant."[29] These seem limited uses that would likely gather more popular support than SCNT strictly for eugenic purposes—particularly if the goal of procuring tissue or organs for transplant is accompanied by the further specification of the parental intent to rear the child produced to be a donor. Those familiar with Robertson's work will recognize his characteristic combination here of a wide reproductive liberty with a strong insistence on parental intention to rear—the first, to some extent, dependent on the second.[30]

---

29. "Liberty, Identity, and Human Cloning," 1372. Further references will be given parenthetically. Robertson has also called for appropriate regulation of cloning—not prohibition—in "Human Cloning and the Challenge of Regulation," 119-22.

30. Of the extensive claims Robertson makes for parental liberty in shaping offspring, Francis Fukuyama notes, "It may come as a surprise to many that they have a fundamental right to do something that is not, as yet, fully possible technologically, but such is the wonderfully elastic nature of contemporary rights talk." Fukuyama, of course,

Robertson begins by justifying these relatively limited uses of SCNT but ultimately offers a much broader defense of the practice. Indeed, his position seems to entail the unlimited use of SCNT as long as it is accompanied by the intention to rear. I believe he also understands this to be the implicit direction of his argument—one that would include nearly all SCNT procedures within a notion of wide reproductive liberty, not just those that can clearly be designated therapeutic. He recognizes, quite rightly I believe, that the birth of Dolly shifted decisively the debate over assisted reproduction, putting the "issues of selection and engineering of offspring traits" directly on the table. He also claims, rightly, that ethical decisions about SCNT can only be informed so far by analogies to other cases of assisted reproduction. These are "constitutive decisions" that inevitably include reshaping and defining the very terms involved in making the decision: "individuality, personal identity, family, and reproductive liberty" among them (1371–72).

Without parsing the whole of Robertson's argument, I do want to suggest how it makes clear that reproductive SCNT will be virtually impossible to limit. He begins with perhaps the most innocuous possible use of SCNT: the cloning of embryos "to enhance the fertility of couples" whose egg and sperm are viable and who are in the process of IVF. SCNT here could involve either embryo splitting or "removing the cell or blastomeres of one or more embryos and placing them into enucleated eggs to create additional embryos." Thus in cases where only a limited number of eggs are produced, the procedure could help enable the creation of enough embryos to raise the likelihood of successful pregnancy. It would have the further advantage of eliminating "the high costs and physical burdens of additional hyperstimulated cycles and surgical retrieval" (1378). Gametic insufficiency might also lead to cases in which SCNT might be preferable to other options. Couples faced with this problem might well prefer to use SCNT rather than having to

---

is not opposed to rights talk, but he does want to ground it in a concept of human nature. The genetic technologies of the "posthuman future" threaten this understanding of the natural ground of rights—hence Fukuyama's warnings about it. See *Our Posthuman Future*, 107. Brent Waters has argued that both Fukuyama and Leon Kass have failed to "come to terms with th[e] transformative imperative underlying posthuman discourse" and thus their appeals "to either biological essentialism or innate human dignity are bound to fail." He believes posthuman transformative discourse must be met by the more profound transformative discourse of Christianity. See "What is Christian About Christian Bioethics?"

depend on anonymous sperm donors or "paid or familial" egg donors. Couples at risk of transmitting genetic disease to offspring might similarly rely on SCNT rather than "anonymous commercial sperm or egg donors" (1379). They might choose to clone one of them or a third party, including perhaps an already existing child who is free of the disease in question. This increased control over the child's genetic health will enable the couple to avoid the current means of negative selection: one or another of the available diagnostic measures followed by therapeutic abortion. In addition, lesbian couples might want to use SCNT in order to produce a child who would have a "biologic connection" (1380) to both parents, to one through nuclear DNA and to the other through the egg and mitochrondrial DNA.

Clearly all of these uses of SCNT are difficult to challenge. SCNT here seems preferable to other well-established options, and simple fairness seems to demand the possibility for those fearing genetic disease and those wanting something resembling the biological connection to a child that others take for granted. It is easy to see, however, why it will be impossible to limit SCNT to these kinds of cases. If parents with established genetic risks may use SCNT to avoid transmission of disease to offspring, then why not other parents as well, as surely all reproduction bears some risk of transmitting disease to children? If the superior control over reproduction made possible by SCNT is not extended to all parents, then some will be left with a disproportionate risk of having to care for children with genetically transmitted disease. How, too, will it be possible to keep therapeutic and eugenic reasons for SCNT clearly distinguished? Suppose a couple has a claim to using SCNT to avoid a genetic risk and they already have one child unaffected by the condition and also extraordinarily intelligent. If they use SCNT to produce a delayed twin of this child, will the motive be strictly therapeutic or eugenic? A couple with a similarly brilliant child would also like to use SCNT but has no established genetic risk to qualify them for the procedure. They, then, have a child with genetic disability. Can this be fair? Another reason for SCNT defended by Robertson and others is its making possible the replacement of lost loved ones. But what possible sense could it make to allow some couples to use the DNA of a lost child to produce a "replacement" and deny others SCNT to create a delayed twin of a living beloved child? It's not difficult to imagine the argument in favor of SCNT here. Does one have to lose one's child in order to be eligible to produce one much like it? It must be remembered, too, that negative selection is already a well-established practice and the philosophical and political underpinning for any discussion of eugenic SCNT. Advocates of positive eugenics will always have the advantage of arguing that such practices will reduce the number of abortions.

For Robertson, a broad right to SCNT for eugenic as well as other purposes follows from his strong sense of reproductive liberty. As "the freedom to decide whether or not to have offspring," procreative liberty is a "deeply accepted moral value" whose importance "stems from the impact which having or not having offspring has in our lives." The "desire to reproduce" is "important" because "it connects people with nature and the next generation, gives them a sense of immortality, and enables them to rear and parent children." To deprive persons of this "fundamental personal liberty" is a "major burden and should not occur without their consent" (1389). The seriousness of this right gives infertile couples a claim to the use of reproductive techniques such as IVF and artificial insemination. "Some right to engage in genetic selection" also seems, for Robertson, to follow "from the right to decide whether or not to procreate." This is true because people make the decision to procreate based on the "package of experiences" they believe reproduction will bring them. The "makeup of the package" thus determines "whether or not they reproduce," and thus they should have at least some right to choose the child's characteristics, "either by negative exclusion or positive selection" (1390).[31]

---

31. Just how truly free parental choices of the "package" will be in the era of Germinal Choice Technology remains to be seen. Pondering how the "enhanced" and the "unenhanced" will live with one another in the future, Greg Stock predicts a competitive ratcheting up at both the personal and national levels: "Initially, the differences between the enhanced and the unenhanced would be only statistical, in that those with enhancements would tend to outperform many, but not all, of those without enhancements. But as the technology grew more potent, less overlap would exist between the two populations, and as this became clear to parents, many of the children of those who had shunned the technology would likely enhance their own children, to keep them from being at a disadvantage. A similar story would be played out globally, as countries that initially blocked GCT gradually felt compelled to amend or appeal their laws and accept it." Stock seems undistressed by this Hobbesian prediction. See *Redesigning Humans*, 191. For an account of how the inevitable gap between the GenRich and the Naturals will lead to subspeciation, see Silver, *Remaking Eden*, 240–50. Silver seems troubled by this possibility but, as Fukuyama points out, he has no grounds on which to be: "Since there is no stable essence common to all human beings, or rather because that essence is variable and subject to human manipulation, why not create a race born

As long as the couple intends to rear, eugenic SCNT seems to Robertson a rightful exercise of procreative liberty. He considers a number of different SCNT scenarios, based mostly on the identity of the donor to be replicated: a couple's embryos, one's children, third parties, oneself. In each case, Robertson finds SCNT justifiable because the couple may not reproduce otherwise. They make their exercise of procreative liberty contingent, in other words, on the ability to use SCNT to determine the genetic identity of their offspring. Apart from a significant showing of harms to others, there is no reason to treat SCNT as radically different from other forms of reproductive choice. SCNT could be disallowed if it did significant harm to the child herself, but the conceptual problem here returns us to the harm conundrum. Being "born with the DNA of another" is not likely to have "such devastating effects on the child that it is better off, once it exists, in not continuing life" (1406). As the only way for this particular child to be born was through SCNT, it is difficult to argue it was harmed by the practice. Surely it is not harmed by existence, and there was no other way for it to exist.[32]

I will make three arguments against Robertson's position. The first insists that we can understand the child as being harmed in some ways, though certainly not by its existence. My second claim is that Robertson's

---

with metaphorical saddles on their backs, and another with boots and spurs to ride them? Why not seize *that* power as well?" See *Our Posthuman Future*, 154. H. Tristram Engelhardt displays a similar concern that germ-line genetic engineering will eventually bring about the fracturing of *Homo sapiens* into several species. The loss of human nature "as a source of perennial guidance and constraints" (507) promises to be tremendously dislocating to humanity, yet there are no "general secular, rationally discoverable content-full norms" available to justify restrictions on such engineering (515). Apart from the content-full moralities of particular communities, the most one can hope for will be sensible regulation guided by formal constraints like those against using persons without their permission. Yet even here I wonder why one would expect the GenRich of Silver's fantasy, for instance, to abide by principles of permission or consent in their relations to the Naturals. At the very least, there would surely be tension in such relations between the principle of permission and the requirement to maximize the good. If the GenRich are so much more capable of good than the Naturals, why allot living space to the Naturals for their sustenance and reproduction? See "Germ-Line Genetic Engineering and Moral Diversity," 503–16.

32. Glenn McGee challenges the claim of a positive right to use SCNT as a form of assisted reproduction. For McGee, the new genetic technologies challenge the traditional paradigm of family based on the seeming rightness of "sameness" between parents and child. This depriveleging of "sameness" undermines the claim of a positive right to SCNT and points to a much reduced status for assisted reproduction in the allotting of research funding. See *Beyond Genetics*, 197–210.

position allows for injustice between the generations—assuming SCNT becomes widely practiced, as I think the desire for standardization of reproductive products makes inevitable. My third claim is that what I will call the hostage argument is perhaps the one thing we must never allow ourselves to believe or invoke. Claiming that a child could not have been born otherwise than the way we willed it to be holds the child hostage in a way we would never will for ourselves.

First, I believe existence in nearly every case is a blessing. Apart from unbearable suffering to the person herself, existence is a good. Thus it is difficult to argue that life for the child produced by SCNT can be anything but a net benefit. Yet it seems possible to speak of the child being inevitably harmed by being deprived of the very thing that makes the exercise of procreative liberty an important experience: possession of a unique genetic code. This is not to engage in genetic determinism but only to say that uniqueness for all of us involves living out a mortal existence as a person of specific genetic inheritance. Nurture seems to me more important than nature, but the ways nurture shapes me are always either limited or enabled by my specific genetics. The phenomenon of twinning affects this not one whit. The problem for the child of SCNT is that she will never be independent of her parents in the same way as the rest of us; being a person in her own right will never mean what it means to us. She will always know her being born was not based on any expectation that she would be of worth in herself. This points to a crucial difference between SCNT or genetic enhancement and other forms of character formation—education, religion, socialization. All of those can be undone; the child can reject every bit of all that and challenge the parents to love her on her own account. The child created through genetic selection can never do that. He is bound too closely to his parents with a binding that cannot be undone.

My second point relates closely to the above. The exercise of procreative liberty through SCNT undermines the very reasons the liberty is important. Surely the basis for our strong commitment to procreative liberty lies in our recognition that the desire for children is closely related to our knowledge of mortality. When I teach the opening chapters of Genesis, I like to refer to children as "plan B." Plan A was the garden, but after death came to be experienced as coercion, genesis becomes the next best option. The Lord provides, and what he provides are children. Our freedom to procreate is important to us because we die as the specific unrepeatable histories we are. Our unique genetic inheritance is an important part of that specificity. The child produced through reproductive cloning is denied precisely the condition of genetic uniqueness that makes procreative liberty important. She will not, it seems to me, experience death in the same way as the rest of us: it will not be for her, to the same degree, the death of all that she is as a particular embodied being—because she will never have the sense of particularity we now take for granted. Thus widespread use of reproductive SCNT should be seen as a matter of generational injustice. Our exercise of reproductive liberty undermines the ability of the next generation to exercise the same liberty. If children come to be regarded primarily as packages of desirable experiences for their parents, it seems hard to believe that procreative liberty could last for many generations. Or that anyone would care.

To see why we must never invoke the hostage argument, we need to imagine the parent and child face-to-face. The parent says to the child, "You exist only because I allowed you to do so and I only allowed you to do so because I designed you to fulfill my expectations." Who, as a child, could hear this from a parent and live? What complicates the matter is that the first part of the statement is true: children do exist only because parents allow them to do so. That reality makes possible the extraordinary tyranny of one generation over another, and I would suggest that the hostage argument be read as a version, an underpinning, of such tyranny. It might help to consider whether the child created through SCNT, or any child, could give retroactive consent to its existence if it understands itself to have been conceived as a hostage. Consent or choice would seem to be meaningful only where there are real alternatives, but here there is no alternative for the child. The child is coerced to say, in effect, "Yes, existence is such a good thing that I am glad to have it on any terms." The possibility of nonexistence ought never to be used against a child that way, for since the child does exist, nonexistence can only seem like death. In fact, for the child to say "no" in the hostage situation seems tantamount to suicide. He has only been allowed to exist on one condition; the condition and existence are inextricably bound together; to reject the condition means to reject existence. The child cannot say this "no" without rejecting his own life.

Our repugnance at cloning, then, is an expression of our fear that the clone will never be able to hear the affirmation that Josef Pieper has called the authentic form of love: "It is good that you exist."[33] I have no doubt that most parents of clones will love their children and believe that it is good for them to exist. What is less clear is how the word "you" will resonate for them. Whether they will understand themselves as fully other to their producers is difficult to say. Whether love will be for them a bond that retains difference is something we non-clonants can only ponder. One thing that seems more certain is that reproductive cloning will surely alter the relationships among the generations. Parents of clones seem unlikely to see their children as new beginnings of the world. Children will be designed in accord with correct forms of responsible relationship within horizontal networks of care. What may increasingly be lost is the narrative sense of life: that each of us lives a unique, unrepeatable history toward an open future. Perhaps it is unbearable to live history in that sense, where each step is irretrievably lost, without what the Abrahamic traditions have known as faith. For Christians the "yoke is easy, and [the] burden is light" (Matt 11:30)—the burden being something like I spoke of earlier as learning to give our deaths. For the Christian this is part of the work of love in those necessarily connected dimensions: the vertical relationship to God and the horizontal one of care and responsibility for the neighbor. Death remains the enemy, but, through the cross, it can come to be seen as a kind of gift, the condition of a love that sees the other truly as other. Nourished by the infinite love of God, Christian parents can come to understand that their work and joy is not to rear images of themselves but to be, with their children, images of God.

---

33. Pieper, *About Love*, 26.

Bibliography

Adams, Mark B. "Eugenics in Russia, 1900–1940." In *The Wellborn Science: Eugenics in Germany, France, Brazil, and Russia*, edited by Mark B. Adams, 153–216. New York: Oxford University Press, 1990.

———. "Toward a Comparative History of Eugenics." In *The Wellborn Science: Eugenics in Germany, France, Brazil, and Russia*, edited by Mark B. Adams, 217–31. New York: Oxford University Press, 1990.

Adams, Robert M. "Must God Create the Best?" *Philosophical Review* 81 (1972) 317–32.

Agar, Nicholas. *Liberal Eugenics: In Defense of Human Enhancement*. Malden, MA: Blackwell, 2004.

Akron v. Akron Center for Reproductive Health. In *Abortion Decisions of the United States Supreme Court: The 1980's*, edited by Maureen Harrison and Steve Gilbert, 71–104. Beverly Hills, CA: Excellent, 1993.

Allen, David B., and Norm Fost. "Growth Hormone Therapy for Short Stature: Panacea or Pandora's Box?" *Journal of Pediatrics* 117 (1990) 16–21.

Allen, Garland. "Genetics, Eugenics and Society: Internalists and Externalists in Contemporary History of Science." *Social Studies of Science* 6 (1976) 105–22.

Anscombe, G. E. M. *Contraception and Chastity*. London: Catholic Truth Society, 1975.

———. "Who Is Wronged?" *The Oxford Review* 5 (1967) 16–17.

———. "You Can have Sex without Children: Christianity and the New Offer." In *Ethics, Religion, and Politics*, 82–96. Vol. 3, *The Collected Philosophical Papers of G.E.M. Anscombe*. Oxford: Blackwell, 1981.

Aquinas, Thomas. *On the Truth of the Catholic Faith: Summa Contra Gentiles. Book Two: Creation*. Translated by James F. Anderson. Garden City, NY: Image, 1956.

———. *Summa Theologiae*. Ia2ae. 90–97. Vol. 28. Translated by Thomas Gilby, O.P. Cambridge: Blackfriars, 1966.

Arendt, Hannah. *The Human Condition*. 2nd ed. Chicago: University of Chicago Press, 1998.

———. *Totalitarianism: Part Three of the Origins of Totalitarianism*. New York: Harcourt, Brace, 1985.

Aristotle. *The Ethics of Aristotle: The Nicomachean Ethics*. Translated by J. A. K. Thomson. London: Penguin, 1976.

Arneson, Richard J. "What, if Anything, Renders All Humans Morally Equal?" In *Singer and His Critics*, edited by Dale Jamieson, 103–28. Oxford: Blackwell, 1999.

Asch, Adrienne. "Can Aborting 'Imperfect' Children Be Immoral?" In *Ethical Issues in Modern Medicine*, edited by J. D. Arras and B. Steinbock, 386–89. Mountain View, CA: Mayfield, 1995.

Augustine. *The City of God against the Pagans*. Translated and edited by R. W. Dyson. Cambridge: Cambridge University Press, 1998.

———. *Confessions*. Translated by R. S. Pine-Coffin. Baltimore: Penguin, 1961.

———. *De civitate Dei libri XXII.* Vol. 1. Edited by Bernardus Dombart et Alfonsus Kalb. Darmstadt: Wissenschaftliche Buchgesellschaft, 1981.

Aukerman, Dale. *Darkening Valley: A Biblical Perspective on Nuclear War.* New York: Seabury, 1981.

Bacon, Francis. "Of Marriage and Single Life." In *Essays, Advancement of Learning, New Atlantis, and Other Pieces,* edited by Richard Foster Jones, 21–22. New York: Odyssey, 1937.

Balkany, Thomas, et al. "Ethics of Cochlear Implantation in Young Children." *Otolaryngology—Head and Neck Surgery* 114 (1996) 748–55.

Banner, Michael. *Christian Ethics and Contemporary Moral Problems.* Cambridge: Cambridge University Press, 1999.

Baron, Jonathan. *Against Bioethics.* Cambridge: MIT Press, 2006.

Barth, Karl. *Church Dogmatics.* Vol. III, *The Doctrine of Creation: Part Four.* Edited by G. W. Bromiley and T. F. Torrance. Translated by A. T. Mackay et al. Edinburgh: T. & T. Clark, 1961.

Beauchamp, Tom L., and James F. Childress. *Principles of Biomedical Ethics.* 2nd ed. New York: Oxford University Press, 1983.

———. *Principles of Biomedical Ethics.* 5th ed. Oxford: Oxford University Press, 2001.

Beckwith, Francis J. "Arguments from Bodily Rights: A Critical Analysis." In *The Abortion Controversy: A Reader,* edited by Louis P. Pojman and Francis J. Beckwith, 155–74. Boston: Jones and Bartlett, 1994.

Bedate, Carlos A., SJ, and Robert C. Cefalo. "The Zygote: To Be or Not Be a Person." *Journal of Medicine and Philosophy* 14 (1989) 641–45.

Beehler, Rodger. *Moral Life.* Oxford: Blackwell, 1978.

Bentham, Jeremy. *The Theory of Legislation.* Dobbs Ferry, NY: Oceana, 1975.

Berry, Wendell. "Are You All Right?" In *Fidelity: Five Stories.* New York: Pantheon, 1992.

———. "Economy and Pleasure." In *The Art of the Commonplace: The Agrarian Essays of Wendell Berry,* edited by Norman Wirzba, 207–18. Washington: Counterpoint, 2002.

———. *Hannah Coulter: A Novel.* Washington: Shoemaker & Hoard, 2004.

———. "Racism and the Economy." In *The Art of the Commonplace: The Agrarian Essays of Wendell Berry,* edited by Norman Wirzba, 47–64. Washington: Counterpoint, 2002.

———. *Remembering.* In *Three Short Novels,* 119–222. Washington: Counterpoint, 2002.

———. "Two Economies." In *The Art of the Commonplace: The Agrarian Essays of Wendell Berry,* edited by Norman Wirzba, 219–35. Washington: Counterpoint, 2002.

———. "The Whole Horse." In *The Art of the Commonplace: The Agrarian Essays of Wendell Berry,* edited by Norman Wirzba, 236–48. Washington: Counterpoint, 2002.

Biesecker, Leslie G. "Clinical Commentary: The Law of Unintended Ethics." *Journal of Law, Medicine & Ethics* 25 (1997) 16–18.

Bole, Thomas J., III. "Zygotes, Souls, Substances, and Persons." *Journal of Medicine and Philosophy* 15 (1990) 637–52.

Boonin, David. *A Defense of Abortion.* Cambridge: Cambridge University Press, 2003.

Boothroyd, Arthur. "Profound Deafness." In *Cochlear Implants: Audiological Foundations,* edited by R. S. Tyler, 1–33. San Diego: Singular, 1993.

Boyle, Mary. *Re-Thinking Abortion: Psychology, Gender, Power and the Law.* London: Routledge, 1997.
Brock, Dan W. "The Non-Identity Problem and Genetic Harms—The Case of Wrongful Handicaps." *Bioethics* 9 (1995) 269-75.
Brown, Eric. "The Dilemmas of German Bioethics." *New Atlantis: A Journal of Technology & Society* 5 (2004) 37-53.
Brown, Peter. *The Body and Society: Men, Women and Sexual Renunciation in Early Christianity.* New York: Columbia University Press, 1988.
Buchanan, Allen, et al. *From Chance to Choice: Genetics and Justice.* Cambridge: Cambridge University Press, 2000.
Burggraf, Shirley. "How Should the Costs of Child Rearing Be Distributed?" *Challenge* 36:5 (1993) 48-55.
Burley, Justine. "The Ethics of Therapeutic and Reproductive Human Cloning." *Seminars in Cell & Developmental Biology* 10 (1999) 287-94.
———. "Morality and the 'New Genetics.'" In *Dworkin and His Critics with Replies by Dworkin,* edited by Justine Burley, 170-92. Malden, MA: Blackwell, 2004.
Cahill, Lisa Sowle. "Catholic Sexual Ethics and the Dignity of the Person: A Double Message." *Theological Studies* 50 (1989) 120-50.
———. *Theological Bioethics: Participation, Justice, and Change.* Washington: Georgetown University Press, 2005.
Calabresi, Guido. *Ideals, Beliefs, Attitudes, and the Law: Private Law Perspectives on a Public Law Problem.* Syracuse: Syracuse University Press, 1985.
Carter, Stephen L. *The Culture of Disbelief: How American Law and Politics Trivialize Religious Devotion.* New York: Doubleday, 1994.
Casal, Paula. "Environmentalism, Procreation, and the Principle of Fairness." *Public Affairs Quarterly* 13 (1999) 363-76.
Cassell, Eric. *The Healer's Art: A New Approach to the Doctor-Patient Relationship.* Philadelphia: Lippincott, 1976.
Cather, Willa. *Death Comes for the Archbishop.* New York: Knopf, 1927.
Chapman, Audrey R. *Unprecedented Choices: Religious Ethics at the Frontiers of Genetic Science.* Minneapolis: Fortress, 1999.
Cherry, April L. "A Feminist Understanding of Sex-Selective Abortion: Solely a Matter of Choice?" *Wisconsin Women's Law Journal* 10 (1995) 161-223.
Childress, James F. "Comments of James F. Childress." *Journal of the Society of Christian Ethics* 24 (2004) 195-204.
———. "Just-War Criteria." In *War or Peace? The Search for New Answers,* edited by Thomas A. Shannon, 40-58. Maryknoll, NY: Orbis, 1980.
Clemens, Samuel L. *The Mysterious Stranger.* In *Selected Shorter Writings of Mark Twain,* edited by Walter Blair, 306-88. Boston: Houghton Mifflin, 1962.
Cohen, Cynthia B. "'Give Me Children or I Shall Die!': New Reproductive Technologies and Harm to Children." *Hastings Center Report* 26:2 (1996) 19-27.
Cohen, Noel L. "The Ethics of Cochlear Implants in Young Children." *The American Journal of Otology* 15 (1994) 1-2.
Cole-Turner, Ronald, and Brent Waters. *Pastoral Genetics: Theology and Care at the Beginning of Life.* Cleveland: Pilgrim, 1996.
Cudd, Ann E. "Sensationalized Philosophy: A Reply to Marquis's 'Why Abortion is Immoral.'" *Journal of Philosophy* 87 (1990) 262-64.
Daniels, Norman. *Just Health Care.* New York: Cambridge University Press, 1985.

Davis, Dena S. *Genetic Dilemmas: Reproductive Technology, Parental Choices, and Children's Futures.* New York: Routledge, 2001.

———. "Religious Attitudes Toward Cloning: A Tale of Two Creatures." *Hofstra Law Review* 27 (1998–1999) 509–21.

Davis, Dena S., and Laurie Zoloth, *Notes from a Narrow Ridge: Religion and Bioethics.* Hagerstown, MD: University Publishing Group, 1999.

Davis, Michael. "Fetuses, Famous Violinists, and the Right to Continued Aid." *Philosophical Quarterly* 33 (1983) 259–78.

Dawkins, Richard. "What's Wrong with Cloning?" In *Clones and Clones: Facts and Fantasies about Human Cloning*, edited by Martha C. Nussbaum and Cass R. Sunstein, 54–66. New York: Norton, 1998.

Deane-Drummond, Celia. *Genetics and Christian Ethics.* Cambridge: Cambridge University Press, 2006.

Derrida, Jacques. *The Gift of Death.* Translated by David Wills. Chicago: University of Chicago Press, 1995.

Dewey, John. *The Quest for Certainty: A Study of the Relation of Knowledge and Action.* New York: Minton, Balch, 1929.

Diamond, James J. "Abortion, Animation, and Biological Hominization." *Theological Studies* 36 (1975) 305–24.

Dickinson, Emily. *The Complete Poems of Emily Dickinson.* Edited by Thomas H. Johnson. Boston: Little, Brown, 1960.

Dolnick, Edward. "Deafness as Culture." *Atlantic Monthly*, September 1993, 37–53.

Dombrowski, Daniel A., and Robert Deltete. *A Brief, Liberal, Catholic Defense of Abortion.* Urbana: University of Illinois Press, 2000.

Donceel, Joseph, SJ. "Abortion: Mediate v. Immediate Animation." *Continuum* 5 (1967) 167–71.

———. "Immediate Animation and Delayed Hominization." *Theological Studies* 31 (1970) 76–105.

Dorlodot, Canon Henry de. "A Vindication of the Mediate Animation Theory." In *Theology and Evolution*, edited by E. C. Messenger, 259–83. London: Sands, 1949.

Duster, Troy. "Persistence and Continuity in Human Genetics and Social Stratification." In *Genetics: Issues of Social Justice*, edited by Ted Peters, 218–38. Cleveland: Pilgrim, 1998.

Dworkin, Ronald. *Life's Dominion: An Argument about Abortion, Euthanasia, and Individual Freedom.* New York: Knopf, 1993.

———. "Playing God: Genes, Clones, and Luck." In *Sovereign Virtue: The Theory and Practice of Equality*, 427–52. Cambridge: Harvard University Press, 2000.

———. "Ronald Dworkin Replies." In *Dworkin and His Critics with Replies by Dworkin*, edited by Justine Burley, 339–95. Malden, MA: Blackwell, 2004.

Emerson, Ralph Waldo. *Nature.* In *Selected Writings*, edited by Brooks Atkinson, 1–42. New York: Modern Library, 1940.

Engelhardt, H. Tristram. *Bioethics and Secular Humanism: The Search for a Common Morality.* London: SCM, 1991.

———. "Controversies, Conflicts, and Consensus: A Concluding, Untheological Postscript." *Christian Bioethics* 7 (2001) 291–95.

———. "The Dechristianization of Christian Hospital Chaplaincy: Some Bioethics Reflections on Professionalization, Ecumenization, and Secularization." *Christian Bioethics* 9 (2003) 139–60.

———. *The Foundations of Bioethics*. 2nd ed. New York: Oxford University Press, 1996.
———. "The Foundations of Bioethics and Secular Humanism: Why Is There No Canonical Moral Content?" In *Reading Engelhardt: Essays on the Thought of H. Tristram Engelhardt, Jr.*, edited by Brendan P. Minogue et al., 259–85. Dordrecht: Kluwer, 1997.
———. *The Foundations of Christian Bioethics*. Lisse: Swets & Zeitlinger, 2000.
———. "Genetic Enhancement and Theosis: Two Models of Therapy." *Christian Bioethics* 5 (1999) 197–99.
———. "Germ-Line Genetic Engineering and Moral Diversity: Moral Controversies in a Post-Christian World." In *Ethical Issues in Biotechnology*, edited by Richard Sherlock and John D. Morrey, 503–16. Lanham, MD: Rowman & Littlefield, 2002.
———. "Public Discourse and Reasonable Pluralism: Rethinking the Requirements of Neutrality." In *Handbook of Bioethics and Religion*, edited by David E. Guinn, 169–94. Oxford: Oxford University Press, 2006.
———. "What is Christian About Christian Bioethics? Metaphysical, Epistemological, and Moral Differences." *Christian Bioethics* 11(2005) 241–53.
English, Jane. "Abortion: Beyond the Personhood Argument." In *The Abortion Controversy: A Reader*, edited by Louis P. Pojman and Francis J. Beckwith, 295–304. Boston: Jones and Bartlett, 1994.
Evans, John Hyde. *Playing God?: Human Genetic Engineering and the Rationalization of Public Bioethical Debate*. Chicago: University of Chicago Press, 2002.
———. "Who Legitimately Speaks for Religion in Public Bioethics?" In *Handbook of Bioethics and Religion*, edited by David E. Guinn, 61–79. Oxford: Oxford University Press, 2006.
Ewart, Wendy R., and Beverly Winikoff. "Toward Safe and Effective Medical Abortion." *Science* 281 (1998) 520–21.
Feinberg, Joel. "The Child's Right to an Open Future." In *Freedom and Fulfillment: Philosophical Essays*, 76–97. Princeton: Princeton University Press, 1992.
———. *Harm to Others*. New York: Oxford University Press, 1984.
———. "Wrongful Life and the Counterfactual Element in Harming." In *Freedom and Fulfillment: Philosophical Essays*, 3–36. Princeton: Princeton University Press, 1992.
Fins, Joseph J., et al. "Clinical Pragmatism: A Method of Moral Problem Solving." In *Pragmatic Bioethics*, edited by Glenn McGee, 30–44. Nashville: Vanderbilt University Press, 1999.
Fitzgerald, F. Scott. *The Great Gatsby*. New York: Scribners, 1953.
Fletcher, Joseph. *The Ethics of Genetic Control: Ending Reproductive Roulette*. Garden City, NY: Anchor, 1974.
Foertsch, Jacqueline. "The Right, the Wrong, and the Ugly: Teaching Shelley's Several Frankensteins." *College English* 63 (2001) 697–711.
Foot, Phillipa. "Killing and Letting Die." In *Killing and Letting Die*, 2nd ed., edited by Bonnie Steinbock and Alastair Norcross, 280–89. New York: Fordham University Press, 1994.
———. "The Problem of Abortion and the Doctrine of the Double Effect." In *Virtues and Vices and Other Essays in Moral Philosophy*, 19–32. Oxford: Basil Blackwell, 1978.
Foucault, Michel. *The History of Sexuality*. Vol. 1. Translated by Robert Hurley. New York: Vintage, 1980.

Frankena, William K. *Ethics*. Englewood Cliffs, NJ: Prentice-Hall, 1963.
Franks, Angela. *Margaret Sanger's Eugenic Legacy: The Control of Female Fertility*. Jefferson, NC: McFarland, 2005.
Frier, B. W. "Roman Life Expectancy: Ulpian's Evidence." *Harvard Studies in Classical Philology* 86 (1982) 213–51.
Frost, Robert. *The Poetry of Robert Frost*, edited by Edward Connery Lathem. New York: Holt, Rinehart and Winston, 1969.
Fukuyama, Francis. *Our Posthuman Future: Consequences of the Biotechnology Revolution*. New York: Farrar, Straus, Giroux, 2002.
Gauthier, David. *Morals By Agreement*. Oxford: Clarendon, 1986.
George, Rolf. "On the External Benefits of Children." In *Kindred Matters: Rethinking the Philosophy of the Family*, edited by Diana T. Meyers et al., 209–17. Ithaca: Cornell University Press, 1993.
———. "Who Should Bear the Cost of Children?" *Public Affairs Quarterly* 1 (1987) 1–42.
Gill, Robin. *Health Care and Christian Ethics*. Cambridge: Cambridge University Press, 2006.
Gilligan, Carol. *In a Different Voice: Psychological Theory and Women's Development*. Cambridge: Harvard University Press, 1982.
Glover, Jonathan. *What Sort of People Should There Be?* New York: Penguin, 1984.
Godwin, William. *An Enquiry Concerning Political Justice 1793*. Vol. 1. Oxford: Woodstock, 1992.
Grabowski, John S. *Sex and Virtue: An Introduction to Sexual Ethics*. Washington: The Catholic University of America Press, 2003.
Graham, Peter W., and Fritz H. Oehlschlaeger. *Articulating the Elephant Man: Joseph Merrick and His Interpreters*. Baltimore: Johns Hopkins University Press, 1992.
Green, Ronald M. *Kierkegaard and Kant: The Hidden Debt*. Albany: State University of New York Press, 1992.
———. "Much Ado About Mutton: An Ethical Review of the Cloning Controversy." In *Cloning and the Future of Human Embryo Research*, edited by Paul Lauritzen, 114–31. Oxford: Oxford University Press, 2001.
———. "Parental Autonomy and the Obligation Not to Harm One's Child Genetically." *Journal of Law, Medicine & Ethics* 25 (1997) 5–15.
Grisez, Germain, et al. "'Every Marital Act Ought to Be Open to New Life': Toward a Clearer Understanding." In *The Teaching of "Humanae Vitae": A Defense*, by John C. Ford, S.J., et al., 33–116. San Francisco: Ignatius, 1988.
———. "A New Formulation of a Natural-Law Argument Against Contraception." *The Thomist* 30 (1966) 343–61.
Hanson, Mark J. "Indulging Anxiety: Human Enhancement from a Protestant Perspective." *Christian Bioethics* 5 (1999) 121–38.
Hare, R. M. *Essays in Bioethics*. Oxford: Clarendon, 1993.
Harris, John. *Clones, Genes, and Immortality: Ethics and the Genetic Revolution*. Oxford: Oxford University Press, 1998.
Hau, Michael. *The Cult of Health and Beauty in Germany: A Social History, 1890–1930*. Chicago: University of Chicago Press, 2003.
Hauerwas, Stanley. *Against the Nations: War and Survival in a Liberal Society*. Minneapolis: Winston, 1985.

———. *A Community of Character: Toward a Constructive Christian Social Ethic.* Notre Dame: Notre Dame University Press, 1981.

———. "Epilogue: A Pacifist Response to the Bishops." In Paul Ramsey, *Speak Up for Just War or Pacifism: A Critique of the United Methodist Bishops' Pastoral Letter "In Defense of Creation,"* 149–82. University Park: Pennsylvania State University Press, 1988.

———. "Explaining Christian Nonviolence: Notes for a Conversation with John Milbank and John Howard Yoder." In *Performing the Faith: Bonhoeffer and the Practice of Nonviolence,* 169–83. Grand Rapids: Brazos, 2004.

———. "Foreword." In *Heal Thyself: Spirituality, Medicine, and the Distortion of Christianity,* by Joel James Shuman and Keith G. Meador. Oxford: Oxford University Press, 2003.

———. "Must a Patient Be a Person to Be a Patient? Or, My Uncle Charlie Is Not Much of a Person But He Is Still My Uncle Charlie." In *Truthfulness and Tragedy: Further Investigations in Christian Ethics,* 127–31. Notre Dame: University of Notre Dame Press, 1985.

———. *Naming the Silences: God, Medicine, and the Problem of Suffering.* Grand Rapids: Eerdmans, 1990.

———. "Not All Peace is Peace: Why Christians Cannot Make Peace with Tristram Engelhardt's Peace." In *Wilderness Wanderings: Probing Twentieth-Century Theology and Philosophy,* 111–23. Boulder: Westview, 1997.

———. *The Peaceable Kingdom: A Primer in Christian Ethics.* Notre Dame: University of Notre Dame Press, 1983.

———. "Postscript: A Response to Jeff Stout's *Democracy and Tradition.*" In *Performing the Faith: Bonhoeffer and the Practice of Nonviolence,* 215–41. Grand Rapids: Brazos, 2004.

———. "Sacrificing the Sacrifices of War." *Journal of Religion, Conflict, and Peace* 1 (2007) n.p. Online: http://www.plowsharesproject.org/journal/php/archive/archive.php?issu_list_id=8

———. "Salvation and Health: Why Medicine Needs the Church." In *Suffering Presence: Theological Reflections on Medicine, the Mentally Handicapped, and the Church,* 63–83. Notre Dame: University of Notre Dame Press, 1986.

———. *Sanctify Them in the Truth: Holiness Exemplified.* Nashville: Abingdon, 1998.

———. *Suffering Presence: Theological Reflections on Medicine, the Mentally Handicapped, and the Church.* Notre Dame: University of Notre Dame Press, 1986.

Hauerwas, Stanley, Richard Bondi, and David Burrell. *Truthfulness and Tragedy: Further Investigations in Christian Ethics.* Notre Dame: University of Notre Dame Press, 1985.

Heaney, Stephen J. "Aquinas and the Presence of the Human Rational Soul in the Early Embryo." *The Thomist* 56 (1992) 19–48.

Heyd, David. *Genethics: Moral Issues in the Creation of People.* Berkeley: University of California Press, 1992.

Hobbes, Thomas. *Leviathan.* London: Dent, 1973.

Hollinger, David. *Postethnic America: Beyond Multiculturalism.* New York: Basic, 1995.

Holmes, Helen Bequaert. "Choosing Children's Sex: Challenges to Feminist Ethics." In *Reproduction, Ethics, and the Law,* edited by Joan Callahan, 148–77. Bloomington: Indiana University Press, 1995.

Horn, Richard M., et al. "Audiological and Medical Considerations for Children With Cochlear Implants." *American Annals of the Deaf* 136 (1991) 82-86.

Hume, David. *An Enquiry Concerning the Principles of Morals*. In *Hume's Ethical Writings: Selections from David Hume*, edited by Alasdair MacIntyre, 21-156. Notre Dame: University of Notre Dame Press, 1965.

Huxley, Aldous. *Brave New World*. New York: Harper, 2006.

James, William. *Pragmatism*. Cambridge: Harvard University Press, 1975.

Jeffreys, Derek S. "Euthanasia and John Paul II's 'Silent Language of Profound Sharing of Affection': Why Christians Should Care About Peter Singer." *Christian Bioethics* 7 (2001) 359-78.

Jenson, Robert. "How the World Lost Its Story." *First Things* 36 (1993) 19-24.

John Paul II. *Familiaris Consortio*. Online: http//www.vatican.va/holy_father/john_paul_ii/apost_exhortations/documents/hf_jp-ii_exh_19811122_familiaris-consortio_en.html.

———. *The Gospel of Life: Evangelium Vitae*. Boston: Pauline Books & Media, 1999.

———. *The Original Unity of Man and Woman: Catechesis on the Book of Genesis*. Boston: St. Paul, 1981.

———. *Reflections on Humanae Vitae*. Boston: St. Paul, 1984.

Johnson, Mark. "Delayed Hominization: Reflections on Some Recent Catholic Claims for Delayed Hominization." *Theological Studies* 56 (1995) 743-63.

Jonas, Hans. "Biological Engineering: A Preview." In *Philosophical Essays: From Ancient Creed to Technological Man*, 141-67. Englewood Cliffs, NJ: Prentice-Hall, 1974.

———. *Philosophical Essays: From Ancient Creed to Technological Man*. Englewood Cliffs, NJ: Prentice-Hall, 1974.

Jonsen, Albert, and Stephen Toulmin. *The Abuse of Casuistry*. Berkeley: University of California Press, 1992.

Kamm, Frances M. "Abortion and the Value of Life: A Discussion of *Life's Dominion*." *Columbia Law Review* 95 (1995) 160-221.

———. *Creation and Abortion: A Study in Moral and Legal Philosophy*. New York: Oxford University Press, 1992.

———. "Harming, Not Aiding, and Positive Rights." *Philosophy and Public Affairs* 15 (1986) 3-32.

———. "Killing and Letting Die: Methodological and Substantive Issues." *Pacific Philosophical Quarterly* 64 (1983) 297-312.

———. "Ronald Dworkin's Views on Abortion and Assisted Suicide." In *Dworkin and His Critics: With Replies by Dworkin*, edited by Justine Burley, 218-40. Malden, MA: Blackwell, 2004.

Kamrat-Lang, Debora. "Healing Society: Medical Language in American Eugenics." *Science in Context* 8 (1995) 176-96.

Kant, Immanuel. *The Doctrine of Virtue*. In *The Metaphysics of Morals*. Translated by Mary Gregor. Cambridge: Cambridge University Press, 1991.

———. *Foundations of the Metaphysics of Morals*. Translated by Lewis White Beck. London: Macmillan, 1985.

Kass, Leon R. "Cloning and the Posthuman Future." In *Life, Liberty and the Defense of Dignity: The Challenge for Bioethics*, 141-73. San Francisco: Encounter, 2002.

———. "'Making Babies': The New Biology and the 'Old Morality.'" In *Toward a More Natural Science: Biology and Human Affairs*, 43-79. New York: Free, 1985.

———. *Toward a More Natural Science: Biology and Human Affairs*. New York: Free, 1985.

———. "The Wisdom of Repugnance." In *The Ethics of Human Cloning*, Leon R. Kass and James Q. Wilson, 3–59. Washington: AEI, 1998.

Kavka, Gregory S. "The Paradox of Future Individuals." *Philosophy and Public Affairs* 11 (1982) 93–112.

Keenan, James F., SJ. "Whose Perfection is it Anyway?: A Virtuous Consideration of Enhancement." *Christian Bioethics* 5 (1999) 104–20.

Kerr, Anne, et al. "Eugenics and the New Genetics in Britain: Examining Contemporary Professionals' Accounts." *Science, Technology & Human Values* 23 (1998) 175–98.

Kevles, Daniel J. *In the Name of Eugenics: Genetics and the Uses of Human Heredity*. New York: Knopf, 1985.

Khushf, George. "Thinking Theologically About Reproductive and Genetic Enhancements: The Challenge." *Christian Bioethics* 5 (1999) 154–82.

Kierkegaard, Søren. *Works of Love: Some Christian Reflections in the Form of Discourses*. Translated by Howard and Edna Hong. New York: Harper & Row, 1962.

Kluge, Eike-Henner W. *Biomedical Ethics In A Canadian Context*. Scarborough, Ontario: Prentice-Hall, 1992.

Lane, Harlan. "Constructions of Deafness." *Disability & Society* 10 (1995) 171–89.

———. *The Mask of Benevolence: Disabling the Deaf Community*. New York: Knopf, 1992.

———. *When the Mind Hears: A History of the Deaf*. New York: Random House, 1984.

Lane, Harlan, and Michael Grodin. "Ethical Issues in Cochlear Implant Surgery: An Exploration into Disease, Disability, and the Best Interests of the Child." *Kennedy Institute of Ethics Journal* 7 (1997) 231–51.

Laslett, Peter. "Necessary Knowledge: Age and Aging in the Societies of the Past." In *Aging in the Past: Demography, Society, and Old Age*, edited by David I. Kertzer and Peter Laslett, 3–77. Berkeley: University of California Press, 1995.

Le Guin, Ursula K. "The Ones Who Walk Away from Omelas." In *The Wind's Twelve Quarters: Short Stories by Ursula K. Le Guin*, 275–84. New York: Harper & Row, 1975.

Levin, David S. "Thomson and the Current State of the Abortion Controversy." *Journal of Applied Philosophy* 2 (1985) 121–25.

Lewis, C. S. *The Abolition of Man*. New York: Macmillan, 1947.

———. *The Screwtape Letters*. Rev. ed. New York: Macmillan, 1982.

Lifton, Robert Jay. *The Nazi Doctors: Medical Killing and the Psychology of Genocide*. New York: Basic, 1986.

Ludmerer, Kenneth M. *Genetics and American Society: A Historical Appraisal*. Baltimore: The Johns Hopkins University Press, 1972.

Lunnenborg, Patricia. *Abortion: A Positive Decision*. New York: Bergin & Garvey, 1992.

Lysaught, M. Therese. "And Power Corrupts . . .: Religion and the Disciplinary Matrix of Bioethics." In *Handbook of Bioethics and Religion*, edited by David E. Guinn, 93–123. Oxford: Oxford University Press, 2006.

MacIntyre, Alasdair. "How Can We Learn What *Veritatis Splendor* Has to Teach?" *The Thomist* 58 (1994) 171–95.

———. *Three Rival Versions of Moral Enquiry: Encyclopaedia, Genealogy, and Tradition*. Notre Dame: University of Notre Dame Press, 1990.

MacKenzie, Donald. "Eugenics in Britain." *Social Studies of Science* 6 (1976) 499–532.

MacKinnon, Catharine A. "Privacy v. Equality: Beyond *Roe v. Wade*." In *Feminism Unmodified: Discourses on Life and Law*, 93–102. Cambridge: Harvard University Press, 1987.

———. "Sex and Violence: A Perspective." In *Feminism Unmodified: Discourses on Life and Law*, 85–92. Cambridge: Harvard University Press, 1987.

Malm, H. M. "Killing, Letting Die, and Simple Conflicts." *Philosophy and Public Affairs* 18 (1989) 238–58.

Marcel, Gabriel. *Man Against Mass Society*. Translated by G. S. Fraser. Chicago: Regnery, 1962.

———. "The Mystery of the Family." In *Homo Viator: Introduction to a Metaphysic of Hope*, 68–97. Translated by Emma Craufurd. Gloucester, MA: Peter Smith, 1978.

Maritain, Jacques. *The Dream of Descartes, Together with Some Other Essays*. Translated by Mabelle L. Andison. New York: Philosophical Library, 1944.

Marquis, Don. "Fetuses, Futures, and Values: A Reply to Shirley." *Southwest Philosophy Review* 11 (1995) 263–65.

———. "A Future Like Ours and the Concept of Person: A Reply to McInerney and Paske." In *The Abortion Controversy: A Reader*, edited by Louis P. Pojman and Francis J. Beckwith, 354–69. Boston: Jones and Bartlett, 1994.

———. "Why Abortion is Immoral." In *The Abortion Controversy: A Reader*, edited by Louis P. Pojman and Francis J. Beckwith, 320–37. Boston: Jones and Bartlett, 1994.

Marteau, Theresa M., and Harriet Drake. "Attributions for Disability: The Influence of Genetic Screening." *Social Science and Medicine* 40 (1995) 1127–32.

May, Arnd T. "Physician-Assisted Suicide, Euthanasia, and Christian Bioethics: Moral Controversy in Germany." *Christian Bioethics* 9 (2003) 273–83.

May, William E. "Contraception, Gateway to the Culture of Death." *Faith* 31: 4 (2001) n.p. Online: http//www.christendom-awake.org/pages/may/contraception/htm.

Mayberry, Rachel, and Ellen Eichen. "The Long-Lasting Advantage of Learning Sign Language in Childhood: Another Look at the Critical Period for Language Acquisition." *Journal of Memory and Language* 30 (1991) 486–512.

McDonagh, Eileen L. *Breaking the Abortion Deadlock*. New York: Oxford University Press, 1996.

McGee, Glenn. *Beyond Genetics: Putting the Power of DNA to Work in Your Life*. New York: Morrow, 2003.

———. Introduction to *Pragmatic Bioethics*. Edited by Glenn McGee. Nashville: Vanderbilt University Press, 1999.

———. *The Perfect Baby: Parenthood in the New World of Cloning and Genetics*. 2nd ed. Lanham, MD: Rowman & Littlefield, 2000.

McInerney, Peter K. "Does a Fetus Already Have a Future-Like-Ours?" *Journal of Philosophy* 87 (1990) 264–68.

McKenny, Gerald P. "Enhancements and the Quest for Perfection." *Christian Bioethics* 5 (1999) 99–103.

———. *To Relieve the Human Condition: Bioethics, Technology, and the Body*. Albany: State University of New York Press, 1997.

———. "Utopia, Nihilism, and Quest for Responsibility." In *To Relieve the Human Condition: Bioethics, Technology, and the Body*, 39–75. Albany: State University of New York Press, 1997.

McMahan, Jeff. *The Ethics of Killing: Problems at the Margins of Life*. Oxford: Oxford University Press, 2002.

———. "Killing, Letting Die, and Withdrawing Aid." *Ethics* 103 (1993) 250–79.
———. "Wrongful Life: Paradoxes in the Morality of Causing People to Exist." In *Bioethics*, edited by John Harris, 445–75. Oxford: Oxford University Press, 2001.
Meilaender, Gilbert. *Bioethics: A Primer for Christians*. Grand Rapids: Eerdmans, 1996.
———. *Body, Soul, and Bioethics*. Notre Dame: University of Notre Dame Press, 1995.
———. "Comments of Gilbert Meilaender." *Journal of the Society of Christian Ethics* 24 (2004) 191–95.
Mellor, Anne K. *Mary Shelley: Her Life, Her Fiction, Her Monsters*. New York: Methuen, 1988.
Melville, Herman. *Billy Budd, Sailor and Other Stories*. New York: Penguin, 1986.
Michaels, Meredith W. "Abortion and the Claims of Samaritanism." In *Abortion: Moral and Legal Perspectives*, edited by Jay L. Garfield and Patricia Hennessey, 213–26. Amherst: University of Massachusetts Press, 1984.
Mill, John Stuart. *On Liberty*. In *Utilitarianism, On Liberty, Considerations on Representative Government*, edited by H. B. Acton, 69–185. London: Everyman's, 1991.
Miller, Richard B. *Interpretations of Conflict: Ethics, Pacifism, and the Just-War Tradition*. Chicago: The University of Chicago Press, 1991.
Moers, Ellen. *Literary Women*. Garden City, NY: Doubleday, 1976.
Moreno, Jonathan D. "Bioethics Is a Naturalism." In *Pragmatic Bioethics*, edited by Glenn McGee, 5–17. Nashville: Vanderbilt University Press, 1999.
Muller, H. J. *Out of the Night: A Biologist's View of the Future*. New York: Garland, 1984.
———. *Studies in Genetics: The Selected Papers of H. J. Muller*. Bloomington: Indiana University Press, 1962.
Murphy, Jeffrie G. "The Killing of the Innocent." In *War, Morality, and the Military Profession*, edited by Malham M. Wakin, 343–69. Boulder: Westview, 1979.
Nagel, Thomas. *Mortal Questions*. Cambridge: Cambridge University Press, 1979.
National Bioethics Advisory Commission. *Cloning Human Beings*. Online: http://www.bioethics.gov/reports/past_commissions/nbac_cloning.pdf.
Noonan, John T., Jr. "How to Argue About Abortion." In *Morality in Practice*, edited by James P. Sterba, 134–44. Belmont, CA: Wadsworth, 1984.
———. *A Private Choice: Abortion in America in the Seventies*. New York: Free, 1979.
Norcross, Alastair. "Killing, Abortion, and Contraception: A Reply to Marquis." *Journal of Philosophy* 87 (1990) 268–77.
Nussbaum, Martha C. "Little C." In *Clones and Clones: Facts and Fantasies about Human Cloning*, edited by Martha C. Nussbaum and Cass R. Sunstein, 338–46. New York: Norton, 1998.
Oates, Joyce Carol. "Frankenstein's Fallen Angel." *Critical Inquiry* 10 (1984) 543–54.
O'Donovan, Oliver. *The Just War Revisited*. Current Issues in Theology 2. New York: Cambridge University Press, 2003.
Oehlschlaeger, Fritz. *Love and Good Reasons: Postliberal Approaches to Christian Ethics and Literature*. Durham, NC: Duke University Press, 2003.
Padden, Carol, and Tom Humphries. *Deaf in America: Voices from a Culture*. Cambridge: Harvard University Press, 1988.
Parfit, Derek. "Comments." *Ethics* 96 (1986) 832–72.
———. "Future Generations: Further Problems." *Philosophy and Public Affairs* 11 (1982) 113–72.
———. *Reasons and Persons*. Oxford: Clarendon, 1984.

———. "Rights, Interests, and Possible People." In *Moral Problems in Medicine*, edited by S. Gorovitz et al., 369–75. Englewood Cliffs, NJ: Prentice-Hall, 1976.
Parkin, Tim G. *Demography and Roman Society*. Baltimore: Johns Hopkins University Press, 1992.
Paske, Gerald H. "Abortion and the Neo-Natal Right to Life: A Critique of Marquis's Futurist Argument." In *The Abortion Controversy: A Reader*, edited by Louis P. Pojman and Francis J. Beckwith, 343–53. Boston: Jones and Bartlett, 1994.
Paul VI. *Gaudium et Spes*. Online: http://www.vatican.va/archive/hist_councils/ii_vatican_council/documents/vat-ii_cons_19651207_gaudium-et-spes_en.html.
———. *Humanae Vitae*. Translated by Janet E. Smith in *Humanae Vitae: A Generation Later*, 269–95. Washington: The Catholic University of America Press, 1991.
Paul, Diane B. *The Politics of Heredity: Essays on Eugenics, Biomedicine, and the Nature-Nurture Debate*. Albany: State University of New York Press, 1998.
Pellegrino, Edmund D., and Alan I. Faden, editors. *Jewish and Catholic Bioethics: An Ecumenical Dialogue*. Washington: Georgetown University Press, 1999.
Pence, Gregory E. "Arguments against Human Asexual Reproduction." In *Who's Afraid of Human Cloning?*, 119–50. Lanham, MD: Rowman and Littlefield, 1998.
———. *Brave New Bioethics*. Lanham, MD: Rowman and Littlefield, 2002.
———. *The Elements of Bioethics*. Boston: McGraw Hill, 2007.
———. "Will Cloning Harm People?" In *Flesh of My Flesh: The Ethics of Cloning Humans. A Reader*, edited by Gregory E. Pence, 115–27. Lanham, MD: Rowman and Littlefield, 1998.
Pernick, Martin S. "Eugenics and Public Health in American History." *American Journal of Public Health* 87 (1997) 1767–72.
Peters, Ted. *For the Love of Children: Genetic Technology and the Future of the Family*. Louisville: Westminster John Knox, 1996.
Pickens, Donald K. *Eugenics and the Progressives*. Nashville: Vanderbilt University Press, 1968.
Pieper, Josef. *About Love*. Translated by Richard Winston and Clara Winston. Chicago: Franciscan Herald, 1974.
Pius XI. *Casti Connubii: Christian Marriage*. Boston: Pauline, n.d.
Plato. *The Republic*. Translated by Francis Cornford. New York: Oxford University Press, 1966.
Poovey, Mary. *The Proper Lady and the Woman Writer: Ideology as Style in the Works of Mary Wollstonecraft, Mary Shelley, and Jane Austen*. Chicago: University of Chicago Press, 1984.
Porter, Jean. "Individuality, Personal Identity, and the Moral Status of the Preembryo: A Response to Mark Johnson." *Theological Studies* 56 (1995) 763–70.
President's Council on Bioethics. *Human Cloning and Human Dignity: An Ethical Inquiry*. Online: http://www.bioethics.gov/reports/cloningreport/index.html.
Proctor, Robert. "Genomics and Eugenics: How Fair is the Comparison?" In *Gene Mapping: Using Law and Ethics as Guides*, edited by George J. Annas and Sherman Elias, 57–93. New York: Oxford University Press, 1992.
———. *Racial Hygiene: Medicine Under the Nazis*. Cambridge: Harvard University Press, 1988.
Quinn, Warren. "Actions, Intentions, and Consequences: The Doctrine of Doing and Allowing." *Philosophical Review* 98 (1989) 287–312.

Rachels, James. "Active and Passive Euthanasia." In *Current Issues and Enduring Questions: A Guide to Critical Thinking and Argument, with Readings*, 5th ed., edited by Sylvan Barnet and Hugo Bedau, 560-66. Boston: Bedford, 1999.
Rae, Scott B., and Paul M. Cox, editors. *Bioethics: A Christian Approach in a Pluralistic Age*. Grand Rapids: Eerdmans, 1999.
Ramsey, Paul. "The Case for Making 'Just War' Possible." In *The Just War: Force and Political Responsibility*, 148-67. New York: Scribner's, 1968.
———. *Fabricated Man: The Ethics of Genetic Control*. New Haven: Yale University Press, 1970.
Rawls, John. *Political Liberalism: Expanded Edition*. New York: Columbia University Press, 2005.
———. *A Theory of Justice*. Cambridge: Belknap, 1971.
Regan, Donald H. "Rewriting *Roe v. Wade*." *Michigan Law Review* 77 (1979) 1569-1646.
Reinders, Hans S. *The Future of the Disabled in Liberal Society: An Ethical Analysis*. Notre Dame: University of Notre Dame Press, 2000.
Renteln, Alison Dundes. "Sex Selection and Reproductive Freedom." *Women's Studies International Forum* 15 (1992) 405-26.
Rhonheimer, Martin. "Contraception, Sexual Behavior, and Natural Law: Philosophical Foundation of the Norm of 'Humanae Vitae.'" *Linacre Quarterly* 56:2 (1989) 20-57. Online: http://www.pusc.it/fil/p_rhonheimer/texts/Contraception_Sexual_Behavior_Natural_Law.pdf.
———. "'Intrinsically Evil Acts' and the Moral Viewpoint: Clarifying a Central Teaching of *Veritatis Splendor*." *The Thomist* 58 (1994) 1-39.
———. *Natural Law and Practical Reason: A Thomist View of Moral Autonomy*. Translated by Gerald Malsbary. New York: Fordham University Press, 2000.
Rifkin, Jeremy. *Algeny: A New Word—A New World*. New York: Penguin, 1983.
Robertson, John A. *Children of Choice: Freedom and the New Reproductive Technologies*. Princeton: Princeton University Press, 1994.
———. "Human Cloning and the Challenge of Regulation." *New England Journal of Medicine* 339 (July 9 1998) 119-22.
———. "Liberty, Identity, and Human Cloning." *Texas Law Review* 76 (1998) 1371-1456.
Roe v. Wade. In *Abortion Decisions of the United States Supreme Court: The 1970's*, edited by Maureen Harrison and Steve Gilbert, 1-54. Beverly Hills, CA: Excellent, 1993.
Roemer, John E. "Equality of Talent." *Economics and Philosophy* 1 (1985) 151-81.
Roll-Hansen, Nils. "Geneticists and the Eugenics Movement in Scandinavia." *BJHS* 22 (1989) 335-46.
Rowland, Robin. *Living Laboratories: Women and Reproductive Technologies*. Bloomington: Indiana University Press, 1992.
Saatkamp, Herman J., Jr. "Genetics and Pragmatism." In *Pragmatic Bioethics*, edited by Glenn McGee, 152-67. Nashville: Vanderbilt University Press, 1999.
Sanger, Alexander. *Beyond Choice: Reproductive Freedom in the 21st Century*. New York: Public Affairs, 2004.
Shakespeare, Tom. "Choices and Rights: Eugenics, Genetics, and Disability Equality." *Disability & Society* 13 (1998) 665-81.
Shelley, Mary. *Frankenstein*. New York: Bantam, 1981.
Shirley, Edward S. "Marquis's Argument Against Abortion: A Critique." *Southwest Philosophy Review* 11 (1995) 79-89.

Shuman, Joel James. *The Body of Compassion*. Boulder: Westview, 1999.
———. "Desperately Seeking Perfection: Christian Discipleship and Medical Genetics." *Christian Bioethics* 5 (1999) 139–53.
Shuman, Joel James, and Keith G. Meador. *Heal Thyself: Spirituality, Medicine, and the Distortion of Christianity*. Oxford: Oxford University Press, 2003.
Silver, Lee M. *Remaking Eden: Cloning and Beyond in a Brave New World*. New York: Avon, 1997.
Singer, Peter. "Animal Liberation." In *Current Issues and Enduring Questions: A Guide to Critical Thinking and Argument, with Readings*, 5th ed., edited by Sylvan Barnet and Hugo Bedau, 138–51. Boston: Bedford, 1999.
———. *A Darwinian Left: Politics, Evolution, and Cooperation*. New Haven: Yale University Press, 2000.
———. "Equality for Animals?" In *Practical Ethics: Second Edition*, 55–82. Cambridge: Cambridge University Press, 1993.
———. *The Expanding Circle: Ethics and Sociobiology*. New York: Farrar, Straus & Giroux, 1981.
———. "A German Attack on Applied Ethics: A Statement by Peter Singer." *Journal of Applied Philosophy* 9 (1992) 85–91.
———. "On Being Silenced in Germany." In *Practical Ethics: Second Edition*, 337–59. Cambridge: Cambridge University Press, 1993.
———. *Practical Ethics: Second Edition*. Cambridge: Cambridge University Press, 1993.
———. "A Response." In *Singer and His Critics*, edited by Dale Jamieson, 269–335. Oxford: Blackwell, 1999.
———. "The 'Singer-Affair' and Practical Ethics: A Response." *Analyse & Kritik* 12 (1990) 245–64.
Smith, Janet E. *Humanae Vitae: A Generation Later*. Washington: The Catholic University of America Press, 1991.
Sobsey, Dick. "Family Transformation: From Dale Evans to Neil Young." In *Conference Proceedings: Through the Lifespan*, edited by R. Friedlander and D. Sobsey, 13–16. Kingston: National Association for Persons with Developmental Disabilities and Mental Health Needs, 1996.
Song, Robert. "Christian Bioethics and the Church's Political Worship." *Christian Bioethics* 11 (2005) 333–48.
Stacey, Meg. "The New Genetics: A Feminist View." In *The Troubled Helix: Social and Psychological Implications of the New Human Genetics*, edited by Theresa Marteau and Martin Richards, 331–49. Cambridge: Cambridge University Press, 1996.
Steffen, Lloyd. *Life/Choice: The Theory of Just Abortion*. Cleveland: Pilgrim, 1994.
Steinbock, Bonnie. *Life Before Birth: The Moral and Legal Status of Embryos and Fetuses*. Oxford: Oxford University Press, 1992.
———. "The Logical Case for 'Wrongful Life.'" *Hastings Center Report* 16:2 (1986) 16–20.
Steinbock, Bonnie, and Ron McClamrock. "When Is Birth Unfair to the Child?" *Hastings Center Report* 24:6 (1994) 15–21.
Stock, Greg. *Redesigning Humans: Our Inevitable Genetic Future*. Boston: Houghton Mifflin, 2002.
Stout, Jeffrey. "Comments of Jeffrey Stout." *Journal of the Society of Christian Ethics* 24 (2004) 187–91.
———. *Democracy and Tradition*. Princeton: Princeton University Press, 2004.

Suarez, A. "Hydatidiform Moles and Teratomas Confirm the Human Identity of the Preimplantation Embryo." *Journal of Medicine and Philosophy* 15 (1990) 627–35.
Taboada, Pauline. "Human Genetic Enhancement: Is It Really a Matter of Perfection? A Dialog with Hanson, Keenan, and Shuman." *Christian Bioethics* 5 (1999) 183–96.
Tate, Allen. "The Angelic Imagination." In *Essays of Four Decades*, 401–23. Chicago: Swallow, 1968.
Thobaden, James R. "'Pleased to Make Your Acquaintance': A Review of Kevin Wm. Wildes' *Moral Acquaintances: Methodology in Bioethics*." *Christian Bioethics* 7 (2001) 425–39.
Thom, Deborah, and Mary Jennings. "Human Pedigree and the 'Best Stock': From Eugenics to Genetics?" In *The Troubled Helix: Social and Psychological Implications of the New Human Genetics*, edited by Theresa Marteau and Martin Richards, 211–34. Cambridge: Cambridge University Press, 1996.
Thomasma, David C. "The Sanctity-of-Human-Life Doctrine." In *Jewish and Catholic Bioethics: An Ecumenical Dialogue*, edited by Edmund D. Pellegrino and Alan I. Faden, 54–73. Washington: Georgetown University Press, 1999.
Thomson, Judith Jarvis. "A Defense of Abortion." In *The Abortion Controversy: A Reader*, edited by Louis P. Pojman and Francis J. Beckwith, 131–45. Boston: Jones and Bartlett, 1994.
Thoreau, Henry David. "Civil Disobedience." In *Walden and Civil Disobedience*, 385–413. New York: Penguin, 1983.
Tolmein, Oliver. "The Case of Peter Singer." Online: http://www.tolmein.de/pub02_eng.html.
Tooley, Michael. *Abortion and Infanticide*. Oxford: Clarendon, 1983.
Toulmin, Stephen. "The Tyranny of Principles." *Hastings Center Report* 11:6 (1981) 31–39.
Traherne, Thomas. *Centuries of Meditations*. London: Bertram Dobell, 1908. Online: http://www.ccel.org/ccel/traherne/centuries.i_1.html.
Trammell, Richard L. "Saving Life and Taking Life." *Journal of Philosophy* 72 (1975) 131–37.
Tribe, Laurence H. *Abortion: The Clash of Absolutes*. New York: Norton, 1990.
Tucker, Bonnie Poitras. "Deaf Culture, Cochlear Implants, and Elective Disability." *Hastings Center Report* 28:4 (1998) 6–14.
Veeder, William. "The Negative Oedipus: Father, *Frankenstein*, and the Shelleys." *Critical Inquiry* 12 (1986) 365–90.
Verhey, Allen. *Reading the Bible in the Strange World of Medicine*. Grand Rapids: Eerdmans, 2003.
———, editor. *Religion and Medical Ethics: Looking Back, Looking Forward*. Grand Rapids: Eerdmans, 1996.
Verhey, Allen, and Stephen E. Lammers, editors. *Theological Voices in Medical Ethics*. Grand Rapids: Eerdmans, 1993.
Walzer, Michael. *Arguing About War*. New Haven: Yale University Press, 2004.
———. *Just and Unjust Wars: A Moral Argument with Historical Illustrations*. New York: Basic Books, 1977.
Waters, Brent. "What is Christian About Christian Bioethics?" *Christian Bioethics* 11 (2005) 281–95.
Weil, Simone. "Human Personality." Translated by Richard Rees. In *The Simone Weil Reader*, edited by George A. Panichas, 313–39. Mt. Kisco, NY: Moyer Bell, 1977.

———. "Spiritual Autobiography." In *The Simone Weil Reader*, edited by George A. Panichas, 10–26. Mt. Kisco, NY: Moyer Bell, 1977.

Weiss, Sheila Faith. "The Race Hygiene Movement in Germany." *Osiris* 3 (1987) 193–236.

Wenz, Peter S. *Abortion Rights as Religious Freedom*. Philadelphia: Temple University Press, 1992.

Wikler, Daniel, and Jeremiah Barondess. "Bioethics and Anti-Bioethics in Light of Nazi Medicine: What Must We Remember?" *Kennedy Institute of Ethics Journal* 3 (1993) 39–55.

Wildes, Kevin Wm. *Moral Acquaintances: Methodology in Bioethics*. Notre Dame: University of Notre Dame Press, 2000.

Wilson, James Q. "The Paradox of Cloning." In *The Ethics of Human Cloning*, Leon R. Kass and James Q. Wilson, 61–74. Washington: AEI, 1998.

Winnett, Susan. "Coming Unstrung: Women, Men, Narrative, and Principles of Pleasure." *PMLA* 105 (1990) 505–18.

Wittgenstein, Ludwig. *Philosophical Investigations*. 3rd ed. Translated by G. E. M. Anscombe. Oxford: Blackwell, 2001.

Wojtyla, Karol. "The Anthropological Vision of *Humanae Vitae*." Translated by William E. May. Online: http://www.christendom-awake.org/pages/may/anthrop-visionjpII.htm.

———. *Love and Responsibility*. Translated by H. T. Willetts. New York: Farrar, Straus, Giroux, 1981.

Woodward, James. "The Non-Identity Problem." *Ethics* 96 (1986) 804–31.

Zimmerman, Lee. "*Frankenstein*, Invisibility, and Nameless Dread." *American Imago* 60 (2003) 135–58.

Zoloth-Dorfman, Laurie. "Mapping the Normal Human Self: The Jew and the Mark of Otherness." In *Genetics: Issues of Social Justice*, edited by Ted Peters, 180–202. Cleveland: Pilgrim, 1998.

Zupan, Daniel S. *War, Morality, and Autonomy: An Investigation in Just War Theory*. Aldershot, Hampshire: Ashgate, 2004.

Index

abortion, 3, 4, 5n8, n9, 11, 11n21, 12, 12n22, n23, 13–14, 216, 235, 236n7, 242n13, 255–56, 258n25, 265, 271, 273–80, 280n16, 281, 281n17, 282–88, 294, 296, 302, 326, 342–43; and "conception criterion," chapter 3 (72–103); bad Samaritan defense of, 11, 106–8, 117–37, 145–46, 158; Boonin's defense of Thomson on, 12, chapter 5 (145–69); connection to sacred/sacrifice, 4, chapter 2 (47–71), 132–36, 138–39; derivative objection to, 55–58, 70–71; detached objection to, 55–58, 70–71; just war analogy, 11, 108, 136–44; Singer on, 50–52, 302, 306–9, 313–16; Thomson on, 11–12, 106–9, 117–31, chapter 5 (145–69)
achondroplasia, 263n35, 293–96
active euthanasia, 109n10, 110, 300n2
Adams, M., 207n13, 208n15, 212n19
Adams, R. M., 248n18
Agar, N., 202–3n8, 204n9, 210–11n18
aging; and sexuality, 34–39; as factor in our response to death, 67–70; of societies, 28–35
Akron v. Akron Center, 82, 82n12, 91n20
Allen, D., 220n27
Allen, G., 207n13
Anscombe, G. E. M., 37, 37n29, 38, 38n30, 109–10n10
Aquinas, T., 21–22, 22n7, 74–75, 79, 84–85, 85n16, 86, 86n18
Arendt, H., 81n10, 174n7, 338, 338n26
Aristotle, 41n33, 82–85, 87n19
Arneson, R., 311n11
artificial contraception, 11, chapter 1 (19–46), 148, 216, 234

Asch, A., 281n17
ASL, 288, 292n26
Augustine, 34, 74–75, 79, 79n8, 80–81, 81n10, 324, 324n10, 338n26
Aukerman, D., 12n23

Bacchetta, M., 172
Bacon, F., 3n6, 189, 189n23, 270, 270n6, 271
Balkany, T., 288n20
Banner, M., 2n5
Baron, J., 272n8
Barondess, J., 207n13
Barth, K., 10n19, 190, 190n25
Beauchamp, T., 2n3, 109, 109n9
Beckwith, F., 92n22, 124n19, 152
Bedate, C., 86n18
Beehler, R., 337, 337n24
Beethoven, L. 210
beneficence, 2n3, 109, 135, 239, 242–43, 245, 326
Bentham, J., 303, 303n6, 305
Berry, W., 4, 4n7, 63, 63n15, 147n2, 193, 193n28, 194, 226n29, 290n24
Biesecker, L., 263, 263n34, 264
Blacker, C. P., 207n14
Blackmun, H., 82, 134
Boas, F., 209n16
Bole, T., 86n18
Bondi, R., 268n1
Boonin, D., 11, 11n21, 12, 74, 91–92, 92n21, 92–93n23, 93–96, 96n25, 97–102, chapter 5 (145–69), 236n7
Boothroyd, A., 288n20
Boyle, M., 47n1, 52, 52n7, 53–54
Brewer, H., 207n14
Brock, D., 196, 260, 260n30, 261–62
Brown, E., 300n2
Brown, P., 28–29, 29n17

Buchanan, A., 14n25, 184n21, 196, 196n1, 200n4, 202-3, 205n11, 206n12, 207n13, 217
Burggraf, S., 147n2
Burley, J., 327n15
Burrell, D., 268n1

Cahill, L., 3n5, 10n19, 44, 44n38, 54n9, 182n20
Calabresi, G., 49n3
capital punishment, 53
Carter, S., 104, 104n1, 106
Casal, P., 147n2
Cassell, E., 269, 269n5
casuistry, 2n4, 106, 112n11, 113, 116, 129, 131, 257n24
Cather, W., 112, 112n12
Cefalo, R., 86n18
Chapman, A., 2n5
charity, 28, 35, 112n11, 167-68, 174n9, 297, 330, 331n21
chastity, 24n11, 25-27, 35-36, 38, 38n30, 41
Cherry, A., 280n16
child survival, 28-43, 46
Childress, J., 1, 2n3, n4, 109, 109n9, 158n10
church, 10n19, 59, 175; Catholic opposition to eugenics, 216; Hauerwas on, 9n18, 15, 171, 191, chapter 9 (268-98); service to medicine, 15, chapter 9 (268-98)
civil disobedience, 8n17, 61n12, 181n18, 241, 241n12
Clemens, S. (Mark Twain), 99, 99n26
cloning, 2n4, 15, 42, 173, 177, 185, 189, 201, 271, 272n8, chapter 11 (319-47)
cochlear implantation, 288, 288n20, 292, 292n26
Cohen, C., 255, 255n23, 256-57, 256-57n24, 257n25, 259
Cohen, N., 292n26
Cole-Turner, R., 272n8
combatant-non-combatant distinction, 140, 159, 159n11, 160, 160n11, 161, 161-62n13, 162-65, 311
commodification of children, 21, 180, 314
compassion, 18, 43, 49, 59, 118, 260n31, 261-62, 301n3, 308, 311n11, 313

compulsory sterilization, 205, 209, 209n17, 210, 214, 214n21, 217, 218n25, 231
contralife will, 19n2, 39n31
1 Corinthians 15:26, 258n27
Cox, P., 3n5
the cross, 89, 135, 191, 286, 297n28, 324n11, 347
Cudd, A., 92n22
culture of death, 19, 19n2, 20, 157, 254
curiosity, 323, 324, 324n10

Daniels, N., 181, 182n19, 196, 199-200n4
Darwin, C., 186, 206, 208, 211, 300n2, 302n5, 320n3
Davis, D., 3n5, 15, 15n28, 232n1, 271, 271n7, 272-74, 287n19, 288-89, 289n23, 290-91, 291n25, 292-94, 294n27, 295, 321, 321n6, 328n16
Davis, M., 121n17
Dawkins, R., 320, 323-24, 324n10
deafness, 256n24, 263n35, 294; as culture, 272n9, 274, 287, 287n19, 288, 288n20, 291-92, 292n26, 293, 295-98
Deane-Drummond, C., 3n5, 174n9, 208n15, 209n16, 210n18, 212n19
death, 3n6, 4-5, 16-17, 182, 199-200, 213n20, 218n25, 271, 320-21, 324, 328-32, 332n22, 333-36, 339, 345-46; and unique personal reality, 70, 73-74, 323, 346; and wrongful life, 254-56, 256n24, 257; as power, 52-53, 108, 144, 333; badness of, 257-58n25, 258, 258n26, n27, 259-60; forgetting of, 115, 124-25; fear of, 144; gift of, 323, 323n9, 324, 324n11, 325; rates, 28-29, 31-32; risk of, 115, 120, 134, 240
delayed hominization, 74-75, 79, 84, 85n13, n15, n17, 86, 86n18
Deltete, R., 11, 11n21, 74, 74n3, 75-79, 85n14, 86-87, 91
democracy, 170-71, 172n2, 191, 193, 195
demographic transition, 28, 28n16, 29
Derrida, J., 323, 323n9
Dewey, J., 170-71, 175-77, 186, 193, 195, 209n16

Diamond, J., 86n18
Dickinson, E., 154–55, 155n6
difference principle (Rawls), 218, 219, 219n26, 226
disability, 200n4, 203, 272n8, 342; and harm conundrum, chapter 8 (232–67); and liberal society, 15, chapter 9 (268–98); designing for, 15, 263n35, 272, 274–75, 287, 287n19, 288, 288n20, 289–92, 292n26, 293–98; Singer on, chapter 10 (299–318)
discrimination (just war), 159–60n11, 162n13
distinction between person and condition, 15, 273, 273n11, 274–85
Dolnick, E., 288n20
Dombrowski, D., 11, 11n21, 74, 74n3, 75–79, 85n14, 86–87, 91
Donceel, J., 84–85, 85n13, n15, n17, 86n18
Dorlodot, H., 85n17
Down syndrome, 110, 195, 265, 271–72, 272n8, 275–78, 279n13, 283, 303, 310
Drake, H., 272n8
Duster, T., 209n17
Dworkin, R., 4, 5n8, 11, 13, 47n1, 54–57, 57n11, 58, 60–61, 61n12, 62, 62n13, 63, 63n14, 64, 64n16, 65–66, 66n17, 67–70, 279, 280n14, 325–26, 326n13, 327, 327n14, n15

Eichen, E., 292n26
Einstein, A., 311n11
Emerson, R. W., 170–71, 179, 179n15
Engelhardt, H. T. Jr., 3n5, 6, 6n12, 6–7n13, 8, 8n15, 8–10n18, 10n19, 174n7, 269n4, 291n25, 344n31
English, J., 128n22
Epicurus, 198n2
equal opportunity, 208, 222, 224–27, 288; as rationale for treatment, 196–202
equal protection, as rationale for abortion, 107, 131–32
eugenics, 14, 196–97, 205, 206n12, 208n15, 209–13, 213n20, 216n24, 243; and McGee, 183–88, 204n9; in Nazi Germany, 205, 205n11, 206, 207n13, 209n16, 211, 214–15, 215n22, n23, 216–17; in Sweden, 207n13, 213–15, 215n22, 216; in United States, 206, 207n13, 209n16, 215n23; incompatibility with justice, 197, 206, 217–19, 227, 230–31; liberal, 202–03n8, 204n9, 210–11n18; main-line, 206–7, 207n14; reform, 207, 207n14, 208
euthanasia, 4, 15, 109n10, 110, 115, 269n4, 299–300, 300n2, 303–5, 308, 308n9
Evangelium Vitae, 20, 20n4
Evans, J., 1, 1–2n3, 2n4, 10n19
Ewart, W., 50n4
Exodus: 1:15–21, 253n20; 22:21–24, 257n24

Faden, A., 3n5
Familiaris Consortio, 24, 24n10, 41, 46, 46n43
Feinberg, J., 204n10, 235n6, 241n12, 256n24, 289, 289n22, n23, 329, 329n18
Fenelon, F., 336, 336–37n23, 337, 337n25, 338
Fins, J., 172, 172n4
Fitzgerald, F. S., 268
Fletcher, J., 213, 213n20
Foertsch, J., 329n20
Foot, P., 109–10n10, 112n11, 155, 155n7, 156, 156n8, 157–58
Fost, N., 220n27
Foucault, M., 9n18, 52, 52n8, 53–54, 64, 200, 200n5
fourth age, 32
fragile X, 278, 283–85
Frankena, W., 1, 1n1
Frankl, V., 247n16
Franklin, B., 61, 61n12
Franks, A., 205n11, 206n13, 210n18
friendship, 28, 36, 37, 41, 41n33
Frier, B., 31n23
Frost, R., 73, 73n2
Fukuyama, F., 307n8, 340–41n30, 343–44n31
"future like ours" argument, 11, 72, 72n1, 92, 92n22, 93–96, 98, 101–2, 145

Galileo, 175
Gaudium et Spes, 40, 40n32, 44n37, 45, 45n40
Gauthier, D., 198n2, 227, 227n30
gender inequality, 14, 14n24, 54, 60, 79n8
generational injustice, chapter 11 (319–47)
generocentrism, 241n11
Genesis: 1:27, 87n19;
   38:8–10, 34
genetic design, 184, 193, 204, 217, 225–26, 255, 296
genetic engineering, 1, 20, 174, 178n14, 179, 224, 227, 272n8, 280n16, 327n15, 344, 344n31
genetic enhancement, 6n13, 8, 14, chapter 6 (170–95), 202n8, 204n9, 225–26, 255n22, 270n6, 271, 329, 345
genetic selection, 293, 343, 345
genetic therapy, chapter 9 (268–98)
"Geneticists Manifesto" (1939), 208, 208n15
Genovese, K., 124, 125, 129, 133
George, R., 147n2
Gill, R., 3n5, 6–7n13
Gilligan, C., 62, 62n13
Glover, J., 229, 229n31
Godwin, W., 329n20, 336–37, 337n25, 338
Golem, 328n16
Grabowski, J., 19n2, 24n11, 45n39
Graham, P., 1n2
Graham, R., 210n18
Green, R., 262, 262n33, 263, 263n35, 264–65, 265n36, 266, 266n37, 267, 267n38, 321n4
Grisez, G., 19n2, 23n8, 39n31
Grodin, M., 292n26
Gulf War, 107n7, 160n12
Gustafson, J., 3n6

Haldane, J. B. S., 207n14
Hanson, M., 174n7
Hare, R. M., 309n10
harm, 109–10, 112n11, 129n23, 136, 138–39, 143, 152, 158n10, 159n11, 162n13, 196, 199–200, 291–95, 321n6, 322, 322n7, 325–26, 340, 344–45

harm conundrum, 14, chapter 8 (232–67), 344
Harris, J., 204n9
Hau, M., 207n13
Hauerwas, S., 3n6, 6, 6n11, 8, 8–10n18, 15, 15n27, 27, 27n15, 49, 64n16, 76, 76n5, 135, 164, 164n14, 170–71, 173, 191, 195, 268, 268n1, n3, 269n4, 270, 286, 339, 339n28
Hawthorne, N., 179
Heaney, S., 85–86, 86n18
Hegel, G. W. F., 170
Heyd, D., 240n10, 241n11, 253n20, 263
Hitler, A., 206, 299
Hobbes, T., 144, 144n27, 198n2, 343n31
Hollinger, D., 172n2
Holmes, H., 280n16
homunculus, 75, 86–87
Horn, R., 292n26
Humanae Vitae, 20n3, 21, 21n5, 23–24, 24n9, n11, n12, 25, 39n31, 45n42
Hume, D., 185, 192, 192n27, 198n2
Humphries, T., 288n20
Huxley, A., 201n7, 226
Huxley, J., 207, 207n14

immediate hominization, 11, 75, 85–87
infant mortality, 30
infanticide, 67, 69, 83, 112n11, 142, 152n11, 300, 302–6, 306n7, 307, 307n7, n8, 308–9, 313, 316–17
investment thesis (Dworkin), 60–64, 64n16, 65–69, 147n2, 188, 204–5
Iraq War, 139
Isaiah 1:18, 273n11

James, H., 321n5
James, W., 175, 180, 180n16, 183
Jeffreys, D., 308n9
Jennings, M., 207n13
Jenson, R., 17n33
Jeremiah: 6:14, 7;
   20:14–15, 258, 258n26
Jesus Christ, 3, 13n23, 21, 70, 89, 135, 143, 167–68, 190–91, 232–33, 258n27, 259, 285–86, 296, 297n28, 311n11, 335
Job 3:3, 258, 258n26

John 12:24, 258n27
John Paul II, 19, 19n1, 21, 23, 24n10, n11, n12, 46, 46n43, 157, 254, 308n9
Johnson, M., 86n18
Jonas, H., 3n6, 174–75, 175n10, 176–77, 181, 321, 321n6, 325, 338–39
Jonsen, A., 257n24
just war, 11, 108, 136–44, 158, 158n10, 159, 159–60n11, 160, 160–61n12, 161, 161–62n13, 164–65
justice, 2n3, 8, 10n19, 14, 53, 69, 119–20, 128, 130–31, 135–36, 160, 168, 172, 191–92, 192n27, 280n16, 329; and harm conundrum, 235, 238, 241–42, 246n16, 247, 247n17, 249–50, 252, 254, 259–60, 262, 264–66; as self-interested reciprocity, 197–98, 198n2, 221, 223, 226–230; as virtue, 24, 28, 35, 37, 39n31, 41, 41n33, 122, 174n9; designing subjects of, 14, chapter 7 (196–231); generational, 340–47; Godwin on, 336, 336–37n23, 337–38; Rawlsian, 10n18, 170–71, 195, 198, 218–19, 219n26, 241n12; subject-centered, 197–98, 198n2, 226–230; Thomson on, 121–23, 126–27, 127n21

Kafka, F., 211
Kamm, F., 4, 5, 5n8, n9, 57n11, 63n14, 108, 108n8, 111–12n11, 129n23, 257n25
Kamrat-Lang, D., 207n13
Kant, I., 6n13, 10n18, 22, 105, 162n13, 198n2, 267n38, 293–94
Kass, L., 3n6, 174–75, 175n11, 176–77, 319, 319n2, 320–21, 321n6, 339, 340n30
Kavka, G., 245–46n15, 252–53n20
Keenan, J., 174n7
kenosis, 191
Kerr, A., 205n11
Kevles, D., 206, 207n13, n14
Khushf, G., 174n7, 270n6
Kierkegaard, S., 42, 42n34, 167–68, 168n15, 169, 259, 259n28, 267, 267n38
killing–letting die distinction, 109, 109n10, 110–11, 111–12n11, 112–13,

113–14n15, 114–17, 123, 129–31, 153–55, 155n7
Kluge, E., 278, 278n12
Kuhse, H., 299

Lamarckianism, 208n15
Lammers, S., 2n5
Lane, H., 287n19, 288n20, 292n26, 297n29
Laslett, P., 28, 28n16, 29, 29n18, 30n20, n21, n22, 32, 32n25, 34
last resort criterion (just war), 141
Lebenshilfe, 299
Leder, D., 3n6
legitimate authority (just war), 140, 142–43, 160
Le Guin, U., 253n20
Leibniz, G., 87–88
Lenin, V., 210–11
Leonardo, 210
Levin, D., 126n20
Lewis, C. S., 260n31, 337, 337n25
life expectancy, 29–30, 31n23, 34–35, 43, 147n2
Lifton, R., 207n13, 217, 218n25
Lotze, R. H., 180n16
Ludmerer, K., 207n13, 209n16
Luke: 10:30–35, 124n18, 167–69; 11:11–12, 232; 17:33, 45; 22:25, 246n15
Lunnenborg, P., 47n1

MacIntyre, A., 19n1, 170, 173, 176, 176n13, 191
MacKenzie, D., 207n13
MacKinnon, C., 14n24, 54, 54n9, 60–61, 79n8, 83n12
Malm, H., 112n11
Marcel, G., 43n35, 187, 187n22, 190, 190n26, 294n27
Maritain, J., 16n32
Marquis, D., 11, 11n21, 72n1, 92, 92n22, 93, 93n24, 94–95, 97, 101–2
marriage, 11, 19, 20–21, 27–29, 31, 34–36, 38–41, 41n33, 42–43, 45–46, 95, 189, 189n23, 216n24, 223, 292, 320, 330, 335–36
Marteau, T., 272n8

Index

Marx, K., 210
Matthew 7:9–11, 233n2
    11:30, 347
May, A., 300n2
May, W., 19, 19n2
Mayberry, R., 292n26
McClamrock, R., 256n24
McDonagh, E., 47n1
McGee. G., 18n34, 173, 173n6, n7, 174, 174n8, n9, 175, 175n10, n11, 176–78, 178n14, 179–82, 182n19, 183–87, 191–93, 195, 204n9, 322, 322n8, 344n32
McInerney, P., 92n22
McKenny, G., 3n6, 5, 5n10, 174n7, 270, 270n6
McMahan, J., 14, 66n17, 113–14n15, 117n16, 235, 235n5, 240n10, 242–45, 246n15, 247, 247n17, 248–52, 258n25
Meador, K., 6n11
Meilaender, G., 2n4, n5, 257n24, 339n27
Mellor, A., 328n17
Melville, H., 259, 259n29
Mendelian-Darwinism, 208n15
mercy, 20, 118–19, 124n18, 167–69
Merrick, J., 1
Michaels, M., 107n6, 132n24
Michelangelo, 65
Milbank, J., 170
military draft, 107, 132–33, 136
Mill, J. S., 289n23, 290
Miller, F., 172
Miller, R., 162n13
Moers, E., 328n17
moral acquaintances, 7, 7n14, 257n24
moral friends, 6, 7, 7n14
moral patiency, 77, 81
moral strangers, 6, 6n13, 7, 7n14
Moreno, J., 172, 172n3
Mother Theresa, 311n13
Muller, H. J., 207, 207n14, 208, 208n15, 209–10, 210n18, 211–12, 212n19, 213, 217, 224
Murphy, J., 162n13

Nagel, T., 257n25

natural law, 11, 11n20, 20–22, 22n6, n7, 23–24, 24n9, 25, 25n13, 27, 27n14, 35n28, 37, 46
Nazism, 205, 205n11, 207n13, 209n16, 211, 214–15, 215n22, 217–18, 218n25, 247n16, 300, 300n2, 301n3
negligence, 149, 243, 245, 247–49, 249n19, 250, 263–65, 267
Newton, I., 210
Niebuhr, R., 143
Nietzsche, F., 6n13, 312
no-difference view (Parfit), 238n8, 244–45
non-identity problem, chapter 8 (232–67)
non-maleficence, 109–10, 326
Noonan, J., 48, 48n2, 124n19
Norcross, A., 92n22
Nussbaum, M., 321n5

Oates, J. C., 332n22
O'Connor, S. D., 82, 82–83n12, 84, 91n20
O'Donovan, O., 159–160n11
Omar Khayyam, 210
open future, 15, 185, 204, 204n10, 272, 274, 289, 289n22, 290–91, 293, 322, 325, 329, 329n18, 347
Osborn, F., 207n14

pacifism, 158n10, 164
Padden, C., 288n20
parable of the Good Samaritan, 167–69
parental liberty, 256, 340n30
parenthood, 21, 23–24, 27, 51, 173, 177, 180, 185, 189–90, 314, 321–22
parenting, 41, 178, 180, 185, 187, 190–91
Parfit, D., 14, 232, 232n1, 233, 235–36, 236n7, 238n8, 239–40, 240n10, 242, 244–45, 245–46n15, 252, 254, 260n30, 263–64
Parkin, T., 31n23, n24
Paske, G., 92n22
passive euthanasia, 109n10, 110
Pasteur, L., 210
Paul VI, 40, 40n32, 44, 44n37, 45, 45n40
Paul, D., 207n13, 212n19
Pellegrino, E., 3n5
Pence, G., 214n21, 322, 322n7
"perfect baby", 177–79, 272n8
Pernick, M., 207n13

personal identity, 87–89, 128n22, 341
personhood, 11, 20, 57n11, 72, 74–76,
    76n5, 77–78, 78n7, 84, 90, 104n1,
    105–6, 128n22, 129n23, 131, 134,
    141–42, 146, 152, 236, 302, 308–9,
    311n11, 316
Peters, T., 180n17
Pickens, D., 207n13, 209n16
Pieper, J., 346–47, 347n33
pity, 201, 261, 312–13
Pius XI, 216n24
Plato, 85, 187, 201n7
playing God, 325
Poe, E., 16n32
Pojman, L., 92n22
Poovey, M., 329n20
Porter, J., 86n18
potential, in abortion debate, 72, 81–83,
    83n12, 84
pragmatism, 8, 14, 170–72, 172n4, 173,
    173n5, 174–78, 180n16, 182,
    184–85, 187, 191–93, 195
preconception nonexistence, 255, 256n24,
    257–58
preformationism, 75, 86–87
President's Council on Bioethics, 280n15,
    319, 319n2, 321n6
principle of permission, 6, 6n13, 10n18,
    344n31
principlism, 2n3, n4, 257n24
processional knowledge, 28, 32
Proctor, R., 207n13, n14, 209n16
progressivism, 191, 209, 209n16
prudence, 35–36, 41, 51, 174n9
public education, 183, 185–87, 208
Pushkin, A., 210
Pygmalion, 179

Quinn, W., 109n10, 117n16

Rachels, J., 106, 108–09, 109n10, 110–11,
    111–12n11, 112–16, 123–24, 142
racism, 214–15, 215n23, 217, 290n24, 302,
    302n4, 306, 310, 317, 320
Rae, S., 3n5
Ramsey, P., 162n13, 174–75, 175n12, 176
Rawls, J., 8n15, 10n18, 195, 198, 218–19,
    219n26, 241n12

Regan, D., 11, 12n22, 105, 105n2, 107–8,
    131–32, 132n24, 133–35, 137,
    236n7
Reinders, H., 15, 15n26, 272–73, 273n10,
    274–76, 281–86
Reno, R., 9n18
Renteln, A., 280n16
replaceability, 50, 189, 235, 237, 308,
    309n10, 310, 315
Repository for Germinal Choice, 210n18
repugnance, 319, 319n2, 320, 322, 346
Rhonheimer, M., 11, 11n20, 19n1, 21–22,
    22n6, 23–24, 24n9, 25, 25n13,
    26–27, 27n14, 28, 35, 35n28, 36
Rifkin, J., 174, 174n8, 176–77
Robertson, J., 204n9, 236n7, 254, 254n21,
    255–56, 256n24, 261n32, 325,
    325n12, 339n27, 340, 340n29, n30,
    341–44
Roe v. Wade, 12n22, 50, 72, 82, 82n11,
    105n2, 131, 133–34
Roemer, J., 224n28
Roll-Hansen, N., 207n13, 215n22
Rorty, R., 170
Rowland, R., 174, 174n9, 176

Saatkamp, H., 172–73, 173n5
sacred, 4, 47, 54–56, 60, 62–64, 64n16,
    65–66, 70, 315–16
sacrifice, 25, 29, 38, 64, 64n16, 70, 107,
    107n7, 113, 133–35, 135n25, 136,
    138–39, 167, 238, 338
Saint Paul, 28–29, 258, 258n27
Saint Thecla, 28
sanctity of life, 60, 66n17, 299, 316, 316n14
Sanger, A., 47n1
Sanger, M., 205n11, 207n13, 210n18
Schemm, H., 207n14
SCNT, 15, 16, 319n1, 320–21, 321–22n6,
    322, 322n7, 325, 327, 327n15,
    328–29, 338–44, 344n32, 345–46
Seailles, G., 43
separation of church/state, 56, 74–75, 90
sex ratios at birth, 280n15
sex selection, 280, 280n15, n16, 281,
    281n17
Shakespeare, T., 272n8

Shelley, M., 15, 80, 325, 327, 328n17, 329, 329n20, 332, 336; *Frankenstein*, 15, 80, chapter 11 (319–47)
Shirley, E., 92n22
Shuman, J., 6n11, 16, 16n30, 173–74n7, 297n28
Silver, L., 343–44n31
Singer, P., 14, 15, 15n29, 50, 50n5, 51, 142, 232, 232n1, 233–34, 234n3, 235–38, 240, 254, 263–64, 299, 299n1, 300, 300–301n2, 301, 301n3, 302, 302n4, n5, 303–7, 307n8, 308, 308n9, 309, 309n10, 310–11, 311n11, 312–14, 314n12, 315–16, 316n14, 317, 317n15, n16
Smith, J., 19n2, 21n5, 24, 24n11, 25, 39n31, 45, 45n42
Smith, S., 157, 157n9, 158
Sobsey, D., 284, 284n18
social constructionism, 49n3, 181, 222–23
Song, R., 10n19, 269n4
species-typical functioning, 181, 200n4, 221–23
speciesism, 302, 302n4, 310, 317
Stacey, M., 279n13
Stalin, J., 212, 212n19
State v. Garber, 289n23
Steffen, L., 11, 12n22, 47n1, 108, 136–37, 137n26, 138–44
Steinbock, B., 148, 148n3, 256–57n24
Stock, G., 343n31
Stout, J., 2n4, 8, 8n16, 10, 170–72, 172n2, 173, 173n7, 176, 191, 193, 193n28
Suarez, A., 86n18
suffering, 3n6, 4n7, 5, 15–17, 20, 46, 51, 68, 81, 129n23, 130, 182–83, 199, 220, 222, 236n7, 256n24, 260, 260n30, n31, 261, 261n32, 262–63, 267–68, 268n1, n3, 269, 269n4, 270, 278, 286–87, 297n28, 301–3, 308n9, 313–14, 314–15n12, 315–17, 345
Sun Yat Sen, 210
supererogation, 59, 136, 146, 147n2, 167, 236n7

Taboada, P., 174n7, 178n14
tacit consent, 148–49, 150n4
Tate, A., 16n32

temperance, 26–27, 35–36, 41, 112, 174n9
therapy-enhancement distinction, 197, 219–24
third age, 32–33, 37
Thobaden, J., 7n14
Thom, D., 207n13
Thomasma, D., 316n14
Thomson, J., 11–12, 12n22, 92, 104–5, 105n3, 106–7, 107n6, 108–9, 117–21, 121n17, 122–24, 124n18, n19, 125–26, 126n20, 127–28, 128n22, 129, 129n23, 130–31, 133, 135–36, 145–46, 148, 150, 152, 154, 165–69, 236n7
Thoreau, H. D., 8, 8n17, 61n12, 113, 113n13, 170, 180, 226
Tillich, P., 213
Tolmein, O., 301n2
Tooley, M., 112n11, 142, 151n5, 152, 306n7
Toulmin, S., 257n24
Traherne, T., 337n25
Trammell, R., 113n14
Tribe, L., 47n1, 104n1
Trinity, 190
trolley problems, 117n16, 155, 157
Tucker, B., 292n26

unitive meaning of sexuality, 24, 38
utilitarianism, 73, 187, 198n2, 237–38, 302–3, 309–10, 312, 316, 318, 336

Van Rijn, Rembrandt, 4, 5, 65
Veeder, W., 331n21
Verhey, A., 2n5, 77n6, 260n31
Vietnam War, 107, 107n7, 133–34, 136, 139
virtue ethics, 174n9
virtues, 24, 26–28, 36–37, 41, 84, 88, 165, 173, 191, 268

Walzer, M., 160n12, 162n13
war, 9n18, 11, 51–55, 64, 64n16, 65, 107, 107n7, 108, 132–37, 139–43, 158, 158n10, 159, 159–60n11, 160, 160–61n12, 161, 161–62n13, 164–65, 187, 215, 269, 311
Waters, B., 269n4, 272n8, 341n30
Weil, S., 315–16, 316n13
Weiss, S., 207n13

Wenz, P., 11, 74–78, 78n7, 79, 81–82,
    82–83n12, 83–84, 90–91
Whitman, W., 170–71
Wikler, D., 196, 207n13
Wildes, K., 7, 7n14, 257n14
Wilmut, I., 319
Wilson, J. Q., 319n2
Winnett, S., 327n14
Winnikoff, B., 50n4
Wisconsin v. Yoder, 289, 289n23, 290
Wittgenstein, L., 128n22
Woodward, J., 247n16

wrongful life, 232n1, 235n5, n6, 246n15,
    250, 254–57, 256–57n24

Yoder, J. H., 9n18

Zaner, R., 3n6
Zenderland, L., 206
Zimmerman, L., 331n21
Zoloth-Dorfman, L., 3n5, 328n16

Zupan, D., 162n13

www.ingramcontent.com/pod-product-compliance
Lightning Source LLC
Chambersburg PA
CBHW020606300426
44113CB00007B/532